Homemaker/Home Health Aide
On the Job Companion

Homemaker/Home Health Aide On the Job Companion

Audree Spatz

Suzann Balduzzi, RN, BSN, MSED

Prepared by Sandra Holter, RN, BS, MS

THOMSON

DELMAR LEARNING

Australia Canada Mexico Singapore Spain United Kingdom United States

THOMSON

DELMAR LEARNING

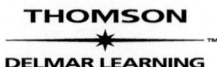

Homemaker/Home Health Aide On the Job Companion
by Audree Spatz and Susann Balduzzi

Vice President, Health Care Business Unit:
William Brottmiller

Editorial Director:
Cathy L. Esperti

Acquisitions Editor:
Marah Bellegarde

Developmental Editor:
Debra Flis

Editorial Assistant:
Erin Adams

Marketing Director:
Jennifer McAvey

Marketing Channel Manager:
Tamara Caruso

Marketing Coordinator:
Kim Duffy

Project Editor:
Natalie Wager

Senior Art/Design Specialist:
Jay Purcell

Production Coordinator:
Kenneth McGrath

Library of Congress Cataloging-in-Publication Number

Spatz, Audree.
  Homemaker/home health aide on the job companion / Audree Spatz, Suzann Balduzzi.
    p. cm.
    ISBN 1-4018-3145-1
  1. Home health aides. 2. Home care services. 3. Care of the sick. I. Balduzzi, Suzann. II. Title

RA645.3S66 2004
610.73'43--dc22
                            2004047822

Notice to the Reader

CONTENTS

INTRODUCTION TO THE LEARNER

Homemaker/Home Health Aide On the Job Companion is a handbook for learners and practicing home health aides. It is designed as a reference to provide essential information to assist in caring for clients in the home, assisted living arrangements, and group homes. It is also a useful tool in helping the learner transition from the classroom setting to practice. All of the procedures from the text are included for ready access.

The book is divided into eight sections: Section 1, Becoming a Home Health Aide; Section 2, Stages of Human Development; Section 3, Preventing the Spread of Infectious Disease; Section 4, Understanding Health; Section 5, Body Systems and Common Disorders; Section 6, Clients Requiring Special Care; Section 7, Maternal/Infant Care; and Section 8, Employment. The practical applications of procedures required by OBRA are included in each unit. The procedures are presented in a step-by-step format, and are illustrated with photographs to assist the learner in understanding the various steps. Note: Agencies and states differ in what procedures they allow home health aides to perform. Always check with your agency for which procedures you are allowed to perform in your state.

Home health aides are key members of the health care team. This handbook will assist home health aides to provide quality care to their clients.

LIST OF PROCEDURES

Becoming a Home Health Aide

Unit 1
Home Health Services

Unit 2
Home Health Aide Responsibilities and Legal Rights

Unit 3
Developing Effective Communication Skills and Documentation

Unit 4
Safety

Unit 5
Homemaking Service

SECTION 1

UNIT 1

Home Health Services

THE DEVELOPMENT OF HOME HEALTH SERVICES

The first homemaker service was established by a social service agency in the United States in 1903. Its main purpose was to provide child care. In the early 1920s employment agencies advertised for mature, practical women experienced in child care and household management. During the Depression of the 1930s the Work Projects Administration funded a program to train the unemployed as "housekeeping aides." They received formal training and some on-the-job training as well. In 1959, the National Conference on Homemaker Service met in Chicago. It was decided that homemaker service should be given to families with children, chronically ill persons, or older adults. It was advised that these individuals should receive care in the home whenever possible, without regard to family income. In 1960, at another conference, personal care and health care were seen as added duties of a homemaker's job; the term home health aide came into use. Home health aides were expected to work only under direct nursing supervision.

Today, all states have guidelines and laws setting minimum standards for home health aide training programs and requirements for home health aides to be listed on their state registry. In 1987, the Omnibus Budget Reconciliation Act, known as **OBRA,** was passed, which mandates national standards for federally funded nursing homes and home health agencies. Once an individual completes both the training program and competency test, she or he is placed on the state Nurse Aide Registry in which they reside. The state in which the test was administered will issue this individual a card stating they are listed on that state's registry. In order to stay on the state Nurse Aide Registry, the home health aide will need to work a minimum number of hours in his or her field within a two-year period. Another requirement to remain on the home health aide registry is to complete 12 hours of continuing education each year, once employed. If you have any questions on your state's requirements, you need to talk with someone from your state nursing assistant registry office. The primary goal of OBRA regulations is to improve care both for individuals in long-term care facilities and for those in their own homes.

3

INCREASE IN NEED FOR HOME CARE SERVICES

Home care is now one of the fastest growing businesses in this country.

There are a number of reasons for the increase in the need for home care. One of the main reasons is that older adults, the main recipients of home care, are the fastest growing population in the country. People are living longer due to advances in health care and modern technology.

A second reason for the increased need for home care services is the high cost of hospital care and the trend on the part of providers and payers to keep costs down. As a result of this trend, clients are often sent home from the hospital as soon as medically possible. Many of these clients still need follow-up care by a home health agency. This trend has led to the tremendous growth in the field of home health care.

A third reason for the increase in home care is that most individuals prefer to remain in their own homes when they become ill or frail, rather than moving to an unfamiliar setting, such as a nursing home. They wish to sleep in their own beds, eat at their own kitchen tables, and talk on their own telephones. They want to have control over their own lifestyles—when they get up in the morning and go to bed at night, what they have for dinner, and who they let into their homes. They want to be near their loved ones, friends, and neighbors.

A fourth reason for the steady increase in home care services is the growing acceptance of the home as a place to die. Hospice services are becoming more available to help a terminally ill client die with dignity in their own home. Health care providers, nurses, home health aides, social workers, and volunteers work as a team to make this possible. Bereavement counseling is also offered to family members.

TYPES OF HOME CARE WORKERS

Home care workers play key roles in their clients' lives. They perform many of the duties that are necessary for their clients to remain at home. Their duties may fall into two main categories—care of the person and care of the home. Care of the person includes assistance with activities of daily living, such as bathing, dressing, toileting, and simple nursing tasks, such as taking blood pressure or assisting with exercises. Care of the home includes light housekeeping, cooking, shopping, and other homemaking duties.

Care of the person requires more training than care of the home. Some workers do all of the above; others may have more limited roles. The role depends on the amount of training that the worker has had and how the person is classified on the state registry (Figure 1-1). The case manager designs a separate care plan to be followed for each client. The care plan specifically outlines the home care worker's responsibilities.

The following are some of the more commonly used titles for home care workers.

> *Companion*—Keeps the client company or maintains safety; usually does not provide personal or homemaking services.
>
> *Homemaker*—Performs household duties, such as laundry and cooking, as well as light housecleaning.
>
> *Personal care worker*—Assists with a minimal level of daily living activities, such as meal preparation and

A. Routine homemaker functions or tasks include the following:
1. Washing dishes
2. Doing light housekeeping, i.e., dusting, scrubbing floors, vacuuming rooms that the client uses
3. Maintaining needed supplies
4. Preparing and serving meals
5. Doing laundry
6. Shopping for client if no other arrangements can be made
7. Accompanying client to medical clinic or other activity

B. Routine home health aide functions done for the client:
1. Under the supervision of a registered nurse or case manager arranging the schedule so that the client follows the care plan, such as increased physical activity or other activity of daily living
2. Recording care and observations on client's record
3. Measuring vital signs and weight
4. Assist with toileting needs
5. Assist with oral care
6. Assist with dressing and undressing
7. Assist with eating
8. Assist with transfer of client from bed to chair and vice versa
9. Assist with repositioning a client
10. Remind clients to take medications on schedule
11. Reinforce or change unsterile simple dressings
12. Assist with care of ostomy bags or urinary drainage bags
13. Measure and record intake and output
14. Assist with grooming—care of hair including shampooing, shaving, and nail care
15. Making and changing bed linens
16. Assist client with walking and other prescribed exercises
17. Assist with applications of prosthetic devices, i.e., hearing aids and braces
18. Assist with rehabilitation measures
19. Assist with skin care
20. Applying elastic support hose
21. Notifying case manager of any notable change in the client's condition

Figure 1-1   Home health functions approved by most states

companionship, as well as minimal assistance with personal care.

Home health aide—Provides substantial assistance with personal care, such as bathing and dressing, as well as supervised health assistance, such as assistance with rehabilitation activities and self-administered medication.

Homemaker/home health aide—Assists in general household tasks, as well as those listed above for the home health aide.

Home care aide—Works with the client with the goal of assisting the client with independent living under professional supervision.

The Health Care Team

Home health care can be defined as all those services that promote, maintain, and/or restore physical, social, or emotional health to clients in the home setting. The home health aide is one member of the health care team who sees the client more frequently than other members of the team. Although members may not see each other on a regular basis, the team still exists. A variety of workers are necessary to carry out the various needs of the client. Teamwork, observation skills, and communication are essential. The entire health care team relies on the home health aide to provide vital observations, documentation, and communication. Other health care personnel who are part of the health care team include:

Case manager (CM)—Assesses overall needs of the client and decides what services should be provided; usually

performed by a nurse or social worker; may supervise the home care worker. (Many home care agencies combine the role of the case manager and the registered nurse.)

Enterostomal therapist (RN, ET)—A specialist who works with clients who have ostomies or clients who require special skin or wound care.

Health care provider—A general term for an agency, institution, or member of the health care team who provides medical care for the consumer.

Licensed practical nurse (LPN)—Provides direct care to the client, such as treatments and medication; may supervise home care workers.

Nurse practitioner (NP)—Specializes in additional training in physical examination and assessment, and works under a health care provider's supervision. The nurse practitioner may work with children, infants, clients who are pregnant, older adults, and clients with cancer.

Occupational therapist (OT)—Evaluates client's ability to perform skills necessary for independent daily living, such as bathing, dressing, cooking; works with client to improve abilities; develops plan of care to be assisted by family and home health aide.

Physical therapist (PT)—Evaluates the home environment in preparation of the client's return, assists with safety adaptations and instructs an appropriate exercise program and usage of special equipment.

Registered dietitian (RD)— Provides information regarding prescribed (by health care provider) dietary needs of the client. Assists in meal planning adjustment according to the medical condition of the client.

Registered nurse (RN)—Initiates the plan of care ordered by the health care provider, performs assessment, planning, and interventions for the necessary home care skills and teaching, and evaluates effectiveness of the plan. Acts as the case manager for the client.

Respiratory therapist (RRT)— Assists the client with any breathing problems. Works with the client with breathing equipment and checks the equipment to see if it is functioning properly.

Social worker (BSW, MSW)— Provides information about community services, financial resources, long-term planning, and respite care. Helps the client and family with psychosocial (emotional, social, and financial) problems.

Speech therapist (ST)—Assesses client's ability to communicate— hear, speak, understand, and write; works with client to improve abilities. Also assesses swallowing difficulties and works with the client to improve swallowing functions.

Registered nurses monitor the client on a continuous basis. Nursing visits are planned according to the level of care and education needed for the client and family members. Emergency support nursing care is available 24 hours a day, 7 days a week through a certified home health care agency. The frequency of social worker visits ranges from once a week to once a month. The social worker role is to assist the client and the family with their financial, legal, and funeral needs. The social worker uses skill as a clinician for problem solving and crisis intervention. A vital part of a home health aide's responsibility is to be an active participant of the health care team. The case manager assesses the client and develops a plan of care, which the home health aide follows. The entire health care team relies on the home health aide for keeping them informed on day-to-day changes occurring with the client.

HEALTH CARE WORKPLACES OUTSIDE THE HOSPITAL OR LONG-TERM CARE FACILITY

Home care agencies differ in many ways: types of service provided, fees for services, policies and procedures, and administrative structures. They can be large or small; nonprofit or for-profit; Medicare certified or non-Medicare certified; and private, religiously affiliated or publicly operated.

Adult Day-Care Centers

Adult day-care centers provide care for adults who need minimal care or supervision during the day. The health care worker in this setting will assist the client in eating, bathing, and recreational activities. The client might come every day or only once a week to the center. These centers are great for a spouse who is a primary caregiver and needs a break for a day from the stress of constant caregiving.

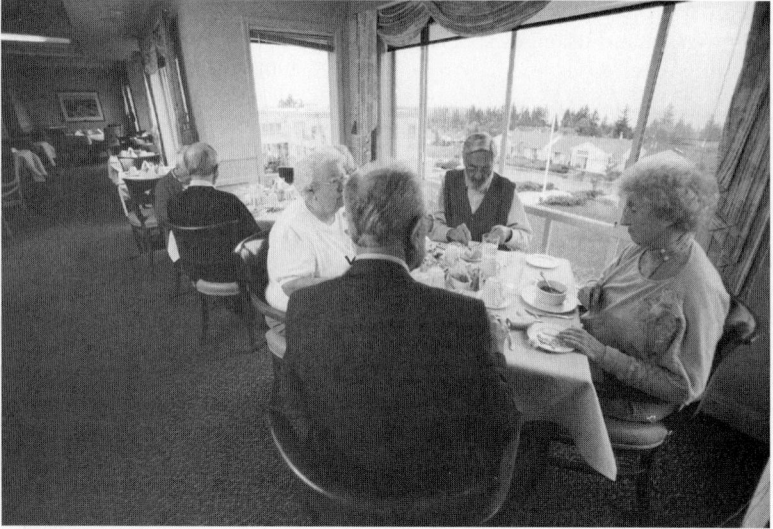

Figure 1-2   An assisted living complex

These types of centers often are equipped with specialized bathing equipment to bathe a client, if their primary care giver is unable to do this task or the client's home does not have the proper equipment to do it.

Assisted-Living Facility

Assisted living centers vary from a two-bedroom condominium to a private room with a shared dining room and central dayroom (Figure 1-2). Individuals can elect to have all meals prepared or eat one meal a day in the central dining area. Generally, these facilities offer a supervised medication program, cleaning and laundry services, and minor assistance in activities of daily living (ADLs). The client pays according to the services requested.

Homemaker/Home Care Agencies

These agencies provide a variety of nonmedical home support services.

They provide companions, homemakers, and personal care workers for the client. These workers are employed to help the client with cleaning, cooking, minimal assistance in personal care, shopping, and companionship.

Home Health Care Agencies

Home health care agencies, some of which are affiliated with hospitals, focus on the medical or nursing aspect of care. Their professionally trained personnel (e.g., registered nurses, speech therapist, physical therapist, etc.) can do dressing changes, monitor vital signs, and perform other tasks ordered by the health care provider. The majority of them offer services of the home health aide. Their services may be paid for by the client, private insurances, Medicaid, or Medicare.

Self-Employment

Self-employed workers have the benefits of working independently, but have some challenges as well. They must find their own clients. If their clients are temporarily hospitalized or placed in a long-term care facility, they are out of work. Unless these workers obtain a private professional liability insurance policy at their own expense, they will not be financially protected from claims and lawsuits if their clients are injured while under their care. Additionally, they will be responsible for filing federal and state estimated income tax returns as well as their year-end returns. They will be responsible for the payment of 100% of their Social Security taxes unless advance arrangements are made with their clients to pay the employer's portion of the tax.

REIMBURSEMENT ISSUES INFLUENCING HEALTH CARE

In the year 2000, the Prospective Payment System (PPS) was implemented in home care and it has great influence on how home health agencies are paid. This system is based on the Outcome and Assessment Information Set (OASIS). Today, a registered nurse performs an assessment of the client and then completes the Outcome and Assessment Information Set form and enters data into the computer for transmission to each state. In 2000, these assessments became the basis of payment and are required in order to bill for services. Information on this admission/OASIS form will determine how much the insurance or Medicare will pay for care of this client within a 60-day period. The reimbursement for services and supplies to a client for 60 days can range from $1,200 to $5,200 (in 2003) and is based on the OASIS assessments completed at the start of care and every 60 days afterwards. *In order for an agency to receive ade-* *quate reimbursement for care of their clients, it is crucial that the home health aide report and document any change in the condition of each individual client.*

Medicare

There are two parts to Medicare. Part A (Hospital Insurance) covers inpatient care in hospitals and skilled nursing facilities. It covers hospice care and some home health care. There is no charge for Part A. Medical Insurance (Part B) helps cover health care provider services and outpatient hospital care (e.g., diagnostic tests, durable medical equipment, and diabetic supplies). In 2004, if you enrolled in Part B when you were first eligible, the premium for Part B was $66 a month. Medicare insurance pays for part of the cost of health care, but certainly not all. The new "Medicare Personal Plan Finder" helps a person to narrow down the Medicare health plan choices and choose the best plan. One can also get important information about special programs that might help pay for health care costs that Medicare does not pay for.

Hospice Medicare Benefits (HMB) are available for clients who have Medicare Part A and have less than six months to live. Medicare will pay hospice for home health aide services, supplies, equipment, some medications, ambulance, respite care, and outpatient care.

To qualify for Medicare reimbursement for home health, an individual must be:
- Confined to home
- Under the care of a doctor who certifies the need for care
- In need of skilled nursing care, physical therapy, or speech therapy
- Receiving services from a Medicare-certified agency as provided by a registered nurse

Medicaid

Medicaid is a federally and state-funded program that pays for health care services for persons whose income is below a certain amount. The coverage provided to recipients and the minimum income level that makes one eligible varies from state to state. The purpose of these programs is to prevent seniors from moving into long-term care facilities before it is absolutely necessary. A person can qualify for both Medicare and Medicaid or other community support programs. Medicare and Medicaid offerings vary from state to state, as no two states offer the same coverage.

Whenever government funding is involved, the federal or state government can regulate the health care industry and demand that certain standards be maintained with regard to health care facilities, health care workers, and educational requirements. The home health aide must be aware of these standards.

LONG-TERM CARE INSURANCE

A new type of insurance, called long-term care insurance, provides help in paying for long-term care. The time covered may be from 12 months up to 5 years. This insurance may cover costs for home health care, respite care, adult day services, assisted living facilities, and long-term care facilities. There is usually a waiting period of six months before the policy starts to pay for care. In order to qualify, a client must be unable to perform some of the activities of daily living (bathing, eating, toileting, walking, or dressing, for example). The cost will vary according to the policy. The premium cost increases with increasing age. One should always do a com-parison study before making a decision regarding this type of insurance. This type of insurance could keep one's estate from being exhausted.

Managed Care

Health maintenance organizations (HMOs) are examples of managed care. This is a method of health care delivery that attempts to cut costs through providing gatekeepers to control access to and use of health care providers, hospitals, nursing facilities, and other forms of care. The goal of this gatekeeper, whether it be a nurse case manager or a health care provider, is to provide the best quality care for the lowest cost. Home care, for example, may be a less costly and more appealing alternative in certain situations. Managed care companies usually offer their patients fewer choices of hospitals, nursing homes, and health care providers. The out-of-pocket cost to the patient, however, is usually lower than with traditional insurance.

These companies often apply the same eligibility restrictions as Medicare, although there has been some expansion in recent years.

THE CLIENT

Home care clients are of all ages, from birth to more than 100 years old. They are typically affected by one or more illnesses or disabilities. Acute illness is one that arises quickly, requires immediate care, and can be expected to go away, such as a cold, flu, or appendicitis. Chronic illness is a long-standing health problem, such as Alzheimer's or Parkinson's disease, or arthritis. Many individuals over the age of 70 are affected by chronic illnesses. Developmentally disabled means the person has a severe chronic emotional or physical disability that occurs before the age of 22, such as cerebral palsy or Down syndrome. Terminal illness is one that is expected to result in death within a limited time period.

Home care clients are truly diverse. They represent different cultures and ethnic groups—Hispanics, Asians, Eastern Europeans, and so forth. They are different races, including African Americans, Caucasians, and Native Americans. They practice different religions—such as Protestantism, Catholicism, Judaism, Muslim, or Buddhism. Throughout this text, you will find examples of this diversity among your clients.

The ethnic makeup of our senior population is rapidly changing. The U.S. Census Bureau expects there will be a large increase in seniors in the Asian and Hispanic populations as compared to the African American and Caucasian populations.

Home health workers cannot expect to know everything about every different culture, race, or religion. It is important, however, to realize that there are differences, to be accepting of them and to be willing to learn about them. Home health aides may learn, for example, that Native American medicine and religion cannot be separated and that they will turn to traditional healing practices from time to time. A home health aide may observe the strength of family ties in

the Hispanic and Asian cultures or learn about the dietary practices of the Orthodox Jewish faith. In addition, the home health aide may be called to do respite care work for the family of a developmentally disabled child, adult, or terminally ill person. This means taking care of the client when the main caregiver needs a break to go shopping, visit with friends, or even rest a bit.

Religious practices, traditions, types of food, and the manner in which food is prepared are very often determined by the culture and religion of the individual. The home health aide must (1) accept the practices of others, (2) be sensitive to the client's needs, and (3) follow the instructions given by the case manager in meeting the needs of the client regardless of religion, color, or belief. An aide must not judge clients, but must allow them the freedom to follow their own practices and beliefs while providing safe and proper care.

In each unit of this text, you will find new words to master and new techniques to learn. As your knowledge grows, so does your confidence as an individual. In becoming a home health aide, you can be proud of your newly acquired skills. Satisfaction comes from being able to use your new knowledge and skills in caring for clients who need your care.

UNIT 2

Home Health Aide Responsibilities and Legal Rights

SKILLS AND QUALITIES OF THE HOME HEALTH AIDE

A career is an occupation or profession for which one has been specially educated. Teacher, lawyer, electrician, and home health aide are examples of careers. In addition to the training and education that are required for each career, certain personal qualities or characteristics make people good at what they do. It is important for a teacher to like children, for a lawyer to be a good communicator, and for an electrician to be cautious and not take risks. Likewise, a number of special qualities make for a good home health aide.

Responsibilities of the Home Health Aide

Punctuality and reliability are very important characteristics for the home health aide. Your client depends on you. If you will be riding the bus, it would be wise to study the bus schedule ahead of time to ensure proper location of the closest bus stop, and to allow adequate time to arrive at the client's home. Or, check your local taxi company for the cost of the ride and the time it might take to arrive at the client's home. If you use your own car, as the majority of home health aides do, be sure to check the location of your client's home and the route to take ahead of time. Check with your agency for their reimbursement policy for mileage to your client's home. The majority of agencies will pay mileage plus salary for travel between clients' homes. This is a good question to ask, once you become employed with an agency, since driving from one home to another can become quite costly and also time-consuming.

It is your responsibility to inform the agency and the family if you cannot report to work as scheduled. Remember that your client is dependent on you, and the agency depends on you to show up for work as scheduled. Check with your agency regarding their policy for being absent or taking time off.

Working Hours. Working hours may be irregular. Primarily the working hours will be during the day, but often a home health aide may be required to work during the night. The aide may be asked to work on varying shifts or on weekends. It is common for a home health aide to be assigned several part-time cases. Due to this irregularity of assignments, a home health aide must be flexible and have access to transportation. This means being able to quickly adjust from one type of situation to another and being able to feel comfortable meeting new people.

Variety of Assignments. The aide must adjust to different family situations and varied health care needs of the clients. No two family situations are the same. This means the aide will have to establish new interpersonal relationships in each case. The medical conditions can range from ill infants to terminally ill clients.

Variety of Settings and Equipment. The aide must adapt to homes that are not as well equipped as others. Some homes have modern equipment and beautiful furnishings. Other homes offer the bare necessities of life. Some homes are spotlessly clean, others are just the opposite. The home health aide will be expected to treat all clients with dignity regardless of their financial position. Each human being is entitled to respectful and dignified care.

Occasionally, you may arrive at the client's home to find the door locked and no one seems to be home. You should go to the nearest phone and call your case manager or inform the agency of the situation. They will give you directions for additional action. It may be that the client needed to be hospitalized or has gone away with his or her family and the agency forgot to notify you.

Ability to Follow Instructions

The being "able" part is what you are learning in this class. At first glance, the role of the home health aide may appear to be simple. It is made up of everyday tasks: keeping a house in order, preparing and cleaning up after meals, and providing for the comfort and safety of a client. Students may feel that they already know how to take care of a house. Most people have been doing housekeeping tasks since early childhood. They think there is nothing new to learn. The student may ask, "Why don't we get to the important things? I want to take care of the sick. Why should I waste my time relearning homemaking skills?" However, everyone can benefit by learning new ways to do certain jobs. Once a new method is learned, the aide can compare it with the old way and may discover a more efficient technique.

By learning to focus on the components of a task, the aide will find understanding comes more easily. Components are the separate parts that make up a whole. Learning how to do something, when to do it, and what should be done first will add up to a more complete understanding.

There are many ways to do some tasks, for example, preparing a meal. There will be certain essential components of the task that if not completed correctly and in the right order will mean the task has been done wrong. For example, you need to wash your hands first. You need to follow the client's dietary requirements. You can toast the bread before or after you slice a tomato, but you must put ingredients away and clean up after preparing food. A procedure is a list of steps used to complete a task.

There are usually two parts to the instruction given to the home health aide. The first is called theory. Theory is the information that forms a basis for action. In classroom lectures and in the assigned readings, the student learns theory. The second component is devoted to practice. Practice is the actual performance of the procedures. Practice is combined with the theory to enable the student to build skills in both areas at the same time. The home health aide learns client care procedures and homemaking procedures.

The student will need to demonstrate a designated list of procedures satisfactorily in front of an instructor. Each procedure will be demonstrated by the instructor before the student performs the procedure. The instructor will give the student a copy of the procedure with all the required steps listed. Use these procedure guidelines in practicing each procedure in the laboratory. Your instructor will determine if you have learned the procedure correctly by giving you an evaluation. An evaluation may consist of written tests or demonstrations where you actually perform the procedure. Evaluation helps the student know which areas require extra study or practice.

Willingness to Follow Instructions

As important as being able to follow the instructions of your supervisor is being willing to follow them. Before taking a case, a home health aide should be sure to ask for all vital information. In addition, the supervisor will provide a home care plan for the client, outlining the specific care to be provided and the aide's responsibilities. This includes duties, client needs, and the name and telephone number of the case manager.

Both ability and willingness to follow instructions affect the home health aide's liability when things go wrong.

Constructive Criticism

The home health aide should develop a nondefensive attitude toward criticism by the professional staff at the agency where he or she is employed. Constructive criticism is a way of achieving additional skills or upgrading present techniques. The aide must be open to new suggestions. Recognizing one's ability to adapt to new ideas presented by more experienced staff members will result in the improvement of your own professional skills. Look kindly on and accept the guidance of your supervising nurse, as this will only benefit your client as well as yourself. Your goal must be to move in a positive direction toward optimum client care.

Legal Terms

The home health aide should be familiar with the following legal terms:

Abandonment is being left without care or support by family or agency.

Aiding and abetting is not reporting dishonest acts that one observed.

Assault is an intentional attempt or threat to touch a person without the person's consent.

Battery is the actual touching of a person's body without the person's consent.

Defamation is stating untrue statements about a person, which would injure this person's name and reputation.

False imprisonment is the unlawful restriction of a

person's freedom of movement.

Invasion of privacy is exposing or making public a person's name, photograph, or private information without the consent of the person.

Liability refers to the degree to which you will be held financially responsible for the damages resulting from your negligence.

Libel is a false written statement about another person.

Malpractice is the failure to exercise reasonable judgment in the application of professional knowledge.

Negligence is an action on your part or your failure to act that either causes or contributes to the cause of a personal injury or property damage to others.

Slander is making a false oral statement about another person.

HEALTH INSURANCE PORTABILITY AND ACCOUNTABILITY ACT OF 1996

The Health Insurance Portability and Accountability Act (HIPAA) was created to develop guidelines for maintaining and transmitting health information that identified individual clients. The HIPAA went into effect in April 2003. This act mandates that all of your client's health information—oral, paper, or electronic—be protected and confidential. This includes any medical information used to make a decision about the client's health care coverage, as well as the client's name, address, and telephone number. HIPAA was de-veloped to allow the flow of health information needed to provide and promote quality health care while assuring proper protection of individual private health information.

The law describes certain individual rights. Upon written request, an individual may view or make copies of his or her protected health information, which is in a designated record set defined by the plan. Individuals may also make a written request to receive an accounting disclosure of their health information on payment of their care (what charges were for health care and what costs were paid for by Medicare or private insurance). Individuals can also make a written request to correct their health information, although the law does not require the health agency to grant all requests it receives.

You might ask, how does this act affect a home health aide? As you work as a home health aide, you have an opportunity to read the client's chart, interact with the family members, know if this client's health care is being paid for by Medicaid, and know the health condition of the client. You must keep all this information confidential. You are allowed to discuss information about your client to other members of the home health care team, and it must be limited to the team members only. Do not discuss your client with your friends or family.

A few of your clients might live in a senior high-rise, and often clients are curious about who else in the building has a home health aide, or what is wrong with that person. You are not allowed to tell another client that you are even caring for someone else in the building. You might tell your client to talk to his or her neighbor to find out the information.

Situations for Home Health Aides to Avoid

Do only and exactly what your case manager instructs you to do. There are some situations you should recognize and avoid.

1. *Doing more than is assigned.* Practice saying "no" in a tactful way, encouraging the client to contact the case manager if more services are wanted. When you do something that was not assigned, you are assuming responsibility (liability) for these acts, and your agency is no longer responsible.

2. *Doing less than is assigned.* This may put the client in danger and lead to a charge of negligence, which means "an action or lack of action that leads to an accident or injury."

3. *Doing hasty, careless, or poor-quality work.* You have received training in the proper way to carry out your work activities. It is your responsibility to work carefully. Sometimes, even with the greatest amount of care being taken, accidents happen: a valuable vase breaks while you are dusting it or a client falls. If you have been carrying out your assigned duties and exercising a reasonable amount of care, you usually are not held liable for the damage or injury that results; agencies carry liability insurance to cover these types of accidents.

4. *Using your car for work activities.* This particularly applies to taking a client in your care, even to the doctor's office or just out for a ride, without letting your car insurance agency know. If an accident occurs, you might be liable for the resulting damage and you may be required to personally pay for those damages, if you do not have proper coverage. Be sure your driver's license is current and in good standing, that your car is in good repair and have approval of your agency to take the client in your car. Also, be sure you will be paid mileage for use of your car by your agency. Before employing an individual, some agencies will require that the home health aide has a valid driver's license, car, and proper automobile insurance.

5. *Failing to do accurate and daily reporting and documentation.* You are in a hurry and decide not to chart today on your client, but plan to do it the next day when you will have more time. The client's daughter comes to visit her mother and sees that nothing is written on the chart that day and immediately assumes that no one was there to care for her mother. The daughter becomes quite upset over this incident, which could have easily been avoided, and calls the home health agency.

6. *Failing to act in an emergency.* You should know what the emergency plan is for each client you care for, and you should be prepared to follow it. In a life-threatening situation, call 911 if available in your area. If 911 service is not available, call for an ambulance before calling your case manager. There are a few exceptions before calling an ambulance in an emergency. In some cases the family wants to be notified before calling an ambulance; or some agencies want to be notified first before calling an ambulance. This information should be clearly stated in the client's care plan. Some agencies

may require you to be CPR/first aid certified before you are hired. Do not try to perform first aid or cardiopulmonary resuscitation (CPR) if you have not been trained to do so.

7. *Attempting to do things that are beyond your abilities.* It is okay to say, "I don't know how to do that. Let's see if we can get someone who does." You are not employed as a nurse, a plumber, an electrician, or a counselor . . . do not try to be one.

8. *Injuring yourself or the client* by doing something you are not assigned or adequately trained to do. If you have been assigned to do something you do not feel comfortable doing, ask for more training. Trying to do something without assignment and adequate training, such as moving a client with a Hoyer lift, can leave you liable for injury that results.

9. *Failing to report* unsafe working conditions that later cause injury to you or another home health aide. Do not take unnecessary risks. Follow the agency procedures for reporting.

ORGANIZATIONAL SKILLS

A successful aide possesses good organizational skills. An aide must manage time well to be able to complete all the tasks required in the allotted time. The instructions may include light housekeeping, laundry and ironing, meal preparation, marketing, and personal care of the client. The aide will have to decide the best way to plan each day's activities. This will require flexibility, practical judgment, and time organization. Some pitfalls to avoid are:

- Not replacing or ordering supplies when needed from your case manager
- Watching television
- Jumping from one task to another and one room to another without organizing priorities
- Putting off unpleasant tasks because they are disagreeable
- Talking to friends on the telephone or doing personal business
- Stopping frequently for a cup of coffee

Prior to starting your work, it is a good idea to make a list of tasks that need to be done for your client that day. Then check to see if you have all the supplies you need to accomplish these tasks. As you work, you can check off the list as you go, this will lessen your chance of forgetting some tasks. After all the routine tasks are completed and the client care procedures are done, then you might start the less important tasks. Each plan should be flexible enough to plan for the unexpected.

A home health aide may be scheduled to work with several clients during a week. It is not unusual to stay with one client only two hours and then be on your way to another client's home for another two hours. It is a good idea to write your own personal notes on each assignment so as not to forget something or other peculiarity of the client. Another suggestion as you work is to record in your notepad any supplies that are getting low and any observations about your client, so once you are ready to chart, you will remember to write this down.

When beginning a new job, the aide must adjust to the client's or family's routine. Aides should not reorganize the entire house or daily schedule to suit themselves. An aide's job is to make the family comfortable and to assist them, not to change their lifestyle. Remember, as a home health aide, you are a guest in the client's home.

INTERPERSONAL SKILLS

When people live, work, or play together, one person acts and the other reacts or responds to the act. This process is called an interaction.

People are expected to handle interactions as a part of everyday life. The feeling and understanding that result from the interactions between two or more persons form what are called interpersonal relationships. To the person entering a service occupation, interpersonal relationships can determine success or failure. Each of the persons involved in these relationships is entitled to be treated with dignity. Everyone should follow the golden rule—treat others as you would like to be treated. This helps to establish good interpersonal relationships.

Home health aides must remember that they are entering a home where an illness or problem already exists. An illness or problem may cause the family members to be unhappy or disorganized. Anger, fear, and other emotional reactions may be obvious. The client may be in pain, cranky, sad, or depressed. The home health aide who is aware of the source of the problem often finds it easier to accept the family's behavior. As a result, awkward interpersonal relationships often can be avoided.

GOOD PERSONAL HEALTH AND HYGIENE

A home health aide must observe the personal hygiene standards expected of any health team member. When working in other people's homes, the aide should reflect the highest standards. This means being clean and well groomed each workday. The person who goes on a job unbathed, with dirty hair and nails, and wearing wrinkled, stained clothes makes a bad impression. A sloppy appearance implies that the person also has a poor self-image and sloppy working habits.

An aide should wear a clean uniform, clean undergarments, and comfortable, polished shoes.

An aide who is appropriately dressed or in the proper uniform creates a more professional appearance and makes the client feel more comfortable. Home care agencies vary greatly in their dress codes. A few agencies do require a designated uniform, whereas others may allow the aide to wear comfortable, clean, untattered street clothes. Most agencies do not allow their home health aides to wear blue jeans or shorts.

Guidelines for Personal Appearance of the Home Health Aide

Following are guidelines the home health aide should follow:

- Bathe daily and use deodorant.
- Do not wear strong perfumes or strong aftershave lotion.
- Brush your teeth regularly and use mouthwash if necessary.
- One is not allowed to smoke while on duty in the client's home, if need be you can smoke on your break outside the client's home. Clients with lung disease, allergies, respiratory illness, or personal distaste for the smell of cigarettes may have an adverse reaction to cigarette smoke.
- Wear makeup moderately; if you have tattoos, cover them with clothing; body piercing jewelry such as in the nose, tongue, and

eyebrows should be removed while on duty.

- For men, shave daily and keep beard or mustache neat and clean.
- Shampoo your hair often; if you have long hair, pull it back so it is off your collar.
- Fingernails are to be clean and short.
- Jewelry should be limited. Small post earrings for pierced ears are usually acceptable.
- Bracelets, dangling earrings and necklaces, and large stone rings are not acceptable, as clients who are confused might grab them and a large ring can tear a client's skin.
- Shoes should be clean and in good repair.
- Wear a watch with a second hand and your name pin from your agency.

ETHICAL BEHAVIOR

Ethics is a standard or code of behavior. It is a code concerned with what is "right" and what is "wrong." Health care providers take an oath when they are licensed in which they promise to help and care for clients without causing unnecessary pain or suffering. Although there is no written code for home health aides, they are expected to uphold a definite set of standards as they practice their profession.

Ethical Standards

- Be honest in your dealings with clients and coworkers. Stealing involves not only the taking of objects or money, it involves falsifying reports of time and activities.
- Never discuss the financial, emotional, family, medical, or other problems of the client with outsiders. Confidentiality is a commitment to keep your client's affairs private. The home health aide must not discuss the client's health, family situation, finances, or any other personal matter with anyone except the supervisor or other agency staff directly involved in the client's care. This includes the worker's family and friends.
- Respect the cultural and religious practices of the client and family.
- Never walk out in the middle of an assignment. Some people may be more pleasant to work with than others. If a personality conflict or the work load is impossible to deal with, the aide should try to finish the shift, then call the case manager and explain the problem. If the aide is working a private case or did not get the job through an agency, the problem should be discussed directly with the employer. Having accepted the duties as an employee, a home health aide is ethically bound to give service for the wages paid.
- Refuse tips and gifts. Some clients may forget that they have given you a gift and accuse you of theft. The family may also resent any gifts that are given to the home health aide.
- Report possible cases of abuse.
- Do not have any sexual contact with a client.
- Safeguard the confidential information you acquired from any source concerning the client.
- Never ask to borrow money from a client.
- Do not adjust the client's care plan without permission of the case manager.

Professional Standards

- Maintain high standards of personal health and appearance.
- Be dependable and reliable.

- Carry out the responsibilities of the job in the best way you possibly can.
- Show respect for the client's privacy and modesty.
- Recognize and respect the right of clients to determine their lifestyle.
- Keep your professional life separate from your personal life. Personal problems of the home health aide should not be discussed with the client or the client's family.
- Control any negative reactions to chronic disability or the living conditions of the client.
- Maintain safe conditions in the working environment.
- Do not use client's medications for your own health problems.
- Do not give your home phone number or mobile cell phone number to the client unless the case manager instructs you to do so. Occasionally, a client may become lonesome and call you continuously just to talk.

CLIENT'S RIGHTS

The home health aide must respect the rights of the clients. The following is a list of common client rights that are mandated by OBRA regulations:

1. Every client shall be treated with consideration, respect, and full recognition of the client's dignity and individuality.
2. Every client shall receive care, treatment, and services that are adequate, appropriate, and in compliance with relevant federal and state law.
3. Every client has the right to be free from mental and physical abuse.
4. Every client shall be informed of these rights in writing and in the language the client can understand.
5. Every client who is responsible for a fee for service shall be given

a statement of the services available by the agency and related charges.

6. Every client shall participate in the development of the plan of care and discharge plan and be informed of all treatments, when and how services will be provided, and the name and functions of any person and affiliated agency providing care and services.
7. Every client has the right to refuse treatment after being fully informed of and understanding the consequence of such actions.
8. Every client shall be informed of the procedure for submitting complaints to the agency. If the client is not satisfied by the agency response, the client may complain to the state Department of Health and Social Services.
9. Every client shall have the right to recommend changes in policies and services to agency staff, the area office representatives of the department, or any outside representative of the client's choice free from restraints, interference, coercion, discrimination, or reprisal.
10. Every client shall receive respect and privacy, including confidential treatment of client records, and the right to refuse release of records to any individuals outside the agency.
11. Every client has the right to privacy.
12. Every client has the right to request change of caregiver.
13. Every client has the right to be informed of the state consumer hotline telephone number.

HOME HEALTH AIDE'S RIGHTS

As an employee of an agency or your client, you also have rights. Examples of your rights are:

1. The right to take pride in a job well done
2. The right to make suggestions and complaints within designated channels without fear of retaliation
3. The right not to be abused physically, verbally, or sexually by clients
4. The right to recommend care plan changes designed to facilitate care delivery and reduce caregiver stress
5. The right to be informed when complaints concerning client treatment are alleged against you
6. The right to a fair hearing with your case manager
7. The right to a confidential investigation
8. The right to be informed of the investigation's outcome
9. The right to be paid for your services by your agency for a predetermined salary and mileage for travel
10. The right to attend continuing education programs offered by your agency at no cost to you
11. The right to work in a safe environment

CLIENT ABUSE

You and your supervisor should not tolerate client abuse, neglect, or mistreatment. All home health aides are expected to use a professional, caring approach with all clients. There are many forms of abuse. Abuse is defined as the willful infliction of physical pain, injury, mental anguish or fear, unreasonable confinement, or the willful deprivation by a caretaker of services that are necessary to maintain mental and physical health. Abuse may be emotional, financial, involuntary seclusion, mental, physical, or sexual.

- *Emotional or verbal abuse* is using depreciative terms or remarks either orally, written, or by gestures to describe someone. The client behaves in an unusual way with this person is present.
- *Financial abuse* is using the client's money inappropriately or stealing money or other valuables. The client might mention that money is missing or the client states that he or she was forced to sign checks for services the client never received.
- *Involuntary seclusion* is placing the client in his or her room without the person's consent or not allowing the individual to visit with others.
- *Mental abuse* is threatening or humiliating a client. Using profanity or obscene words, shouting, teasing, or any other method to humiliate the client. Obvious signs might be passive, withdrawn, and emotionless behavior of the client and lack of reaction to pain.
- *Physical abuse* is hitting, burning, or pinching another person. Another example is forcing a treatment on a client that the client has requested not to be done. Other signs might be frequent, unexplained injuries or complaints of pain without obvious injuries, and burns or bruises suggesting the use of a cigarette or curling iron, etc.
- *Sexual abuse* is making sexual advances to someone or touching a person in inappropriate places. Signs to look for are injury to genital area, difficulty in sitting or walking, fear of being alone with caregivers.

Every state now has a reporting requirement to the state Department of Health if a person has reasonable cause to believe that a child or a disabled adult is in need of protective services. If a home health aide knows or has a reasonable belief that a client is being abused by the client's family, another caregiver, or anyone else, the aide must report the abuse to the client's case manager. It is preferable to document what you saw or other pertinent observation about the abuse. There are criminal penalties imposed by the state if a person fails to make a report. Every state gives legal immunity from civil or criminal liability to the reporting person unless that person acted in bad faith or with a malicious purpose. If the home health aide is self-employed, he or she must report directly to the state Department of Health in the state where the abused person resides. The state sends out an ombudsman who investigates and mediates problems regarding the complaints.

Although it is known that in 90% of all reported elder abuse cases the abuser is a family member, it is not known how many of these abusive family members are also caregivers. Researchers have estimated that anywhere from 5% to 23% of all caregivers are physically abusive. Most agree that abuse is related to the stresses associated with providing care.

UNIT 3

Developing Effective Communication Skills and Documentation

The ability to communicate effectively may be the most important skill that a care provider can learn. Communication is the successful transmission of information from one person to another. A care provider's work with people consists primarily of performing tasks, but it also includes establishing positive relationships. The care provider often must communicate why a certain task needs to be done or perhaps coax the person to help with the task. The care provider may also communicate concern—or frustration—in nonverbal ways. Communication with the client's family may involve explaining the reasons why the care provider cannot do certain tasks the family wants, or the need to encourage the family to offer more assistance.

CULTURAL DIVERSITY

Culture is defined as the behaviors, values, beliefs, habits, and customs of a group of people, which have been passed on from one generation to another. In the United States, we have cultural diversity, which is a mixture of individuals from different cultures. Different cultures require slightly different approaches in their personal care and in communication. It would be ideal if all the caregivers could be of the same culture as their clients, but that is not possible. However, Native Americans do request that only individuals from their own tribe be their caregivers. They do not like caregivers of another culture doing personal care on them. In some cultures, it is considered very disrespectful to have the caregiver look the client directly in the eyes. Another difference with individuals of different cultures is how they deal with pain. Other cultural differences deal with personal approach: two people may need to shake hands or embrace one another before talking. This is their right and we need to adjust care according to their beliefs. If any of these cultural differences do exist, they should be in the client's care plan and explained to you by your case manager. Take time to learn about your clients and beliefs. Always be respectful of and interested in other cultures without being judgmental.

To enhance the communication process with a client who does not speak or understand English, the case manager may make arrangements for an interpreter to visit the client when you are there and assist you with fundamental communication needs.

In summary, when caring for a client of another culture:

- Avoid body language that may be offensive or misunderstood.
- Plan your care based on the communication needs and cultural background of the client.
- Adopt special approaches when the client speaks another language.
- Do not judge your client in any way.
- Communicate with the client in a nonthreatening way.
- Research cultural information as necessary.

STRESSFUL CONDITIONS IN THE HOME

Family can be defined as a group of people living in the same household and usually under one head—including parents, children, relatives, and friends. As a home health aide, you must remember that every family operates differently and no two families are alike. It is wise not to take sides with family members in caring for your client. Often the stress of illness and disability brings changes in the behavior of family members. The financial aspect of care can also become a heavy stressor on families, especially in a chronic long-term illness. The home health aide must respect the confidentiality of the family

and share his or her concerns only with the case manager or another designated health team member.

COMMUNICATION IN THE WORKPLACE

Good communication is essential in the worker-supervisor relationship. A worker who knows what, how, and to whom she should report is an effective team member.

Communicating, something that we all do every day, sounds easy, but it is actually a complicated process. There are three key aspects of communication: how messages are sent and received, active listening, and nonverbal communication.

SEND A CLEAR MESSAGE

Communication is a two-way process. The sender must send a message and the receiver must receive it for communication to occur. However, the communication is not successful unless the meaning of the message sent and the one received are the same. This is not easy to accomplish. At many points something can go wrong.

Problems in communication can begin before words are even spoken. We have all experienced times when our thoughts are unclear. Although we are not sure what we want to say, we say it anyway. The resulting confusion is no surprise. Taking the time to organize our thoughts before speaking is the basis for all clear communication.

For many different reasons, we do not talk to each other, and the result is rarely good. When clear communication of expectations has not taken place, mistakes happen that could have been avoided. Care providers often have thoughts, feelings, and information that the case manager should know about. When the care providers do not

a–before	HS–hour of sleep	PT–physiotherapy,
ac–before meals	Ht–height	physical therapy
ad lib–as desired	I & O–intake and	q2h–every 2 hours
ADLs–activities of	output	q3h–every 3 hours
daily living	IV–intravenous	q4h–every 4 hours
Amb–ambulatory	K–potassium	qd–every day
bid–twice a day	Lab–laboratory	qid–four times a day
BM–bowel	lb–pound	qod–every other day
movement	mg–milligram	ROM–range of
BP–blood pressure	mL–milliliter	motion exercises
BRP–bathroom	Na–sodium salt	s̄–without
privileges	noc–night	SOB–short of breath
C–Celsius	NPO–nothing by	Spec–specimen
c̄–with	mouth	SSE–soap solution
CBR–complete bed	O_2–oxygen	enema
rest	OD–right eye	ST–speech therapy
cc–cubic centimeter	OS–left eye	stat–immediately
c/o–complains of	OT–occupational	Temp–(T)–
CPR–cardiopulmonary	therapy	temperature
resuscitation	OU–both eyes	tid–three times a day
dc–discontinue	oz–ounce	TLC–tender loving
dsg–dressing	p̄–after	care
F–Fahrenheit	pc–after meals	TPR–temperature,
Fe–iron	PO–by mouth	pulse, respiration
gtt–drop	prep–prepare for	VS–vital signs: TPR
H_2O–water	prn–when needed or	and BP
HOB–head of bed	necessary	w/c–wheelchair
HOH–hard of hearing	pt–patient	Wt–weight

Figure 3-1 Standard medical abbreviations must be learned to understand and correctly chart medical orders.

communicate with the case manager problems can occur. The case manager will not know how the worker is feeling unless she mentions it. Only then can she get the support she needs.

OBSERVATION

The home health aide is in a unique position to observe client needs in the home environment. Through frequent observation and interaction with the client, the aide will see changes in the client's behavior and the environment. In this role the aide has two responsibilities: to orient the client and to provide observations to other members of the care team.

Including orientation to space and time as a part of her routine with the client may be helpful to some clients. "Good morning, Mrs. Jones. It's 9 o'clock, time for your breakfast. You

AIDS–Acquired immunodeficiency syndrome	CVA–Cerebral vascular accident (stroke)	MS–Multiple sclerosis
ARC–AIDS-related complex	DJD–Degenerative joint disease	PID–Pelvic inflammatory disease
ASHD–Arteriosclerosis (hardening of the arteries)	DM–Diabetes mellitus	STD–Sexually transmitted disease
CA–Cancer	Fx–Fracture	TB–Tuberculosis
CBS–Chronic brain syndrome	HIV–Human immunodeficiency virus	TIA–Transient ischemic attack (small stroke)
CHF–congestive heart failure	HPV–Human papillomavirus	URI–Upper respiratory infection
COPD–Chronic obstructive pulmonary disease	MI–Myocardial infarction (heart attack)	UTI–Urinary tract infection

Figure 3-2   Abbreviations used in the diagnosis of a condition or disease. Many times more than one diagnosis will be listed for a client.

know, this is the coldest January 5th I can remember." For many homebound ill people, one day is similar to another. Reminders of the day, the time, the season, and life outside their home are helpful. If a client seems unable to remember even after this orientation, the home health aide will report this to other health care team members or the family.

For the work team to be effective, the home health aide must make sure that she is providing as much detail as possible about the client to other members of the health care team. Observing and reporting are key aspects of the care provider's work. She is the eyes and ears of the family and of the employer. Good case notes can help keep families and other professionals up-to-date and informed about the client. Figure 3-1 includes some commonly used abbreviations that may be encountered and used in writing case notes. Figure 3-2 includes a list

of abbreviations used in the diagnosis of a condition or disease of a client. Accurate and clear communication is the goal of these notes.

POSITIVE FEEDBACK

For some reason, many of us have difficulty complimenting others and receiving compliments. We may be thinking a kind thought, but we do not put it into words. Unless the other person is a mind reader, it means nothing. One should always state the positive action that a person is doing first, rather than saying a negative statement. We all like "warm fuzzies" and that compliment will help the client's self-esteem. Your client, Mr. Keane, has just progressed from a walker to a cane. He was able to walk from his kitchen to the bathroom with little difficulty, but very slowly. The aide states, "Mr. Keane, you are doing great without your walker, it is good you are not walking fast the first time, as you may lose your balance." A negative approach for the aide would be, "Mr. Keane, you should be able to walk faster now that you have a cane." Remember compliments and praise are comforting to a client and also for the home health aide.

PUTTING THOUGHTS INTO WORDS

The message being sent often has more than one meaning, and the receiver must try to figure out what the sender really means. There are many common phrases and words that have a wide range of meanings.

There is not likely to be total agreement on many terms that we commonly use. We must be very careful that the understanding of the sender and the receiver is the same. Communication can be difficult when the message is not clear enough and when the person who receives the message does not ask for clarification.

MESSAGE DELIVERY

Any message can be delivered in a variety of ways. Comedians say that the success of a joke depends on delivery. Tone of voice, facial expressions, body language, and gestures all affect how a message is delivered. For example, tone of voice can make a profound difference in the way a message is sent. Nonverbal communication also may include eye contact, posture, and the distance between people.

RECEIVING MESSAGES

Many factors can affect how a message is received. Hearing loss, medications, disabilities, and depression can have major effects on how a client receives a communication. Clients with hearing, speech, or visual impairments need special attention.

The following list of techniques can be used to improve communication with these clients.

- Be sure you have the person's attention before beginning to speak.
- Face the person and make eye contact.
- Lower the pitch of your voice; do not mumble.
- Speak clearly and slowly.
- Use short sentences.
- Avoid background noise, turn off the TV or radio.
- Encourage the use of nonverbal communication, such as touch, or hold the client's hand.
- Use written communication or other visual aid if you are unable to communicate verbally.
- Do not shout; use a normal tone, as shouting makes words less clear.
- Do not speak with something in your mouth or with your hands over your lips.
- Restate your sentence when you are not understood.
- If you do not understand a part of your client's message, restate the part that you do understand and ask for clarification.
- Talk toward the "better" ear because many people hear better out of one ear.
- Recognize that illness or fatigue reduces the ability of a person with a hearing or speech impairment.
- Do not exhaust the person with irrelevant noise or chatter.
- Visual cues may assist the client; use hand gestures when appropriate; provide the opportunity for lipreading.

Touch is an important form of nonverbal communication. In some cultures touching is not appropriate, so talk with your supervisor if you are unsure.

BARRIERS TO THE COMMUNICATION PROCESS

The following techniques hinder good communication rather than improve the process.

Not Listening

One reason that a message may not be received correctly is because of poor listening skills. It is interesting how little we are taught about how to listen. Yet listening is one of the most important factors in communication.

A poor listener shows inattention by various means. Some of the behaviors demonstrated by a poor listener are not paying attention to the speaker, listening passively, preparing an answer before the speaker is through talking, rushing the speaker, interrupting the speaker or changing the subject, and becoming emotional. Another common mistake by a listener is to give advice when it is not asked for.

Changing the Subject

It is often tempting to change the subject because the subject is uncomfortable. The client may be depressed and speaking about things that are discouraging to hear. Stay with the client, who may need to talk about something that is deeply troubling. Changing the subject will not take the problem away, but listening may very well ease the load.

Using Clichés or Platitudes

A platitude is a word or a phrase that people use very often for a lot of different situations.

- "Oh, you'll get over it."
- "Just make the most of it."
- "Tomorrow's another day."
- "It's God's will."

You will offer these words of encouragement from time to time, and, at some point in the conversation, these reassurances may be much appreciated. However, when a person comes to you with a problem, platitudes may completely invalidate her feelings, making her feel that her problems are not important. Platitudes may be useful at a later point in the conversation, after the individual has had the opportunity to express feelings.

Giving Advice

Do not give your client advice or make recommendations. Just listening to your client will usually help the person to arrive at his or her own decision.

Talking About Yourself

Caregiver-client discussion is not restricted, but the caregiver's role is to listen to the clients, not to air her own problems.

Showing Disapproval and Passing Judgment on the Client

It is extremely important to remain nonjudgmental of clients.

Asking "Why" Questions

Often more information is needed before you can understand what someone means. In that case, a "why" question is often used. Care must be taken when asking "why" questions because they can also send the message that you are judging the other person. Such questions include:

- "Why did you do that?"
- "Why are you thinking that?"

These short, direct questions may suggest that you are disapproving or judging the other person. "Mrs. Jones,

I'm not sure why you did that—help me understand so I can do it better next time." Or, "Mr. Smith, why would you think I would do that?" These are softer messages that include the fact that you are inquiring to understand the situation better.

EFFECTIVE LISTENING SKILLS

A person who is an effective listener shows positive behaviors. Paying attention to the speaker, adopting an accepting attitude with a calm, open facial expression and a relaxed non-threatening body position, and allowing the speaker plenty of time are just a few ways to be an effective listener. We are all very susceptible to distraction when asked to be a listener. Our own needs, fears, values, and beliefs can influence our ability to listen and communicate objectively.

The final factor in good communication is one that is often underestimated. That is when we "interpret the message" that has been sent. At this point, we develop our own understanding of what has been said. Active listening is a tool that will allow the home health aide to become very involved in the communication process. The home health aide can make sure that he or she understands not only what the speaker has said, but also how the person feels. We do this by giving the speaker feedback about what we have heard The speaker may then confirm or correct our understanding.

We often assume that we know what a person is saying without checking to make sure that one is correct in those assumptions. When we carefully listen, then check to see if we heard correctly, we are participating in active listening. In **passive listening,** listeners simply sit and

hope that they understand what is being said. However, there are many points along the way during which the message may go wrong, so we should work to become active rather than passive listeners. Active listeners become very involved in the process, constantly checking to see if they are on target in what they understand.

ACTIVE LISTENING BEHAVIORS

There are four active listening behaviors that should be practiced.

- Paraphrasing
- Reflecting the speaker's feelings
- Asking for more information
- Using nonverbal communication

Paraphrasing

Paraphrase what has been said. Paraphrasing involves restating, in your own words, what the other person has said; this gives you a chance to check whether your understanding of what has been said is correct. It also gives the speaker a chance to correct you if you have misunderstood. You might say such things as "Do you mean that . . .?" "I understand you are saying. . . ."

Reflecting the Speaker's Feelings

The feelings behind what is being said are often as important as the words, if not more so. Therefore, it is important to try to understand the underlying feelings, attitudes, beliefs, or values. You might make such statements as "That must have made you upset." "I imagine you were thrilled about that." "Does that worry you?"

Asking for More Information

We often need more information to understand what has been said. In most cases, we simply need to ask for clarification. Responses may include: "I'm interested. Tell me more about that." "What happened after that?" "How did you feel when that happened?"

Using Nonverbal Communication

The average person spends only approximately 5% of the day listening and 30% of the day speaking. These factors can cause us to make assumptions, which may not always be true. As a listener, realize that everyone naturally makes assumptions, but it is important to remain skeptical about these assumptions, until they are proven true.

- Certain behaviors on the part of the listener and the speaker communicate that messages are being received. It is important to both listen and observe as some messages are communicated in ways other than speaking.
- Nonverbal communication reinforces what a client or family member is feeling. It is important to pay attention to facial expressions, posture, and body language. At all times, the health care workers need to be aware of their own facial and body expressions, gestures, and posture.
- Eye contact is another important nonverbal form of communication. It is very important to make and maintain eye contact. This shows the client or family member that you are paying direct attention to him or her.
- Posture, the way you sit or position the body, also demonstrates information. Always try to sit comfortably. Be sensitive to the client's spatial (space) territory. Sitting too close can be an invasion of personal space, while sitting too far away can suggest fear or distrust.
- Verbal input indicates that you are listening and observing. Your response must show that you have listened and can accurately reflect what has been heard and observed.
- Questioning is an excellent way to learn about the client and family. Open questions allow room for response and expression of feelings. Open questions lead to further discussion of a subject or feeling. Examples of open questions include: "Could you describe . . . ?" "Now do you understand that . . . ?" or "Tell me about. . . ." Closed questions generally can be answered with specific information or "yes" or "no." These questions are useful to begin conversations, especially when a client or family member is not very talkative. It is most important to avoid asking leading questions that put words into the client's or family member's mouth.

OBSERVATION SKILLS

In most cases, the client is with the home health aide more than any other person. If there is a problem, the aide may be the only, or at least the most likely, person to notice it. The client may be developing a rash, losing weight, or becoming more disoriented—all indications that there may be a problem. If the problem is noticed and professional assistance is obtained, it may be resolved quickly. If not, the situation may be life-threatening. That it why the home health aide's skills of observation are so important.

All five senses—seeing, hearing, touching, smelling, and tasting should be used in the day-to-day work of the home health aide. Let's consider each sense as follows:

1. Seeing

Look at the client carefully, watching for any change since your last visit. Things you might note are facial expression, posture, skin color, rashes, color of drainage, swelling, way of walking (gait), and steadiness when walking.

Look at the home for safety hazards (overloaded electrical outlet, throw rugs, loose steps or locks), cleanliness, medications sitting out with covers off, spots and stains on furniture or floors.

2. Hearing

Listen to the client. What is being said? How is it being said? Is the client's speech clear or slurred? Is it logical or nonsensical? Are the words sad, angry, friendly, or hostile? Does the client use profane language? Do you hear wheezing, coughing, or gasping for breath?

Listen to the home. Does the faucet drip? Does the furnace or hot water heater make noises? Are the telephone and doorbell loud enough for the client to hear?

3. Touching

Touch the client's hand. Does the skin feel hot, cold, or moist? Is it rough or swollen? What is the pulse rate?

Feel things in the house. Are the sheets dry? Is the bread dried up? Is the water too hot?

4. Smelling

Does the client have bad breath or body odor? Does the odor smell like sweat, urine, feces, alcohol, or fruit? Is there an odor from an open sore or dressing?

5. Tasting

Is the food too salty or too spicy? Is the coffee too strong?

REPORTING

Some important instructions that you need during your orientation to an agency are how to report information, who to report it to, and when to report it. The person who you will most likely report to is either your supervisor or case manager.

You will need to exercise judgment in making these reports. Some things need to be reported immediately, such as a fall. Some things need to be reported when you call the office at the end of your shift. Others can be documented on the chart or talked about at your weekly conference with your case manager. Examples of abnormal signs and symptoms that need to be reported and documented are: shortness of breath, rapid respirations, chills, fever, pain in the chest, bluish color to lips, pain in abdomen, nausea and vomiting, drowsiness, excessive thirst, excessive perspiration, purulent drainage, blood in urine, pain on urinating, or dark urine with strong odor.

Throughout your career as a home health aide, and especially as a beginner, you should remember it is *always* better to report something than to risk endangering the client, the agency, and yourself by not reporting it. Your case manager will help you learn how to sort out the "crisis" from the "unusual," and develop good judgment in reporting. When you talk over your observations and your feelings with the supervisor, you can speak freely and voice your opinions and small details. All of these help your case manager to make decisions; he or she can help you learn to be more concise and accurate in your oral reports as time goes on.

DOCUMENTING

Writing down your observations and actions, or documentation, is an important part of your job. Each agency has their own forms that they want you to use and will tell you how often you need to document something in writing, where to do it, and when to turn it in.

There is a saying that "The job is not over till the paperwork is done." This certainly holds true in home health care. The information you write can be in different forms (e.g., narrative, or story form, observations, notes, or charting). The information contained in client records is of significant importance for the following reasons:

1. It is a lasting record of what was done to, for, and by the client. *If it is not charted, it is considered not to have been done.*
2. It is a record of what was observed about the client.
3. It is a record of how the client reacted to the care that was given.
4. It contains information that can be used by other health team members in evaluating the care that was given and in deciding if changes in the care plan should be made.
5. If the client or family is unsatisfied with services and decide to complain, the client record can be used to show that certain things were done on certain dates and times. It can also show if the client refused to have some treatments done.
6. Always remember that the client record is a legal document. It could be introduced as evidence in a court of law in the event that the client or family sues the home health aide or the agency. A well-documented client record can be the home health aide's best protection against false claims.

When you are recording on your report, it is important that you:

1. *Be factual.* Write only those things that you know to be true.
2. *Chart in ink.* Writing or printing in pencil is not allowed in charting, it must be in either blue or black ink. Your agency will advise you as to their specific requirement.
3. *Be objective.* Record what you actually did, saw, smelled, felt, or tasted. Do not try to interpret the cause or the feelings that went along with the observation. If you feel that you really must put something in the record that is your own interpretation, identify it as such.

   Do not diagnose. If the client complains of pains in his chest and arm, do not write, "Client had a heart attack." Instead write, "Client complains of severe pains in his chest and upper arm. Face is pale and moist."

   If you observed a large discolored area on the client's arm, write a description of it. Do not write, "Mrs. Jones has a big bruise on her arm where I think her husband grabbed her when he got angry with her when she wet the bed." State, "Client has three bruises on her upper right arm. Each bruise, the size of a 50-cent piece." Be specific about the place on the body and size of bruise.

ANSWERING THE TELEPHONE

If the phone rings when you are there and your client asks you to answer it, state "Keane's residence." If need be take the message and relay it to your client, and write the message down. If it is the health care provider and he or she wants to change the client's medication, just state, "I am not allowed to take a health care provider's orders, please call the nurse assigned to this client."

ASSESSMENT AND ADMISSION

After a client is referred to the home health agency, a nurse will make the initial assessment and admission visit. This visit must include a thorough assessment of the client, family, home environment, and physical, emotional, and social needs. The client's living environment is assessed for adaptations that are necessary. Family members are assessed not only for their understanding of the client's illness, but also for their cultural and social needs as they impact the recovery of the client.

Plan of Care

The Plan of Care is a legal document that is constructed by the supervising nurse, in conjunction with the client's health care provider, and implemented by the home health aide and other direct care staff. Based on the

nurse's admission findings, a plan of care is established. All agencies certified to provide home health care are required to use designated forms. These forms must be completed upon admission and signed by a health care provider. Unless a client's condition changes radically, this plan of treatment is effective for 60 days. Health care documentation must include the admission sheet, the OASIS and comprehensive assessment, nursing plan of care, medication assessment record, and progress notes. Interventions are to be implemented by the client, family, or caregivers, and thus all are involved in the treatment plan. The nurse, as the case manager, is responsible to coordinate and evaluate the care.

While each nurse develops his or her own routine for completing a basic assessment, it should be consistent and complete. The admitting nurse will concentrate on the specific system that correlates with the client's diagnosis.

UNIT 4

Safety

COMMON HAZARDS

According to the National Safety Council, at least 4 million people are injured each year in home accidents. This means that about 1 person in 50 suffers some kind of injury as a result of an accident that occurs in the person's home.

Because home health aides care for clients in the home, they should be aware of potential hazards in this environment.

An aide should be aware of the effects of medication on the client. Pain killers or tranquilizers can cause clients to become so unsteady that they may fall if they get up from a chair or bed without assistance. If an aide observes that a client becomes disoriented and loses balance easily after taking medication, the aide should inform the supervisor.

Clients who are disoriented will not remember if they have taken a particular medication. Overmedication can be just as bad as undermedication.

Falls and Risks

As the human body ages, the bones become brittle and break easily. Broken hips are a common injury among the elderly.

Many clients may need canes, walkers, or wheelchairs. Before a client uses a cane, walker, crutches, or other device, make certain that each rubber tip is firmly in place and has not worn through.

Some hazards may be avoided by providing a safer environment. Stairways and landings should be kept uncluttered. Children's toys, such as skateboards, balls, blocks, and roller skates, must be put away after use. Waxed and polished floors and stairways can be very dangerous. Scatter rugs in hallways should have a skidproof backing or be removed completely because they pose a safety hazard in the home. Spills on kitchen and bathroom floors should be wiped up at once so that falls may be avoided.

Do not permit the client to walk about with untied shoelaces. Tripping over the laces can result in serious injury. The home health aide should tie the laces so they do not present a hazard.

The bathroom is one of the most dangerous rooms in the house for accidents. Bath mats should have a rubber backing so they will not skid. Bathtubs should be equipped with nonskid rubber strips to decrease the danger of slipping when getting in and out of the tub. For older adults, special handrails should be installed to assist them as they use the tub or shower. Faucets for hot water should be clearly marked so that accidental scalding will not occur. Special elevated toilet seats and handrails make it easier for clients to use the toilet safely, especially after knee or hip replacement surgery.

Another reason clients may fall is due to poor lighting. Many older adults get up in the middle of the night to use the bathroom; they may not wait a few seconds for their eyes to adjust to the light. It is advisable to keep a night-light on in the bedroom so the adjustment from dark to light is minimal. Another reason for falls by the elderly is due to the loss of peripheral vision (side vision), which means they can see only things straight ahead and not on the sides.

If you recognize any unsafe conditions such as loose handrail on the outside steps or if you have suggestions to make the client's home safer, tell the case manager.

RISKS FOR BURNS

The older adult client may have an altered sensation due to the natural process of aging. This may be due to decreased nerve impulse transmission or altered circulation, which puts the elderly at risk for burn injury. In the older adult, pain sensation is often decreased, their reaction time is slower, their ability to smell diminishes, and their ability to adjust their sight from darkness to light is slower, which makes them very vulnerable to accidents. Burns may be fatal to both the young and the elderly client. Therefore, it is important for the home health aide to feel the bathwater with his or her hand prior to the client entering the tub or shower,

whether the client is young or old. When cooking in the kitchen, if feasible have the client use the front burners. Oven mitts need to be worn to prevent burn injury when removing food items from the oven. When cooking over the stove, be sure that the client has clothing with short sleeves or closed sleeves. If the client is a little unsteady, fill the coffee cup two-thirds full to prevent the hot coffee from scalding the client's hand.

Matches and lit candles need to be out of children's reach. No youngster should be left unattended while in the kitchen to ensure that no injury can occur from the stove.

Fire

Few words are more frightening to hear than "Fire, fire!" The smell of smoke or the flash of flames from the kitchen stove can cause panic. Some people are stunned and unable to function. Others rush around wildly trying to save their belongings. The home health aide should advise the client and the client's family whenever a fire safety problem is noticed. If there are toddlers in the home, electrical outlets should be covered with plugs, as 2- to 3-year-olds like to touch and feel everything in sight. Smoke alarms should be standard equipment in the client's home.

As a home health aide, there are basic rules to follow in case a client's home, or something in it, catches on fire. *Remaining calm* is the first and most important rule. Lives can be saved if an emergency plan has been made beforehand. A home health aide, on entering a client's home, should make note of the nearest outside exit.

The aide must consider the client's condition and decide the best way to move the client in case of a fire.

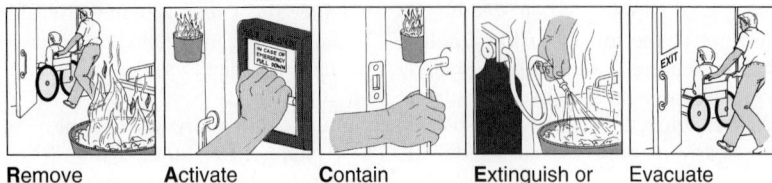

Remove   Activate   Contain   Extinguish or   Evacuate

Figure 4-1   Remember the sequence of critical actions in case of fire.

An aide needs to be aware of any fire danger prior to it happening. A good way to approach a fire situation is to remember the word RACE (Figure 4-1). As an aide, you might want to post this information on the refrigerator door.

R—**remove** the client from harm

A—**activate** the alarm or call 911

C—**contain** the fire

E—**extinguish** the fire

Waiting for the fire department to arrive is difficult for the home health aide and family members. Under no circumstances should the aide return to the burning building. Figure 4-2 lists basic rules in case of a fire. Figure 4-3 explains first aid.

Fire Extinguishers.   Small fires may be extinguished by using a fire extinguisher. There are four main types of fire extinguishers, each of which is used for a specific type of fire.

1. *Class A extinguishers* contain water that is under pressure. They are used to douse fires involving paper, wood, or cloth.
2. *Class B extinguishers* contain carbon dioxide. They are used to put out fires caused by igniting gasoline, oil, paints or other liquids, and cooking fats. These types of

fires would spread if water were used to extinguish them. The carbon dioxide smothers the fire, leaving a white powder residue. These extinguishers should be used with caution because the residue they leave may irritate the skin and eyes. Fumes also may be dangerous to inhale.

3. *Class C extinguishers* contain dry chemicals and are used on electrical fires.
4. *Class ABC* or *combination extinguishers* contain a graphite-like chemical. They can be used on any type of fire. The residue that results from their use can cause irritation of the skin and eyes.

If an aide uses a fire extinguisher on a minor fire, the manufacturer's operating instructions must be followed carefully.

An easy-to-remember method for operating a fire extinguisher is to follow the letters P-A-S-S.

P   **Pull** the pin at the top of the extinguisher that keeps the handle from being pressed. Break the plastic or thin wire inspection band as the pin is pulled.

A   **Aim** the nozzle or outlet toward the fire. Some hose assemblies are clipped to the extinguisher body. Release the hose and point.

Basic Rules in Case of Fire
1. Know the location of the nearest fire alarm box in the area.
2. Know how to phone for the fire department.
3. Remember the location of the nearest exits.
4. Close any door that will tend to confine the fire.
5. See that everyone is out of danger.
6. Know where a fire extinguisher is located and how to operate it. Check batteries of smoke alarms regularly.
7. Never try to fight a fire in a room filled with smoke; the fumes and lack of air are dangerous.
8. Never try to enter a room where much fire is in evidence.
9. Remember that a woolen blanket or other heavy covering will help to smother a small fire.
10. Keep boxes of inexpensive baking soda handy to extinguish kitchen fires. The boxes can be kept in the refrigerator so you will always be able to find them.
11. Use baking soda instead of water to extinguish small grease, oil, paint, varnish, and similar fires, because water spreads such a fire. Dust the flames with baking soda; this smothers the flames physically and chemically with carbon dioxide gas.
12. Smother small grease fires in cooking utensils by covering them with a lid or long-handled pan, or by throwing baking soda on the blaze.
13. Extinguish small broiling pan fires by first turning off oven and then throwing handfuls of baking soda on the blaze.
14. Throw baking soda on small fires in ashtrays, wastebaskets, or upholstered furniture.
15. Do not try to be a hero. If the small fire does not respond to your efforts to extinguish it immediately, remove the client and yourself from the house as quickly as possible. Call the fire department from a neighbor's house, or flag down passing motorists and ask them to call.

Figure 4-2   Basic rules for the home health aide to follow in case of fire in the client's home

S   Squeeze the handle above the carrying handle to discharge the contents of the container. The handle can be released to stop the discharge at any time. Before approaching the fire,

try a very short test burst to ensure proper operation.

S   Sweep the nozzle back and forth at the base of the flames to disperse the extinguishing agent. After the fire is out, watch for

First Aid—What to Do

If you catch on fire:
DON'T PANIC. DON'T RUN—RUNNING WILL INCREASE THE
FLAMES. *Instead:*
1. **Stop.**
2. **Drop** to the ground.
3. **Roll.** Continue to roll until you have completely put out the fire.
4. Remove clothing from the affected area. *Do not* attempt to remove
   clothing that sticks.
5. Flush area with cool water.
6. Cover with a sterile pad or clean sheet.
7. *Seek immediate medical attention.*

If the burn is from a chemical:
1. Follow steps 4–7 and be sure to flush with cool water for 20–30
   minutes.
2. If the eyes are involved, flush the eyes for at least 20 minutes or until medical attention arrives.
3. Remove contact lenses.

If the burn is electrical:
1. Turn off electrical source before touching victim.
2. Check for breathing and pulse. If absent, start Cardiopulmonary
   Resuscitation (CPR), if qualified.
3. Follow steps 4–7.

Home Fire Escape Plan
• Develop a Family Escape Plan.
• Include 2 exits from each room.
• Plan a meeting place outside the home.
• Practice the plan.

(continues)

Figure 4-3 First aid—what to do

remaining smoldering hot spots or possible reflash of flammable liquids. Make sure that the fire is completely out.

Once an extinguisher has been used in a fire, it must be replaced or recharged.

SAFETY CHECKLIST

Just by checking one of the following, may save a life.

• Are all medications in the containers they came in and clearly marked?
• If your client smokes, are there adequate large ashtrays in rooms the client smokes in?

Plan of Escape:
Evacuate!
Do not attempt to fight the fire.
1. If in bed, roll off onto floor.
2. Stay low! Crawl if necessary. Smoke rises, and oxygen will remain near the floor.
3. Cover your mouth and nose with some clothing or material to aid in breathing.
4. Place your hands on any closed door before opening it. If it is hot, *do not open!* Find another exit. If it is not hot, open it slowly, standing to the side. *Do not use elevators.*
5. *If you are trapped in a room:*
   a. Roll a rug or other materials and place across the bottom of the door.
   b. Open a window, both top and bottom, to allow air to enter and smoke to escape.
   c. Telephone for help, if possible.
   d. Attract attention and call for help.

(For further information, call The Burn Center at New York Hospital-Cornell Medical Center, 535 East 68th Street, New York, NY at 212-472-6890.)

Figure 4-3 *(continued)*

- Are there smoke alarms on every level of the house? If client is hard-of-hearing, there is a smoke alarm with a louder alarm.
- Are space heaters placed away from furniture and curtains?
- Are oily rags disposed of correctly?
- Does the home have a carbon monoxide alarm?
- Are cleaning supplies stored in a safe place and clearly marked?
- Are flammable items—gasoline, paint remover—stored in proper containers in a safe place?
- Are the outside steps and side-walks free of ice and snow?
- Do light fixtures have the correct wattage bulb? (As the client ages, they require more light.)
- Do the door locks work?
- Is the furnace in good working order? Have the filters been changed?
- Is the water temperature set at 120 degrees or less?
- Is it easy for the client to get mail?
- Would a night-light be useful?
- Are doorways, hallways, and steps unobstructed?
- Do frequently used steps have nonskid strips?
- Are electrical outlets covered, if there are toddlers in the house?
- Are electrical outlets overloaded? Are electrical extension cords placed in safe areas?
- Are grab bars needed and in place in bathroom?
- Would a sturdy shower or tub bench be beneficial in transferring?

- Would your client benefit from a telephone lifeline?
- Is the client's furniture functional? Can he or she easily sit down and get back up?
- Are guns stored in a locked cabinet with shells removed?
- Do scatter rugs have nonskid backing if client insists on using scatter rugs?

TIPS FOR HANDLING OXYGEN EQUIPMENT

- Do not allow smoking around oxygen, this includes friends and relatives of client.
- Do treat all your oxygen handling equipment with care. Store in clean, dry location. Remember, oxygen is combustible.
- Do maintain your oxygen handling equipment exactly as instructed.
- Don't allow your oxygen equipment near grease or oil. If it gets oil on it, do not use it until it can be properly cleaned.
- Do use plugs, caps, and plastic bags to protect "off-duty" equipment from dust and dirt.
- Turn off oxygen if not in use.

TIPS FOR HOME SAFETY WITH CLIENT WITH DEMENTIA

Here are a few tips to make a home safer for a client with dementia.

- Place additional locks on outside doors preferably high up, so that the client cannot easily locate them.
- Lower the temperature of the hot water to less than 120 degrees to prevent the client from being burned.
- Decorate with solid colors, as patterns make the home more confusing.

- Put safety knobs on stove, so the client cannot turn it on when someone is not there.
- Put safety locks on cabinets or drawers that contain potentially dangerous items such as knives and cleaning supplies.
- Keep a night-light on at night, as this will reduce confusion if the client wakes up.
- Make sure client has an ID bracelet containing medical information and a phone number.
- Remove locks on bathroom doors, as the client might lock it and forget to know how to unlock it.
- Keep furniture in the same place and try to create a clear path for the client to walk.
- Do not overly decorate for holidays, as the decorations can cause further confusion for the client.
- Replace live indoor plants with artificial plants, as the client may like to pick and chew on leaves.

SAFETY OUTSIDE THE CLIENT'S HOME

The home health aide must be aware of safety issues outside the client's home as well as within. The aide must be "streetwise" and safe. To be streetwise each aide must:

1. Be alert.
2. Be observant.
3. Trust own instincts.
4. Know how and when to call 911.

Do's and Don'ts

- Keep your money and identification close to you.
- Wear a fanny pack rather than carry a purse.
- Do not put money or credit cards in shopping bags.
- Do not put your wallet in your back or rear pocket.

- Do not wear flashy jewelry.
- Do not have personal identification on your key chains.

Safety When Walking

- Plan the safest route.
- Choose well-lighted streets, not alleys.
- Avoid vacant lots.
- Take the long way if it is the safest.
- Cross the street and head for a busy, well-lighted area if you are followed.
- Do not hitchhike.

Safety When Driving

- Keep your car in good running condition.
- Plan the safest route.
- Have your keys ready when approaching your car.
- Drive with your doors locked.
- Do not pick up hitchhikers.
- Park in well-lighted areas.
- Stay in your car when you see a street or motorist problem; go to a telephone for help.
- Do not leave valuables in your car.

Buses and Subways

- Have your money or token ready— do not open your purse.
- Try to sit near driver or conductor.
- Do not stand near edge of subway platform.
- Avoid sitting near the exit doors.
- Do not fall asleep.

UNIT 5

Homemaking Service

HOUSEHOLD MANAGEMENT

Many home health aides have a basic knowledge for keeping up a house. The habits developed in their own homes may not be suitable to all working situations.

The home health aide should realize that each home situation may offer different challenges. A professional home health aide must adapt to the physical surroundings of each job. This adjustment requires the use of whatever appliances and supplies the client has available. The home health aide must remember to show as much care for the property of others as is shown for his or her own personal property. The equipment and furnishings used by the home health aide belong to the client. Considerate and cautious care must be used.

If equipment has frayed cords or if appliances do not work, they should be repaired. The aide should notify the case manager or family so that repairs can be made.

When using any cleaning product or appliance, read the labels and directions carefully. This not only makes for proper use, but can limit the number of accidents that might

happen. Using rubber gloves helps avoid skin irritation caused by soaps or household chemical products.

When performing regular household duties, the aide should make a list of any items in short supply.

Always get a receipt for any purchases you make and place the receipts in a special place. If there is any doubt about what an item costs, or if the client has any questions as to where the money was spent, you can quickly verify your expenditures. Honesty in money matters is an absolute necessity.

When you are in a client's home and the client requests a cleaning job done a certain way even though you know a better way, you should follow the client's directions.

A few of the homes you will be going to might be very dirty and unkempt; if you are assigned to work at this home for 3 hours, you will not be able to clean it in that short time and get everything spotless. Your client might think differently. If this situation exists, you need to discuss this with your case manager.

Planning and Organization

An important duty of the aide is to plan, organize, and carry out tasks completely. A home health aide will be given instructions for each assignment. The care of the client is of primary importance, but the household tasks cannot be ignored. The aide should take a few minutes each morning to plan the tasks that should be completed by the day's end.

- Carry a pad and pencil. Make a note of household supplies that may be needed in each room.
- Before starting to clean a room, the home health aide should stop to think which cleaning supplies may be needed. Carry cleaning supplies from room to room in a plastic container or basket.
- Prevent buildup of dirt by tidying rooms, dusting, wiping surfaces, and sponging up spots as soon as possible.
- Keep a sponge in the kitchen and bathroom for quick wipe-ups.
- Schedule major jobs for a certain day of the week.
- Learn how to use and care for the equipment in the home. After using equipment, clean it so it will be ready for the next use. Store small appliances close to where they are used.

Basic Cleaning Supplies

The following is a list of supplies needed to maintain a clean home and do laundry. There are many brands of each available on the market—whatever is available in the client's home is what you will use.

- all-purpose cleaner
- baking soda
- bleach—liquid or powder
- broom and dustpan
- cold-water soap
- commercial stain remover for carpets
- commercial stain remover for clothing—i.e., Spray and Wash

- dishwashing detergent
- disposable gloves
- fabric softener for clothes
- furniture polish—spray or liquid
- glass cleaner
- laundry soap
- paper towels
- scrub pail
- steel wool or small scrubber
- toilet cleaner and brush
- vacuum cleaner
- vinegar

COMBINING CLIENT CARE AND HOUSEHOLD TASKS

The order in which tasks are done is not always important. If one knows just what should be completed by the end of the day the work can be arranged around the client's needs.

MAINTAINING A CLEAN HOME ENVIRONMENT

The home health aide is normally expected to do general cleaning in the living room, dining room, and bedroom. Home health aides set up their own routines for completing daily household tasks. Several factors need to be considered:

- Needs of the client
- Size of the home
- Ages of people living in the home
- Number of people living in the home

DOING THE CLIENT'S LAUNDRY
Sorting Laundry

First check the clothes for stains and sort out the clothes that need to be presoaked (those with stains). Separate the whites from the colors; then separate light colors from dark colors. As you sort, remember to close zippers to prevent snagging and empty pockets. As each item is sorted, check it for spots that may need special care. Collars of shirts and dresses and spots from food or other stains may need special care. Take special precautions if washing red clothes. Liquid bleaches are only used on white cotton. Use only the amount stated on the container.

Loading the Washing Machine

Don't just dump the clothes into the machine. It's important to distribute the clothes evenly. The weight of the clothes should be evenly balanced around the inside cylinder in order to prevent the cylinder from spinning off its track during the wash, and to ensure that the clothes are washed evenly. Be careful not to overload the washer. It is better to do two loads, since in the long run it will save wear and tear on the machine. The detergent goes in first—read the directions on the label to determine how much detergent to use. Most manufacturers include a scoop for powdered detergent and a measured cap for liquid detergent. However, keep in mind that each detergent is different, and hence should be used according to the manufacturer's instructions or the machine's user's manual. Close the machine and turn the dial to the correct setting.

Drying Clothes

Place the clothing into the dryer. Do not put items such as bras, silk pajamas, and other delicates into the dryer, unless your client directs you to do so. Most dryers have a range of minutes you can set, depending upon what types of material are in the dryer.

Once the clothing is dry, remove and fold the laundry and place it in a designated location. Permanent-press clothing needs to be removed right away or it will become quite wrinkled.

Ironing

Today there are very few items that need to be ironed. If you need to iron, turn on your iron to the correct setting according to the fabric you are ironing. Once the iron has reached the desired temperature, start ironing. Spray starch may be used to give the shirt a smoother, nonwrinkled appearance. Finally, place the item on a hanger until thoroughly dried and return it to the closet. Clients may have different ideas about how an item of clothing needs to be ironed, so just listen to their directions and follow their specific way of doing it.

Another problem that could occur is if the client lives in a multiunit apartment building and you must use the commercial machines in the basement of the building. You will need to run back and forth from the laundry room to the client's apartment, which can become time-consuming. Also you need to arrange a time to do the laundry when other individuals are not using the machines. On some occasions you will need to leave the client's home and do the laundry at a Laundromat.

CLEANING THE BATHROOM

Starting with the toilet first, place toilet cleaner in the bowl and with the toilet brush swish the solution around, paying special attention to the area under the rim of the bowl. If time allows, leave the solution set awhile and then flush the toilet. Clean the sink, countertops, and shower or tub with disinfectant. This will help kill the germs. Everything in the bathroom except the mirror can be cleaned this way in just 3 to 4 minutes a day. Rinse and wipe dry. If this does not work, scour with automatic dishwasher detergent or a degreaser or rub with a cloth dipped in vinegar. Use a large sponge and clean the floor with an all-purpose cleaner or spray, unless the floor is carpeted. If the bathroom has an unpleasant odor, place a fabric softener sheet in the wastebasket or add a dab of fragrance on a lightbulb. When the light is on, the heat releases the aroma.

CLEANING THE KITCHEN

The best advice is to clean as you go; work from the cleanest to the dirtiest areas.

Dishes

Separate dishes and wash them in the following order—glasses, silverware, plates and cups, and lastly do the pans. Rinse the dishes under hot water and let them air-dry. If you are unable to wash dishes right after eating, rinse the dishes and soak the pans in warm, soapy water.

Some homes are equipped with dishwashers. Before placing dishes in the dishwasher, scrape and rinse them well. Pour the correct amount of dishwasher detergent into the slot on the door. Close the door tightly and punch the correct button to start the machine. To conserve energy, run the dishwasher only if it is full.

Cleaning Kitchen Countertops

Use a mild dishwashing liquid for laminated plastic and rinse well afterwards to prevent residue from getting on food. For ceramic countertop, clean with solution of warm water, mild soap and vinegar; rinse well and dry with soft towel. After cutting fresh

meat directly on countertop, be sure to wipe off with hot water and soap immediately to prevent the spread of germs.

Cleaning Vinyl Floors

If time and space allows, move chairs and other items on floor before mopping. Sweep floor first, then mop with a mild soap. Rinse with clean, warm water. An old toothbrush works well at rubbing out dirt that may have accumulated in certain areas of the floor.

Cleaning Ceramic Floors

Wipe with warm vinegar water, if need be add a small amount of dish soap. Rinse with clean, warm water. To clean grout around the tiles, us an old toothbrush to scrub the soiled areas.

Cleaning Exterior of Cabinets

The cleaning product used for cabinets will depend on the type of material the cabinets are made of. If wood, clean with a solution of warm water and a small amount of mild soap (like Ivory) on a soft cloth. Dry with another soft cloth. If painted [Formica] or other artificial finish, you may use a mild cleaning solution or spray on the cabinets and dry with a clean cloth. If in doubt, ask your client what you should use to clean the exterior. Remember, kitchen work never ends, but it still can be challenging and satisfying when done well.

CLEANING SAFETY TIPS

Don't mix cleaning products like ammonia and bleach. They can be toxic. If you need to clean up blood on the kitchen floor, use a solution of 1 part bleach to 10 parts water and with your disposable gloves on, wipe up the blood spill. Cleaning supplies should be stored in a place that children and disoriented adults cannot reach.

DAILY CLEANING TASKS

The following are duties that should be done every day. Daily cleaning should not require longer than an hour a day.

- Pick up toys, magazines, newspapers, wet towels, and clothing. Do not discard any of these items without the permission of the client.
- Make the beds.
- Empty ashtrays and wastebaskets. Separate cans and glasses from other garbage.
- Do dishes and wipe off countertops.
- Clean top of stove.
- Sweep kitchen floor.

WEEKLY CLEANING TASKS

Weekly care can be done in more than one way. A load of laundry can be done every day or done all in one day. How and when the laundry should be done will be clearly stated in the care plan. The following tasks need to be done on a weekly basis:

- Change bed linens.
- Water plants.
- Dust furniture—use a flannel or other soft cloth for dry dusting and another for polishing. Pour polish onto the polishing cloth.
- Vacuum floors and carpets, getting under furniture and if need be, move furniture.
- Damp or wet mop the vinyl or ceramic floors in kitchen and bathroom.
- Clean mirrors with glass cleaner.
- Clean television screen with glass cleaner—be sure the TV is turned off before cleaning.
- Wipe off switch plates and door handles with soft, wet cloth.

- Using brush and bowl cleaner, clean the inside and the outside of the toilet. Be sure to scrub the area under the top rim of the bowl and also the toilet seat.
- Wipe out the tub or shower and sink with cleanser and disinfectant.

VARIABLES WHEN CHANGING BED LINENS

If you work in a hospital or long-term care facility, there are usually only one or two different types of beds to change the linens on. Also, there is a supply of clean bed linens readily available for you to change the bed with. In home care, these two things vary greatly. Every home will have a different type of bed and different size and texture of bed linens to work with. In some cultures, they do not sleep in beds but rather on mats that they roll up during the day. In a few homes, you may find regular hospital beds that can either be electrically operated or manually operated. You will need to be flexible and versatile in when and how you change the bed linens. One client may have 10 sets of sheets, whereas the next client will only have one set. As a home health aide, you will never find two homes alike, two clients alike, or two families alike. Every time you start working with a different client, there will always be a different set of variables to work with. Occasionally, you may have a client with respiratory problems such as emphysema or chronic obstructive pulmonary disease (COPD). These clients suffer from dyspnea (difficulty breathing) and shortness of breath. They are unable to sleep in a regular bed and often spend 24 hours a day in a lounge or recliner chair. The chair is their bed, and in this scenario, instead of changing linens on a bed, you will change them right on the chair.

Be sure to ask input from your client on how he or she wants the bed made. If your client is 80 years old and has been making the bed a certain way all of his or her life, follow the client's directions, unless told otherwise. Your supervisor will help to work through each different circumstance, and as you gain more experience, you will be able to problem-solve the situation you are placed in.

Linens

Following is a list of linens generally needed to change a regular bed.
- mattress pad
- fitted sheet
- soaker pad or lift sheet
- flat sheet
- blanket
- bedspread
- two or more pillowcases

Guidelines for Bedmaking

These bedmaking guidelines should be followed by the home health aide.
- Collect the linens in the order you will use them.
- Remember to hold linens away from your clothes.
- When making a bed, do not shake linens as this will just spread germs.
- A flat sheet may be used in place of a fitted sheet on the bottom of the bed.
- If a soaker pad is not available, you may substitute a large plastic garbage bag or plastic tablecloth covered with a flat sheet folded lengthwise.

- Textures of linens vary greatly—they generally are cotton, flannel or jersey knit.
- Bed linens come in a variety of colors—try to match the colors.
- Blankets can be cotton, wool, down, or handmade quilts.
- If the client has an air mattress or foam egg crate mattress on the bed, a fitted bottom sheet will stay in place better than a flat sheet.
- If the bed linens are soiled with urine or vomitus (material vomited), wash the soiled bed linens as soon as possible to prevent germs from spreading and decrease odor in the home.
- Place soiled linens on a chair or in a plastic bag, rather than on the floor.
- To save on bed linens and decrease unpleasant odor in the home, use adult briefs on clients who are incontinent (unable to control urination).
- Plastic protective covers on pillows may be used if the client is incontinent.
- If the pillow has a zippered end, place this end in the pillowcase first.
- A hospital bed can be elevated to the aide's working height when changing bed linens, which will protect the aide's back.
- When finished changing the unoccupied bed, always check to see if the bed looks neat and wrinkle-free.

See Procedure 1 Changing an Unoccupied Bed and Procedure 2 Changing an Occupied Bed.

1 **Procedure**

Changing an Unoccupied Bed

Purpose

- To apply clean and fresh linens to bed
- To add to the client's comfort by removing wrinkled or soiled sheets

NOTE: Complete one side of the bed entirely before moving to the opposite side. If a fitted sheet for the bottom of bed is not available, and the bed is twin size, it is recommended that a full sheet be used for the bottom. The full sheet, once tucked in, will stay in place longer than a flat twin sheet. Remember to use good body mechanics when making a client's bed.

Procedure

1. Strip bed of dirty linens and place in laundry. Do not rub dirty linens against uniform. Roll linens in and away from aide's body. Wear gloves if linens are soiled.
2. Wash hands.
3. Assemble clean linens: top sheet and fitted bottom sheet (if available), pillow cases, mattress pad, bedspread, and blankets if needed.
4. Place mattress pad on bed and then put clean fitted sheet or flat sheet on bed. If flat sheet is being used, unfold the sheet with the long fold at the center of the bed. Place lower hemline even with the bottom of the mattress. If a fitted bottom sheet is used, fit it properly and smoothly around one corner.
5. Open sheet gently; do not shake. Starting at the head of the bed, miter the corner and tuck in that side of the sheet. A great deal of time is saved by working on only one side of the bed at a time. Sizes of bedrooms differ greatly in clients' homes; you will need to adjust this procedure to your client's bed placement in the room.
6. Place top sheet over the bottom sheet wrong side up. Place hem even with the top edge of the mattress. Place the center fold at the center of the bed. Tuck in top sheet at foot of bed and make a mitered corner. **NOTE:** The top sheet, blanket, and spread, if used, may be tucked under the mattress at the same time.
7. Place the blanket back on the bed. Put the top edge 12 inches from the top of the mattress. Place bedspread on the bed.
8. Tuck the blanket and top sheet under the bottom of the mattress at the foot end of the bed. Miter the corner. Fold top sheet over the top edge of the blanket.
9. Walk over to opposite side of bed and make remaining part of the bed.
10. Put pillowcases on pillows. Do not hold the pillow under your chin.
11. Wash your hands.
12. Document completed task.

2 Procedure

Changing an Occupied Bed

Purpose

- To apply clean linens while the client remains in the bed
- To add to the client's comfort by removing soiled and wrinkled sheets

Procedure

1. Wash your hands.
2. Assemble clean linens.
   flat sheet and fitted bottom (if available)
   extra flat sheet or drawsheet if used by client or soaker pad
   pillowcases
   large plastic bag (for soiled linens)
3. Tell client what you plan to do and provide for the client's privacy by closing the bedroom door.
4. Place clean linens on a clean chair or table in room in the order you plan to use them.
5. Loosen bedding from under mattress by lifting the mattress with one hand as you pull out bedding with the other hand.
6. Remove top covers one at a time, folding each to the foot of the bed.
7. Leave top sheet covering the client to prevent chilling and afford privacy.
8. Place two straight chairs against one side of the bed. This helps protect the client from falling out of bed. If the bed has side rails this is not necessary. Simply raise the bed side rail on the opposite side of the bed.
9. Assist the client to turn on the side facing the chairs or side rail. Assist the client to move near the edge of the bed by the chairs. Stand at the other side of the bed.
10. Roll or fanfold (fold in pleats) the soiled bottom sheet to the center of the bed beside the client's back.
11. Fold the clean bottom sheet lengthwise and place the fold at the center of the bed. Fanfold half the clean sheet next to the soiled sheet. Tuck the other half under the mattress. Make a mitered corner at the top. Tuck from the top or head of bed and move toward the foot of the bed.
12. Help client turn toward you onto the clean sheet. Bring the chairs to the other side of the bed for the client's protection (or raise the side rail).
13. Go to the other side and remove soiled sheet. Place soiled linens into large plastic bag.
14. Pull clean sheet across bed and tuck under mattress. Miter corner at top and tuck along side from head to foot of bed. Make certain the sheet is tight and wrinkle-free.
15. Turn client onto the back in center of the bed. Place clean top sheet over the soiled top sheet. Slide the soiled sheet out from under the clean sheet. Have client hold fresh top sheet in place.

16. Place soiled sheet in large plastic bag.
17. Unfold blanket and bedspread and place over top sheet.
18. Tuck in the bottoms of the sheet, blanket, and bedspread at the foot of the bed. Miter the two corners; leave extra room for foot and toe movement.
19. Change the pillowcases and replace pillows under client's head. Put soiled cases in large plastic bag.
20. Be sure client is comfortable and that the room is neat. Remove soiled linens from room.
21. Wash your hands.
22. Document procedure completed.

Stages of Human Development

SECTION 2

UNIT 6

Infancy to Adolescence

BECOMING A FAMILY

An aide who is assigned to care for a newborn infant and the mother is usually going into a happy environment. If it is a first child, both parents may be very attentive toward the baby and watch its every move. Of course, the newness wears off, and suddenly they are faced with a demanding, dependent human being for whom they are entirely responsible. Even so, this is usually a positive assignment.

Pregnancy

Conception is the fertilization of the female egg by male sperm. This union forms the fetus. The time from conception to birth is called the gestation period. When a woman is pregnant, it is essential that she receive prenatal care either from a health care provider or a midwife. Many complications of pregnancy and birth disorders may be prevented by good prenatal care. It is an important duty as a home health aide to encourage your client to seek prenatal care. If the client is pregnant, the aide should encourage the client to eat a balanced diet, not smoke or drink alcoholic beverages, and only take

medication ordered by the health care provider.

Labor and Delivery

Infants are most often delivered by a health care provider in the hospital. However, in some areas, this situation is changing. There has been increasing use of midwives and other birthing options as alternatives to hospital births. Normally, a woman goes into labor and delivers the baby with the assistance of an obstetrician. The baby moves from the uterus into the vagina and passes out of the body. This normal process can be eased, however, by use of medications, health facilities, and trained personnel.

In some cases it may be necessary to deliver the baby by cesarean section. This is a surgical technique in which an abdominal incision is made into the uterus and the infant is lifted out. After a cesarean section, the mother needs extra time to recover. The incision area must be kept clean to prevent infection. The aide may be instructed to assist the mother to clean the incision and apply clean dressings.

Bonding is a process of attachment of mother, father, and infant happening sometime after birth. It is important to remember that each family member bonds differently and at different rates. The newborn infant is placed on the mother's abdomen skin-to-skin so that both parents can make eye contact with the child and feel and cuddle the infant. This initial contact is important because it assists in creating positive emotional ties between the parents and child and the child and the parents. Cuddling and fondling are important in the first few months of the newborn's life. The home health aide needs to encourage a new mother and father to hold, talk, and play with the baby often. The newborn needs to develop a sense of trust and security to develop into a trusting and secure adult.

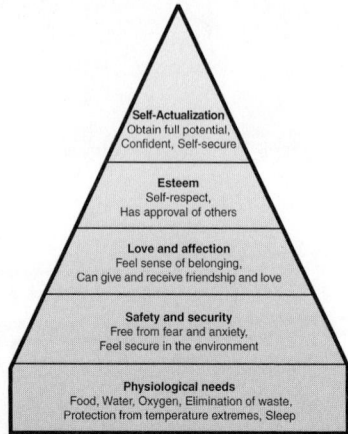

Figure 6-1 Maslow's Hierarchy of Needs

NORMAL INFANT GROWTH AND DEVELOPMENT

As an infant grows, both physical and mental abilities develop. In the first month, infants are quite helpless. They totally depend on others to meet their basic needs. According to American psychologist, Abraham Maslow, all human beings have a hierarchy (ladder) of five basic needs. He suggests that higher types of needs can only be gratified after a person's basic needs have been met. Maslow's hierarchy is best understood by imagining a triangle shape. At the base of the triangle would be the first basic human need, which is physiological in nature, that is, food and shelter. After the physiologic needs are met, the second basic need is for safety. Moving up the hierarchy triangle is the third basic need, the need for love and belonging. The fourth basic need is for esteem, which refers to achievement and recognition. The fifth basic need, at the tip of the triangle, is for self-actualization, the highest human

need, which is the desire to reach one's fullest potential (Figure 6-1).

Maslow's hierarchy of needs shows the importance of meeting basic human needs beginning in infancy and moving throughout the life cycle. For instance, the newborn must be fed, changed, cleaned, kept warm and clothed properly, and be kept safe and secure. Infants also need to be held and cuddled. Giving love to the infant fulfills a basic need. When these needs are met, the child should have every chance to grow up to be a happy, confident, and fulfilled person.

By age 2 months, babies can raise their heads and may cry when they want to be picked up. Crying is the infant's way of communicating that he or she needs something. Through trial and error parents gradually come to understand the needs of their infants. As infants develop, they notice lights and sounds and begin to babble. They get used to certain patterns, especially the time to eat and time to sleep. Usually by the fourth month an infant sleeps 8 to 12 hours at night and naps during the day. Regular schedules of meals, activities, and sleep are needed and should continue through the first year.

Normal Weight Gain

Normally, infants weigh between 5 and 8 lb (2.3 to 3.6 kg) at birth. During the first 5 days, a weight loss of several ounces is expected. Until birth, all the baby's needs are supplied within the uterus through the umbilical cord. Birth is a shock to the baby's system and it takes a few days for the infant's body to adjust. When the body starts to function, a weight gain of 6 to 8 oz (0.17 to 0.23 kg) a week is normal. Birth weight is usually tripled by age 1. In the second year, the weight increases at a rate of 0.5 lb (0.23 kg) per month.

HEALTH PROBLEMS IN INFANCY AND EARLY CHILDHOOD

Some infants are born with diseases, injuries, or malformations. These abnormalities may be inherited through the parents' genes. Conditions also may result from diseases or drugs present in the mother's body during pregnancy. Common abnormal infant conditions are described in Figure 6-2. Children with one of these conditions need special medical and emotional care. The aide may need to help the mother and family members adjust to meeting the child's special needs.

One condition that often causes problems is premature birth. An infant born before full term (before 37 weeks of gestation) is considered premature. Some also judge prematurity by low birth weight. A newborn weighing less than 5 lb may be premature. However, some babies are full term yet weigh less than 5 lb. A

newborn in this condition is called a low birth weight baby.

Another condition of infancy is sudden infant death syndrome (SIDS) where a baby will stop breathing while asleep. This condition occasionally occurs in infants under 1 year of age. It is now recommend that babies be placed on their backs, rather than their stomachs, when sleeping. If breathing disorders are suspected in babies, a monitor may be placed on babies so that an alarm is sounded if the baby stops breathing.

COMMON CHILDHOOD ILLNESSES

Coxsackievirus—Hand-Foot-and-Mouth Disease

The disease is spread by direct contact with fecal material, nasal drainage, or saliva from an infected individual. Clinical manifestations are fever, fussiness, and runny nose followed in a few days by mouth sores and rash on the body or hands and feet. Treat the fever and offer fluids. This disease is seen more in the fall and summer.

Strep Throat

Strep throat is a bacterial infection that is spread via droplets in the air from the nose or throat. A throat culture is usually done to identify the strep organism. If the culture is positive, then the child is placed on a 10-day course of antibiotics. Clinical manifestations may include sore throat, enlarged lymph nodes (swollen glands), headache, and fever. Treatment is necessary to prevent the spread to other individuals, as well as preventing a serious complication known as rheumatic fever. Rheumatic fever can occur 5 to 6 weeks after a strep infection that was

Condition	Description	Treatment
PKU (phenylketonuria)	Body is unable to break down a certain amino acid. Mental retardation, convulsions, and eczema are common.	Specific diet begun early in infancy prevents symptoms. Test for PKU at birth.
Cerebral palsy	Defect, injury, or disease of the brain tissue, which causes lack of muscle coordination and possible paralysis; person has shaking and muscle spasms with poor balance.	No cure, but treatment varies and may include muscle relaxants, orthopedic surgery, use of casts or braces, exercises.
Congenital heart disease	Malformation of vessels, valves, or chambers in the heart; results in faulty circulation and usually cyanosis.	Surgery often is successful in restoring normal functioning.
Down syndrome (trisomy 21)	Chromosome abnormality causing various degrees of retardation and typical physical malformations such as slant eyes, broad hands with short fingers, and protruding tongue.	No treatment, but many persons can be taught to live with some independence.
Hydrocephalus	Defect in the absorption of cerebrospinal fluid; fluid builds up and increases the size of the head.	Common treatment is with surgery. Shunts are commonly used to divert fluid away from brain and into the abdomen.
Sickle cell anemia (thalassemia)	Abnormal sickle-shaped red blood cells break down easily and cannot transport oxygen efficiently; fever, blackouts, and pain. (African American population)	Blood transfusions. No cure.

(continues)

Figure 6-2   Abnormal conditions in infants that may require medical attention, long-term adjustments, and services of the home health aide for the child and family

Condition	Description	Treatment
Leukemia	Overproduction of immature white blood cells, anemia, internal bleeding. Person has increased risk of infection, fever, pain in the joints, and swelling of the lymph nodes, spleen, and liver.	Chemotherapy
Tay-Sachs	Degeneration of the central nervous system; infant does not develop mentally; disease affects those of Jewish ancestry.	No cure; infant usually does not live beyond age 1 year.
Cystic fibrosis	Inherited malfunction of the pancreas, intestine, and sweat glands, and the respiratory system.	No cure; special diet and respiratory care prolong life.
Cleft lip/ cleft palate	Fetal growth incomplete. Infant may have problems feeding. Cleft palate may alter tooth formation and cause speech problems.	Surgical repair; special feeding nipples and special therapy.
Fetal alcohol syndrome (FAS)	Set of signs and symptoms and problems that newborn babies have if the mother drinks during pregnancy: (1) smaller baby, (2) small head, (3) weak heart or kidney problems, (4) failure to thrive, (5) peculiar-appearing flat face with narrow eyes and drooping lips.	No cure—supportive care. The child may experience some degree of mental retardation for the rest of his or her life.
Sudden infant death syndrome (SIDS)	Infant stopped breathing while asleep.	Place monitor on infants with suspected breathing problems.

Figure 6-2   (continued)

untreated. Clinical manifestations of this disease include joint pain and eventually it may affect the valves of the heart. Children can return to day care or regular school after being on the antibiotic for 24 hours with no fever present.

Pinkeye—Bacterial Conjunctivitis

Pinkeye appears as redness of the white part of the eye with development of pus in the eye. There is little or no pain felt by the child. It is treated with antibiotic eyedrops. Pinkeye is highly contagious and children are usually kept out of school or day care until their eyes have had time to heal.

Croup

Croup is caused by several respiratory viruses. Cold symptoms are followed by a "barking" cough, and the child typically wakes at night with cough and some difficulty breathing. Treatment consists of cool, humidified air. For persistent cough at night, take the child outside into the cool night air or open a window in the bedroom (bundle up as needed to prevent chilling). Seek medical help for any labored breathing.

Influenza

This is a respiratory illness that occurs during the winter and early spring. Respiratory symptoms include congestion, cough, sore throat, body aches, headache, and fever. Treatment depends on the degree and severity of symptoms.

Rotavirus (Diarrhea/Vomiting)

Symptoms include vomiting, diarrhea, abdominal cramping, and foul smelling stools. Wash your hands and the child's hands thoroughly. Maintain fluid balance.

Otitis Media (Middle Ear Infection)

Otitis media is caused by an increased amount of fluid and inflammation in the ear, causing the eardrum to bulge. It can be quite painful. A small child may tug his or her ear and be fussy due to the discomfort. Other signs might be drainage from the ear and fever. A mild analgesic such as Tylenol may be given for pain. A culture is taken from the ear and the child is usually placed on a regimen of antibiotics. If untreated, it may lead to hearing loss or other serious complications of the ear canal and brain.

DEVELOPMENTAL DISABILITIES AND LEARNING DISORDERS

Developmental disabilities are mental or physical impairments usually apparent at birth or before the age of 7, which are likely to continue indefinitely and may result in substantial functional limitations that require lifelong or extended care. Examples of these disabilities are cerebral palsy, mental retardation, and autism.

A learning disorder is a condition that affects an individual's ability to either interpret what they see and hear or to link information from different parts of the brain. Examples of these limitations can show up in many ways such as with speaking and writing, coordination, self-control, and attention. Such difficulties extend to schoolwork and can impede learning to read, write, or do math.

Attention-Deficit/ Hyperactivity Disorder

This is a childhood mental disorder that is marked by inattention, hyperactivity, and impulsivity. Children who are inattentive have a hard time focusing their attention and may be bored with a task after only a few minutes. Children who are hyperactive always seem to be in motion; they cannot sit still and may display restlessness. Children who are overly impulsive seem unable to curb their immediate reactions or to think before they act. This disorder is more common in boys than girls.

Autism

Autism is a mental disorder of infants and children that is marked by withdrawal of the individual into a fantasy world of his or her creation. The child has problems with social interaction and communication. The child may be unable to talk and may only utter various sounds. The child with autism likes routine and any change can cause serious behavior problems. Bizarre behavior includes hand flapping and rocking the body. This disorder is also seen more in boys than girls.

RESPONSIBILITIES OF THE HOME HEALTH AIDE

Often a mother must leave one or more children at home while she is at the hospital. The aide may be assigned to attend to the children then, or after the mother has returned home with the newborn. The children are likely to want to be near the mother and may want to play with the baby. Sometimes older children are too rough with the baby even though they do not intend to be. The children also may be jealous of the new member of the family. This jealousy is called sibling rivalry. At these times, the home health aide should give the children extra attention. The aide can make the children feel important by giving them chores to do

for the baby or mother. They should be praised for being helpful. Children may need help adjusting to the role of being a big brother or sister. The aide should be sure that the older children wash their hands before touching the baby to prevent the spread of germs and infections. If they have colds they should be kept away from the baby until they are no longer contagious.

Besides the older children, the aide cares for the mother and the newborn. These duties include:

- Bathing the infant
- Diapering
- Feeding the infant
- Preparing the formula
- Doing added laundry
- Caring for the mother
- Assisting the mother if she is breast-feeding
- Preventing accidents

Handling Visitors

Most mothers are happy to show off their newborn. It is a good idea to plan ahead with the mother as to how to handle visitors. Visitors should not stay too long and should not come in great numbers. The home health aide must encourage the mother to set the standards as to who can and cannot hold the baby. Visitors who have colds or similar infections should be discouraged from going near the baby.

TODDLERS AND PRESCHOOLERS

Ages 1 and 2 are known as the toddler stage. The toddler approaches life with a great deal of interest. A favorite activity is exploring the immediate environment, creating a need for safety precautions. Toddlers want to be more independent and experiment with control—testing their parents' limits and discovering their own. This is a time when children start to show possessiveness with belongings and people close to them. At about age 18 months, their favorite word will often be "No!" As infants grow into toddlers, muscle coordination increases, and physical skills expand and improve greatly. Toddlers can speak several understandable words and can refer to themselves by name. They can recognize themselves in the mirror, they can walk well, and they can feed themselves with a spoon and drink from a cup. By the time the child is 3 years old, he or she should be able to follow simple directions, be toilet trained, and communicate with others in short sentences or phrases. The child's attention span is longer and he or she enjoys playing alone but also likes to play with an adult. Most toddlers like to be outdoors to run and play. Just remember, they need constant supervision whether indoors or outdoors and they love one-on-one attention. The period of time from 3 until 5 years is known as the preschool years. The child has never-ending energy and is always on the go. Preschoolers start playing with other children their age for a longer period of time and are able to do more complex physical tasks such as ride a tricycle, climb a jungle gym, and tie their shoes. They can print their name and begin to recite the ABCs, and they love to ask questions. By the time the child is 5, he or she should be able to hop and skip on one foot, speak clearly, and can be understood by others not in the family. The child can count to 4 and recognize various shapes. The caregiver needs to supervise the child closely, be consistent, firm, and gentle in disciplining the child, and reinforce good social skills. If time allows, the aide may spend time coloring and playing ball or doing other similar activities with the child.

Safety

Keeping a child physically safe is an ongoing responsibility. Accidents are the primary cause of death in children under 5 years of age, the main cause being automobile accidents. Each year 1 million children are brought for medical care due to accidents; 40,000 to 50,000 children suffer permanent damage and 4,000 die. We know that most accidents can be prevented and all accidents can be minimized.

Childhood injury involves three elements: the child, the object that causes injury, and the environment in which it occurs. Here are several safety checks to ensure a safe environment for young children:

1. Infant car seat—Make sure the child rides in the backseat. The backseat is generally the safest place in a crash. If your vehicle has a passenger air bag, it is essential for children 12 and under to ride in the backseat. Make sure infants ride facing the rear until they are about age 1 and weigh at least 20 to 22 pounds. Children over the age of 1 who weigh at least 20 pounds may ride facing forward. Check to see that the safety belt holds the seat tightly in place. Put the belt through the correct slot. The safety belt must stay tight when securing the safety seat. Make sure the harness is buckled snugly around your child. The harness should be adjusted so you can slip only one finger underneath the straps at the child's chest. Keep the straps over the child's shoulder. Have toddlers who weigh over 40 pounds use a booster seat. A belt-positioning booster seat, used with the adult lap and shoulder belt, is preferred for

children weighing 40 to 80 pounds.

2. Fire prevention—Clothes, especially sleepwear, should be flame-retardant. (Check the clothing label to find out.) Install smoke detectors.

3. Choking—Do not put a pacifier or any object on a string around the baby's neck. Check toys for sharp edges or small parts. Check that all foods for an infant be mashed, ground, or soft enough to swallow without chewing.

4. Poisoning—Keep all medications and household cleaning products out of reach. Use safety latches on cupboards or drawers that contain items that might be dangerous.

5. Burns—Always check the water temperature before placing the baby in the bath. Never hold the baby while cooking at the stove or oven, drinking a hot liquid, or smoking.

6. Falls—Use gates at the bottom of stairways. Supervise the baby at all times on the changing table. Never leave a baby unattended on any surface above floor level.

7. Drowning—Never leave a small child alone in the bath or around any container with water in it, no matter how little. This includes buckets, wading pools, and the toilet.

8. Strangulation—Keep strings from window blinds up and out of the way of a crawling or toddling baby. Do not place the baby's crib near window blinds, where the baby can reach the cords.

SCHOOL-AGED CHILDREN

A child beginning school often needs time to adjust to the new situation. The child may one day seem confident and secure and the next day be clingy and dependent. Some children find it difficult to leave the familiarity of home. However, most children enjoy school and being with other children. A school-aged child generally can follow simple instructions and be fairly independent. It is important that children be given small jobs so that they feel a sense of responsibility. They learn that rules are necessary to make groups (family or school) work. Praise for achievements is better than punishments for mistakes. The school-aged child enjoys activities at home and away from home.

ADOLESCENCE

Adolescence often refers to the years between the ages of 13 and 19, during which broad developmental changes occur, including intellectual, emotional, social, and physical changes. Puberty, on the other hand, is the physical process of growing up, which includes the growth spurts, changing body shape, and maturation of the reproductive system. Pubertal changes occur gradually; they may start as early as age 9 or 10 and not be completed until about age 20 or even a little older in some people.

Physical Changes in Puberty

Puberty begins sometime between the ages of 10 and 15 when the endocrine system releases hormones in both boys and girls. At this time, the secondary sexual characteristics begin to mature. In boys, the beard, underarm, and pubic hair starts to grow and the voice deepens. There is usually a marked growth in both height and weight. At puberty, the testes, scrotum, and penis enlarge and the youth is able to produce sperm.

In young girls, the breasts develop and pubic and underarm hair grows.

About every 28 to 35 days the mature female reproductive system releases one or more eggs (ova), and the menstrual cycle begins.

How easily adolescents deal with these changes will partly reflect how closely their bodies match the well-defined stereotypes of the "perfect" body for young men and young women. Adolescents who do not match the stereotypes may need extra support from adults to improve their feelings of comfort and self-worth. If a teenager is dependent on a home health aide for his or her personal care and other needs, this teenager will definitely need emotional support to accept his or her less than perfect physique.

The Teen Years

The teenage years are profoundly influenced by both the physical and mental changes of adolescence. In our society, an adolescent reaches adult status when he or she is financially able to support himself or herself. Today, financial independence is generally not achieved until late adolescence or early adulthood, after the individual has completed some type of education and gained some entry-level work experience. Adolescents start to develop their own set of values and beliefs during this period.

Adolescents face many other challenges. Sexual maturity is difficult because adolescents often confuse sexual feelings with genuine intimacy. Parents need to provide a supportive environment for adolescents to search and explore their identity and their new social role in the community. Status within the community, beyond that of family, is an important achievement for older adolescents. The adolescent should be given an opportunity to make some decisions and be accountable for the consequences of

those decisions. Teenagers are strongly influenced by their peer group (those of the same age). Open communication between parents and teenagers is healthy and important. If teenagers have a previous history of good communication with their parents, they will be willing to share their concerns and feelings with them. Parents and adults have an important role to play and can have a positive impact on the lives of adolescents. If the home health aide is in a home where there is not good rapport between the adolescent and parents, and the teenager wants you to take sides, this may put you in a rather awkward position. The best advice is to stay neutral. Listen to what he or she has to say, which will convey your interest in the teenager's side, and maybe that is all he or she needs. As a home health aide, you rarely will be assigned to care for an adolescent unless there is a physical problem with the youth's health, such as an accident (body in a cast), childhood cancer, or other severe physical condition or behavior problem.

Common Health Problems in Adolescence

Adolescents are at an age of experimentation. They often express their independence by trying new things. For some adolescents, this experimentation leads to smoking, abuse of drugs or alcohol, gang involvement, or sexual experimentation.

Sex-related health problems are especially common with adolescents. An active sex life may pose health and emotional problems. Sexually transmitted diseases (STDs), including the human immunodeficiency virus (HIV) and acquired immunodeficiency syndrome (AIDS), may bring about additional very serious problems. In addition, teenage girls must consider the possibility of becoming pregnant. Sex-related health problems often result from the adolescent having insufficient and inaccurate information.

CHILD ABUSE, MALTREATMENT, AND NEGLECT

All states have child abuse and neglect laws that protect children under the age of 18 years. These laws regulate the conduct of the parent, guardian, custodian, or caretaker.

Most states will define child abuse by a responsible person (parent, caregiver, friend, or relative) who commits any of the following acts:

- Inflicts or allows to be inflicted upon the juvenile a serious physical injury by other than accidental means
- Creates or allows to be created a substantial risk of serious physical injury to the juvenile by other than accidental means
- Uses or allows to be used upon the juvenile cruel or grossly inappropriate vices to modify behaviors
- Commits, permits, or encourages the commission of crimes against the juvenile including, but not limited to the following: rape, any sexual offense, a crime against nature, incest, and preparation of obscene photographs, videos, or motion pictures
- Employs or permits the juvenile to assist in a violation of the obscenity laws or gives obscene material to the juvenile
- Sexually exploits the juvenile including the promoting of prostitution of the juvenile or the taking of indecent liberties with the juvenile
- Creates or allows to be created serious emotional damage to the juvenile

- Encourages, directs, or approves of delinquent acts of the juvenile

There is always a duty to report child abuse, neglect, or maltreatment. Failure to report is itself a criminal act. Accordingly, you must promptly report any such known or reasonably suspect child abuse, neglect, or maltreatment to your employer or your supervisor. If you are self-employed, the law requires you to report directly to the Department of Social Services in the county where the juvenile resides. Every state protects the person who makes these reports by giving the person immunity from any civil or criminal liability so long as the reporting person was acting in good faith. Occasionally, a home health aide will be asked by the child protective service to verify that the family is meeting requirements of the case plan developed jointly by the protective service worker and the family, if prior abuse or neglect has been found in the home.

Examples of maltreatment and neglect of children include cases in which children are:

- Improperly fed, clothed, or deprived of any emotional support
- Allowed to drink alcohol or given illegal drugs
- Chained or locked in a closet
- Kept in an environment where mice, rats, cockroaches, or other pests can harm the child
- Left alone in an apartment or house or locked in a room while the legally responsible adult is away
- Exposed to lead poison from painted walls or furniture

Abusive parents or caretakers may have been raised in abusive families themselves. The husband or wife may abuse the spouse. Life crises such as loss of job, debt, or housing problems, and substance abuse of alcohol or

Avoid contact with parents or other adults
Become upset when other children cry
Be extremely aggressive
Be extremely withdrawn
Suffer mood swings
Fear going into home—run away from home
Be overly demonstrative and loving to abusive parent
Blame themselves for being "clumsy" or "bad"
Wear long sleeves to conceal injuries
Appear to have low self-esteem
Attempt suicide
Grades go down in school

Figure 6-3   Observable patterns of abused or mistreated children

drugs or gambling losses can lead to abusive behavior; physical or mental health problems may cause a parent to become abusive; or parents who are too young themselves may lack self-discipline to deal with their own children. Many of these parents are not aware of the damage they are doing to their children and may need help themselves to develop better parenting skills. Parents of mentally or developmentally disabled children may be unable to cope with their children's

problems. These parents should be encouraged to join support groups with parents with similar problems.

Abuse comes in many forms. It may be categorized as physical, sexual, emotional, or even neglect. Figure 6-3 lists typical behavior for abused or mistreated children. Child abuse may take place in the homes of any group of people, regardless of income, ethnic origin, or religion. It is most important to remember that if you suspect it, you must report it.

UNIT 7

Early and Middle Adulthood

EARLY ADULTHOOD

Early adulthood generally refers to the ages of 20 to 39 years. This is the time when an individual starts planning his or her life and making major decisions that will affect the years to come. The person assumes more responsibility for his or her future. Young adults are no longer required to further their education and must decide whether to complete a college degree, go into the workforce without any additional training, or attend a technical college. This is the time when the majority of people marry or some may elect to live openly as couples without a formal marriage contract. In general, individuals are now delaying marriage and having their first child later in life, compared to the 1950s. The average age of individuals getting married today is in the middle 20s. The average age of first-time mothers is now 24.8. The size of families has been gradually decreasing, with the average woman having only two children. Another recent change in society is that in 1976 there were only 3 million single mothers caring for their children; today there are 10 million single mothers. It is quite difficult for a single mother of a child with a disability to care for this child 24 hours a day, 7 days a week. This mother often relies on a home health care agency to assist her part-time, if she has a child who is emotionally or physically challenging.

During early adulthood, many individuals are interested in establishing a career, joining various social groups, and doing something for their community or country. It is a time in life when many choices are available.

Another big decision is purchasing a home and learning how to manage that home. In the majority of homes today both partners work, and they will need to arrange their personal lives around their jobs. Early adulthood truly is a very busy and active time.

Early Adulthood Adjustments

During early adulthood, the body normally works efficiently. It remains at a high level of health for about 30 or 40 years. The body heals quickly through childhood, adolescence, and early and middle adulthood.

Health problems in early adulthood often accompany parenthood. Normal pregnancy, pregnancy with complications, and reproductive system disorders can occur in the adult woman. If an infant is born with birth defects or serious medical problems, parents may experience considerable stress and financial burdens. Other health problems can result from conditions related to automobile accidents and job-related injuries.

Many health professionals recommend taking certain preventive health measures to maintain a person's health and well-being and to prevent the development of health problems. For example, all persons should have a physical examination at least every 3 years. The early detection of diseases such as cancer, heart disease, diabetes, and emotional stress often leads to a better **prognosis** (outcome).

MIDDLE ADULTHOOD

Society places great demands on a person in middle adulthood from 40 to 65 years of age. It is during this period that people are expected to be highly successful and productive as well as financially secure. If a woman has chosen to remain at home with her children, this may be the time when she decides to reenter the workforce. During the middle adult years, people often assess their accomplishments.

Often during this stage of life, individuals are asked to take responsibility for care of their aging parents. The roles of parent and child often reverse once the parent is unable to manage all of his or her care. The phenomenon of daughters caring for their aging parents and their own children is common. At times this can be a difficult and stressful period in both the parent's and child's lives.

Physically, those in their middle adult years will notice some changes. Their hair may turn gray or recede, and their eyesight may diminish and they may start wearing bifocals. Weight gain may occur as a result of a general slowing of their metabolism and inactivity. Hormonal changes that occur during **menopause,** when a woman's menstrual periods stop, may result in mood swings, changes in sleeping patterns, increased anxiety, or other physical symptoms.

Middle Adulthood Adjustments

People in the middle adult years may have to make several major adjustments. These adjustments are in response to a change in some area of their lives.

Family Relationships. The middle years are generally the time when grown children leave the home. Parents who have been very involved in their children's lives may feel at a loss when this occurs (empty nest syndrome). As the children mature and gain independence, their own roles and responsibilities may become first priorities, and their ties with their family may become more secondary. Another adjustment that can be either a positive or negative experience is when grandparents assume primary custody of their grandchildren. The children's parents no longer want the responsibility of child-rearing and the grandparents either take the grandchildren in or they go to a foster home. All of a sudden the grandparents are tied down to raising a child or children again. This can also be quite a financial burden for the grandparents who are living on a limited income.

Effects of Exercise. It is important during the early and middle years of adulthood to become involved in a regular exercise program. One of the best exercises is walking. Some other alternatives to walking are swimming, riding a stationary or moving bicycle, and dancing.

Leisure-Time Activity

In middle adulthood, the individuals start doing more activities outside of the home, as leisure time is more plentiful than in early adulthood. Couples or individuals might become involved in volunteer work. Some individuals might elect to take short courses at a technical college in computers, photography, or gardening. In general, individuals who keep themselves involved actively do better healthwise than those who become addicted to the television set.

Illness and Disability

It is quite difficult for individuals in this age bracket to accept the fact that they need assistance from others to do their activities of daily living (ADLs) and in some cases may need financial assistance. They see other people their age engaged in full-time work, married and having children, and they become quite frustrated over their condition. In some situations, they are physically unable to have a sexual relationship with another, which can be quite depressing to a young person because intimacy with the opposite sex is an emotional need. Some individuals do rather well accepting their limited abilities, whereas others do just the opposite. As a home health aide, you will encounter some clients who are bitter, irritated, and angry because of their disability. At times, they may try to take their frustrations out on their caregiver.

It is easier for a person with a disability or special needs to remain physically and socially active today

than it was years ago. With modern technology, a client can be transported in specially equipped vans or the public transportation system. Many individuals now have motorized scooters or wheelchairs to assist them in their transportation needs. In some cases, cars are specially made to adapt to a person's specific disability, which makes that person's life more satisfying. Because of new laws and more public awareness, there are also more jobs and training programs available for individuals with special needs. An example of such an agency is the Division of Vocational Rehabilitation (DVR). This agency can set up a training program for individuals with special needs and assist with the costs. The case manager or social worker is the one who can assist the client in searching out these special programs or agencies.

If any of clients you care for are mildly mentally impaired with Down syndrome, local communities often have places for them to work during the day for a small amount of money. These places are government funded and have to meet certain government regulations. The goals of these facilities are to get individuals with disabilities out of the house; teach them a minor skill and good work habits; and offer them an opportunity to socialize with other individuals who have similar disabilities.

Emotional Needs

Two of the most important aspects of care of clients with disabilities or disabling conditions are to keep them physically and mentally active and to try to meet some of their emotional needs. These individuals have the same basic needs as a healthy individual of the same age.

UNIT 8

Older Adulthood

THE AGING POPULATION

Old is defined as having lived or existed for a long time. Old and aging are relative to the individual person and that person's age at that time. Aging is a normal process for all individuals. Chronological age means how long a person has lived. The following classification defines aging (in years): old (65 to 74), middle-old (75 to 84), and old-old (85 and older). Chronological age refers to how the person is functioning at a particular age. Functional age means how well an individual is able to accomplish tasks of daily living.

Developmental Tasks of Older Adults

Individuals go through life facing many problems and achieving either success or failure.

How a person confronts and solves problems earlier in life determines his or her behavior in later years. Successful problem solving leads to satisfaction and growth in one's life. This forms the foundation for happiness in older adulthood.

When a person has not successfully solved problems, this person may show signs of anxiety, depression, and inability for personal growth. Examples of developmental tasks of the older adult are:

- Adjusting to physical changes in one's body
- Adapting to living alone
- Accepting the possibility of moving into a long-term care facility
- Adjusting to new relationships with adult children and their offspring
- Managing leisure time
- Adjusting to physical and emotional stress
- Dealing with the death of friends
- Dissatisfaction with friends
- Accepting the approach of one's own death

Aging Well Characteristics

Research and aging studies have revealed that the following habits are frequently seen in people who age well.

- Exercise three to five times weekly
- Eat a low-fat diet
- Maintain ideal weight
- Do not smoke
- Consume alcohol in moderation
- Have a circle of friends with whom to socialize and see often
- Save enough money to live comfortably in old age

- Be future oriented
- Remain active, learning new things
- Establish conditions for good health—sanitation, immunizations, medical intervention
- Good genes are hereditary

Personalities do not really change over time. If someone calls a person a "mean old codger" they were most likely that way when they were 25—age has nothing to do with it. And as we age, we still like to do things we did when we were younger. Older adults can still drive safely, run in the Senior Olympics, and remain interested in sex. Change is a constant in life and if one lives long enough, there is a lot of it! Think about the number of changes an older adult may experience: retirement, relocation, grandchildren and great-great-grandchildren, physical changes, and technological changes such as the computer. There are at least two common threads in most older adults' lives: change and loss.

Depression

Physical changes that occur naturally as we age can make keeping up with change difficult. Sometimes change is loss: death of a family member or friend, or loss of vision, or change of health status, for example. For a person of any age, these kinds of losses can be serious blows. For some older adults, they can be overwhelming. It may feel as if losses are coming faster than they can handle. The older adult grieves for each loss. Depression may describe the kinds of emotions a person feels after a loss or multiple losses. Depression is a persistent sadness that makes it difficult to do day-to-day tasks. Often a person with depression is not concerned about personal appearance and neglects hair, teeth, and skin care. A person with depression

may look sad without complaining about being sad. If recognized, depression can be readily treated.

Leisure-Time Activities

One of the secrets of keeping emotionally happy is being involved with other people and doing some activities. There are many government, community, and church activities for older adults to become involved in without spending a great deal of money. Local school systems welcome the assistance of older adults to help with the reading and math programs. Many older adults still do some of the same activities they did when they were younger. Some travel extensively, seeing the world, while others might purchase a motor home and travel throughout the country. Many spend more quality time with their grandchildren or other family members. A great deal depends on their financial status, physical health, and individual interests. So the opportunity to keep involved is there, but older adults just need to decide which direction they are going to take in their so-called Golden Years.

PHYSICAL CHANGES DUE TO THE AGING PROCESS

Ear Changes

A condition called presbycusis (gradual loss of hearing) is quite common in the elderly. Hearing ability gradually diminishes from the time a person is 40. Some hearing deficits cannot be helped by hearing aids, and the person's hearing is so poor that verbal communication is difficult. Following are tips you may find useful when working with a client who is hard-of-hearing.
- Be aware that even if sounds can be heard, they may not always be heard correctly.

- Limit the competing stimuli of background noise.
- Find out what optimum tone to use when speaking. Louder is not always better.
- Use writing as a form of communication.
- Encourage the use of nonverbal communication such as a big smile, waving, pointing, or demonstrating.
- Speak slowly and clearly and do not change the subject abruptly.
- Face the person at eye level and have light on your face so that lipreading is possible.
- Try to lower your voice, rather than allowing your voice to become high and shrill.
- A sound system used for music, entertainment, or oral presentation should be adjusted so that base and lower tones are predominant. Some sounds are heard while others are not. Hearing loss is greater for consonants than for vowels. S, Z, T, F, and G sounds are particularly difficult to discriminate.

Clients who are hard-of-hearing (HOH) may have nerve damage affecting the auditory (hearing) nerve, or a disorder called otosclerosis. This condition occurs when the bones of the inner ear harden and sound waves no longer carry in the usual fashion. There is also an increase in cerumen (earwax) in the ears. The majority of clients with hearing loss do wear a hearing aid. Refer to Procedure 3, Inserting a Hearing Aid.

3   Procedure

Inserting a Hearing Aid

Purpose

- To increase the hearing ability of the client
- To ensure the client's optimal use of the hearing aid

Procedure

1. Wash your hands.
2. Check hearing aid appliance to see that the batteries are working.
3. Tell the client what you plan to do. You may need to use gestures because client may not be able to hear spoken words.
4. Check inside of client's ear for wax buildup or any other abnormalities.
5. Check to make sure the hearing aid is off or the volume is turned to its lowest level.
6. Handle the hearing aid very carefully. Do not drop it or allow it to get wet. Be sure hearing aid is clean before giving it to client.
7. Assist the client in inserting the earmold into the ear canal.
8. Store hearing aid in an area away from heat and moisture. Turn hearing aid off when the client is not wearing it, as batteries have a very short life. It is a good idea to have spare batteries in the home.

Behind-the-Ear Hearing Aid

- Place the hearing aid over the client's ear, allowing the earmold to hang free.
- Adjust the hearing aid behind the client's ear.

Behind-the-Ear Hearing Aid and In-the-Ear Hearing Aid
- With volume turned down, gently insert the tapered end of the earmold into the ear canal.

- Gently twist the earmold into the curve of the ear while gently pulling on the earlobe with the other hand.
- Adjust the volume according to the client's desire.

Vision Changes

The eyes appear to be farther back in the eye socket (sunken) and the eyelids seem to droop. The lids are no longer elastic and become baggy and wrinkled. The conjunctiva (membrane that lines the eyelids) becomes thinner and yellow. Fatty pads may form in this area of the eye. The iris (pigmented part of the eye) fades or is irregular in shape. The pupil (lets light into the retina) becomes smaller. That means that less light is let into the back of the eye. Thus, the aging person has difficulty with night vision and depth of objects. The fluid in the eye changes and clients complain of floaters. The term accommodation means the ability of a person to first see objects at a distance and then adjust sight to see something close-up like a newspaper. As a person ages, the lens of the eye loses this accommodation ability and to compensate for this loss the individual may need to start wearing glasses with bifocal lenses. The older eye requires more light than the younger eye. To see clearly, the eye of a 65-year-old person needs more than twice as much light as that of a 20-year-old. The older eye does not adapt quickly to changes in light levels. Abrupt changes can be hazardous and may cause falls and other accidents. Legal blindness occurs most in this age group. Since the change in vision happens slowly, older adults usually are aware of their vision changes.

Following are tips you may find useful when working with a client who has difficulty seeing.
- Provide adequate light.
- Carefully adjust shades throughout the day to avoid glare from windows.
- Have client wear sunglasses outside.
- Have night-light on in bedroom at night.
- Be careful of where you place furniture.
- Have large numbers on clocks, radios, watch, and telephone.
- Contrasting colors make things easier to see.
- Warm colors are easier to see—bright yellow, orange, and red.
- Avoid clutter. It is difficult to see when a space is crowded with items.
- If the client is blind, do not change anything in the home without asking the client.
- Have client use magnifying glass to read mail.
- Talking books and large-print books are available at the public library.
- Identify paper money by folding each type a different way for the client.
- Introduce yourself when you enter the home and then if necessary you can touch the client. Always tell the client when you are leaving.
- Give step-by-step instructions on what you want the client to do.

- When serving food, explain the location of each food and beverage item using the face of the clock. "Coffee is at 9:00; soup is at 3:00."

If the client has an eye removed and has an artificial eye, refer to Procedure 4, Caring for an Artificial Eye.

4   Procedure

Caring for an Artificial Eye

Purpose

- To ensure proper care of client's artificial eye
- To prevent infection or irritation of the eye socket

Procedure

1. Assemble equipment:
   disposable gloves
   eyecup with gauze square
   cleansing solution, if ordered
   washcloth and basin of luke-
      warm water
   cotton balls
   small plastic bag for wastes
2. Wash hands and apply gloves.
3. Tell client what you plan to do.
4. Have client lie down if possible. Position yourself and equipment to be on the same side as the client's artificial eye.
5. With moistened cotton balls clean the outside of the eye from the nose to the outside of the face. Stroke once only with each cotton ball. Place used cotton balls in plastic bag.
6. Remove artificial eye by depressing lower eyelid with your thumb while lifting upper lid with your index finger. If client can remove artificial eye, let the client do it. Carefully take eye and place in gauze-lined eyecup. Place eyecup in a safe

place nearby while you clean the outside of the eye socket.
7. Clean eye socket using warm water and cotton balls. Pat area around eye dry. Observe area for signs of irritation or infection.
8. Carry eyecup to sink. Place washcloth in bottom of sink, as a precaution against breakage. Remove eye from eyecup and gently wash in sink. Remove all debris on outside of the eye. Do not use any cleaner on eye unless ordered.
9. Place clean gauze pad in bottom of eyecup and return to client. Assist the client to insert eye into socket. If eye is moist, it will slide in easier. Position notched edge toward client's nose. You may need to depress the lower eyelid and replace the lid gently over the eye as it slips into the socket.
10. If client does not wish to have eye inserted into socket right away, the eye needs to be placed in water in the eyecup.
11. Return equipment and wastes to correct areas.
12. If client wears glasses, clean the glasses with a cleaning solution, rinse with clear water. Dry with clean washcloth or towel. Handle the glasses only by the

frame. Return glasses to client or place in case.
13. Remove gloves and wash hands.

14. Document procedure completion, your observations, and client's reaction.

Common Diseases of the Eye

Following are some common diseases of the eye in the older adult.

Cataracts. A person is diagnosed with cataracts when there is clouding of the lens of the eye. This once meant a gradual, but steady, march toward blindness. This condition affects 60% of the senior population. Symptoms of cataracts are (1) colors appear dull and hazy, (2) halos seen around lights, (3) difficulty seeing while driving at night, and (4) increasing difficulty in reading. This condition can be easily repaired by surgery. After surgery the client may not even have to wear glasses, as he or she did before the surgery.

Glaucoma. Glaucoma is an insidious eye disease that has no noticeable symptoms until irreversible damage is done. Symptoms of glaucoma may include (1) blurred vision, (2) severe eye pain, (3) headaches, (4) colored halos around lights, and (5) nausea and vomiting. It involves a loss of vision due to raised intraocular (inside) pressure, which damages the optic nerve. Glaucoma if untreated can cause blindness. Eyedrops, laser surgery, and an operative procedure are methods used to help prevent further damage. In some cases oral medication may also be prescribed.

Dry Eye. Dry eye is insufficient lubrication (tears) to keep the eye comfortable. Symptoms of dry eye are (1) stinging or burning of the eye, (2) scratchiness, (3) stringy mucus in or around the eye, and (4) excess tearing. Dry eye is treated by eyedrops called artificial tears. They lubricate the eyes and help maintain moisture. Artificial tears are available without a prescription—many brands are available.

Digestive System Changes

As a person ages, the ability to taste diminishes due to the fact that the taste buds on the back of the tongue are less sensitive to taste. The natural teeth are usually replaced with dentures or the person may lack some teeth, which makes chewing the food a little difficult. The salivary glands produce less saliva, which causes problems in breaking down certain foods and makes the older person thirstier. The sense of smell is decreased, so food does not smell as good as it once did. Some older individuals have problems with an inefficient gag reflex and choke readily on thin liquids. These changes can cause a person to have decreased appetite.

Urinary System Changes

The size of the bladder and kidney decreases and muscle control diminishes. Because of these changes, the person needs to urinate more often and starts having problems such as nocturia (night urination), frequent urination, and leaking.

Immune System Changes

The immune system starts to decline as we grow older. Antibodies, which are like soldiers fighting off invading microorganisms, are not as plentiful in the older adult as in the younger adult. Because of this decline in antibodies, the immune system fails to recognize and destroy diseased cells. This may be the reason for the increase in cancer cells as the person grows older. The antibodies do not respond as quickly in the older adult, thus that person does not recover from infections as fast. Older adults need to be immunized against influenza and pneumonia because of their deficient immune systems.

Musculoskeletal Changes

As one grows older, one's muscles become weaker and sometimes atrophy (wasting away). There is a change in joints and other supportive structures. There is reduced flexibility plus stiffness, particularly in the morning. After the age of 55 a few joints may need replacement because of stiffness and pain. Minerals in bones decrease, which makes the bones more vulnerable to fractures. Pelvis (hip bone), long bones, wrist, and back are the most common places for fractures to occur. The person walks with shorter steps and is more cautious about taking steps, and has wider leg stance to achieve better balance. When an individual has knee pain or damage from an earlier injury, the first surgery done on the knee is usually an arthroscopy (*arthro,* joint, and *scopy,* scope). This is a minor surgery in which the orthopedic specialist repairs the knee joint without a surgical incision using a scope to see the inside of the knee. This surgery does help the person for a few years, but if the knee is badly damaged a more extensive surgery called a knee arthroplasty (replacement of joint) will need to be done. This person will need assistance for

about 6 weeks after the surgery. Often a home health aide is assigned for a short time to care for this client. If the hip needs to be replaced it is called a hip arthroplasty.

Kyphosis. As a person ages, the padding between some of the vertebrae (small bones of the spinal column) shrinks, which causes the vertebrae to bend forward. This condition is called kyphosis.

Osteoporosis. Osteoporosis is often referred to as the *silent disease* because bone loss occurs without any symptoms. Osteoporosis is characterized by a decrease in bone mass due to the decline in the female hormone, estrogen, which helps maintain bone strength. As estrogen levels decrease, bones become more porous and fragile. More than 40% of women over the age of 50 will suffer a fracture in their life due to this condition. While women are at the highest risk level for osteoporosis, it can affect men as well. Oftentimes the condition becomes apparent when one experiences a disabling bone fracture from a bump or fall. The test used to diagnose this condition is called a bone density test. Exercise, calcium supplements, and proper diet can be helpful in prevention of osteoporosis.

Reproductive System Changes

Females have reproductive changes due to lowered estrogen and progesterone (hormones). Pubic hair loss is common and the labia (lip) shrinks. The uterus is reduced in size and there is less lubrication of the cervix. These changes make the person more vulnerable for infection and irritation. Occasionally, an older woman may get an infection of the vagina, which is very difficult to treat, and often the drainage is copious (large amount) and very odorous. The breasts lose their elasticity and become pendulous (hanging loosely). The nipples become flat and smaller. Cancer of the breast, ovaries, and uterus are common cancers of the female.

The male has reduced testosterone hormones and reduced seminal fluid production. As a result, he may have a reduced desire for sexual relations. The testicles will atrophy and thus reduce the production of sperm. The prostate gland enlarges, which can cause problems with urination such as dribbling, frequent urination, and urinary tract infections. In some cases, medication can aid in the reduction of the prostate gland. Transurethral resection (TURP) (surgery) may be indicated to relieve these symptoms.

Sexually Transmitted Diseases. According to 1999 data from the U.S. Centers for Disease Control and Prevention (CDC), people over 50 make up 13% of total HIV cases. A larger senior population is having sex later, a pattern that is enhanced by the popularity of Viagra and the promise of a similar drug for women. Because of this, more seniors are now being screened for HIV.

Integumentary (Skin) System Changes

As a person ages the skin, or integumentary system, becomes thinner and sometimes paper thin like tissue paper. The person no longer has a fatty layer of skin in many parts of the body. This affects the ability of the body to regulate a person's temperature. The older adult's legs may lose their hair and also become shiny and blue due to poor circulation. Age spots occur on various places on the body. If a skin lesion appears either

black or brown with an irregular border, this may be a sign of melanoma (malignant skin cancer) and should be reported to the health care provider. Hair growth decreases in some areas on the body and increases in other areas. Men often become bald, but have increased hair in their ears and eyebrows. Women have increased facial hair. Pubic hair also changes and loss is common due to hormonal changes in the body. The sense of touch diminishes and older adults can burn themselves and not even feel it. There is a lack of oil production and the skin becomes dry and tears easily. The older adult's fingernails become more brittle and the toenails thicken and become difficult to cut.

Endocrine System Changes

There is less production of hormones by the endocrine glands in various systems. Because of less hormone production there is an increase in diabetes and hypothyroidism (thyroid deficiency) in the older adult.

Respiratory System Changes

There is reduced elasticity of the lungs and diminished breathing capacity as the person ages. Because of these changes, the person may have problems with the exchange of oxygen and carbon dioxide. Secretions of the lung usually become thicker, especially if the person smokes. There is greater incidence of cancer of the lung, pneumonia, and emphysema in the older adult.

Circulatory System Changes

Many changes take place in the circulatory system in the older adult. The arteries become harder, less elastic, and fill up with plaque. The veins lose their ability to expand and contract. The valves lose their effectiveness, and the heart cannot pump blood through the body without a great deal of effort. There is a greater incidence of diseases such as arteriosclerosis (hardening of the arteries) and congestive heart failure in the older adult.

Nervous System Changes

As a person ages, circulation of the blood to the brain decreases and there is a gradual reduction of brain cells. Transmission of messages from one part of the body to another does not work as well as it once did. It just takes a little longer for older adults to accomplish a task. Their intelligence does not change, unless they have a form of dementia (loss of memory). Diseases that increase with aging are dementia and Parkinson's disease (a degeneration of nerve cells in the area of the brain that controls muscle movement).

Changes in Sleep Patterns

Generally, as we age, sleep is of shorter duration but the same amount. In other words, we often sleep as many hours as we did when we were younger, but each period of sleep lasts a shorter length of time. It is not uncommon for people to be less physically active as they grow older. Additionally, the bladder gets smaller, so the need to urinate becomes more frequent during the night. These three factors can often leave the older adult feeling as if he or she never gets a good night's sleep.

PAIN

As a person ages, the ability to feel pain diminishes. The older adult may have slight pain in the right lower abdomen and not think it is serious because it is only a dull ache. The

individual would know to seek medical help because the pain, accompanied by nausea, would be a sure sign of appendicitis. This makes the older adult more vulnerable for undiagnosed illness and injury. A home health aide needs to be alert to any behavioral change that might indicate the client is in pain.

A few signs and symptoms to look for are increased vital signs (blood pressure usually goes up when a person is in pain), sweating, facial grimacing, holding or squeezing a particular part of the body, nausea or vomiting, and crying, moaning, or just not talking. If a person has dementia, it is the home health aide who will pick up a few clues that the client is having pain, as the client may not be able to express this in words.

When a client does complain of pain, a home health aide should ask the following questions:

1. Where is the pain? Be as specific as possible—not just the right leg, where on the right leg.
2. When did it start?
3. Describe the pain—is it dull, viselike, sharp, cramping, stabbing, knifelike?
4. Have you had this type of pain before—if so, what helped to relieve the pain?
5. Did you do something prior to the pain starting (e.g., kneel in your garden pulling weeds)?
6. Is the pain constant or does it come and go?
7. Using a pain intensity scale, can you rate your pain (Figure 8-1)?

When documenting the client's pain, it is permissible to use the client's own words in describing his or her pain.

Nursing actions to relieve pain vary. The most common treatment is with drugs. There are mild pain re-

```
                    Pain Intensity Scale
    0    1   2   3   4      5      6   7   8   9      10
   (no                  (moderate               (worst
   pain)                  pain)                 possible
                                                  pain)
```

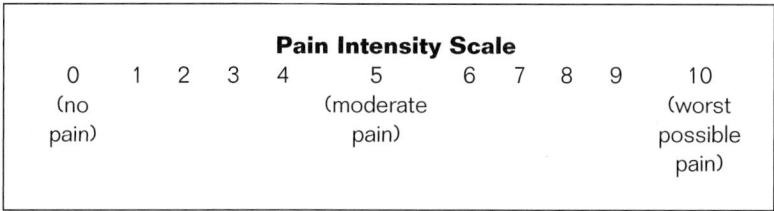

Figure 8-1   Pain levels—have the client use this scale to rate his or her pain

lievers or analgesics such as aspirin or Tylenol and stronger pain relievers such as Percodan and Demerol. The drugs are usually administered before the pain becomes too intense.

MEDICATION

Today, the majority of older adults take some form of medication. At one time, people took medicine just to treat a disease they already had. Today, many medications are given to older adults to prevent diseases. Examples are calcium supplements to prevent osteoporosis and cholesterol lowering drugs to prevent heart problems. There are different types of medicines such as prescription drugs, nonprescription drugs like aspirin, laxatives, and cough medicine. If the client has any allergies, or if the client has had a problem taking a medicine before, that also should be noted. The medication record should indicate what each medicine is for and if it is prescribed by a health care provider. If the client is taking antibiotics, be sure they take the complete 10-to-14-day course even if they feel better and want to stop. Be sure the medicine is given as ordered (e.g., some medicines are given before meals on an empty stomach, others might be given after meals on a full stomach). Because of the expense of drugs, some clients might elect to take half a dosage, if so, this needs to

be documented and reported. Don't mix alcohol or hot drinks with medication administration. They change the effect of the drugs—may destroy the ingredients. Don't combine medications with food unless specifically indicated. Encourage the client to use a special medication reminder container. This will be a handy reminder if the client doubts whether she or he took the medication or not. If the client needs to divide the pill or capsule, it is better to use a special cutter to get a more accurate cut. If the client wants to crush the pill for easier swallowing, check with the nurse to see if it is permissible.

Always be on the alert for drug reactions because they are common occurrences with the older adult. As a home health aide, you might be the first person to notice one or more of the following signs of a drug reaction.

- Tendency to bruise more easily
- Skin rashes
- Diarrhea
- Constipation
- Heartburn
- Dizziness
- Nausea and vomiting
- Fever
- Extreme fatigue

Some drugs are not eliminated from the body as they might be in a younger person, resulting in drug buildup. Given with every prescription bottle today or attached to a bottle when it is refilled is a list of possible side effects of that particular drug. Save these papers just in case you need them for a quick reference. Encourage the client to stay with the same pharmacy so that all of the client's records will be in one place. If you see the prescription bottle is running low, request a refill for the client. Most pharmacies have a call-in system, so all you need to do is call in and the medicine will be ready when you want to pick it up. Some pharmacies might even deliver the drugs for a nominal fee. If your client refuses to have his or her prescription refilled or refuses to take his or her medicines because of financial reasons, do report this to the case manager. The case manager may be able to find funding to assist the client in purchasing required medications.

When a client has an appointment with his or her health care provider it is wise to take a record of all the medicines the client is taking and the dosage. This list of medications can then be brought to the appointment with the health care provider.

Although home health aides do not administer medication, they are allowed to do the following for the client.

a. Remind clients when to take the prescribed medication
b. Assist clients in checking to see if the dosage of medicines is correct
c. Bring the medicine container or prefilled medication container to the client
d. Open the container or bottle and observe the client removing the capsule or liquid from the bottle
e. Shake the liquid medicines if necessary before opening the bottle for the client
f. Check to see if the eyes are clean before the client inserts eyedrops into the eyes
g. Check the ears to see if there is any visible earwax before the client inserts eardrops

Refer to Procedure 5, Assisting the Client with Self-Administered Medications.

5   Procedure

Assisting the Client with Self-Administered Medications

Purpose

- To relieve pain and other symptoms, to help the body fight infections, to prevent diseases, and to treat diseases
- To encourage the client to take the prescribed medication at the right time, in the right dose, in the right amount, and in the right manner

- The following information should be made available to you by your nurse and clearly written down:
  —Name of each medicine
  —What each medication is for
  —Description of medicine— color, form
  —What time(s) of day or night when each medicine is to be taken

—How long the medicine should be taken

—Whether the medicine should be taken with food or other liquid

—Possible side effects

• The home health aide should be aware of common reactions to medications so the nurse can be called if side effects appear.

NOTE: The aide must take special care in assisting clients who are blind or have low vision with their medications. Be sure that medications are coded so that the client can find the correct bottles when they are needed. Medications for the client who is blind must be kept in exactly the same spot so that an error will not be made. Special arrangements should be made by the pharmacist or nurse in setting up the coding.

Procedure

1. Have the nurse or pharmacist prepare a list of medications prescribed and the time they are to be given. Some medications are given 3 times a day (tid), usually before (ac) or after (pc) each meal. Others may be ordered 4 times a day (qid) or every 6 hours (q6h). A medication taken every 6 hours could be given at 6 A.M., noon, 6 P.M., and midnight. The pharmacist usually informs the client at which times the medications should be taken.

2. The nurse will set a schedule to be followed daily. After each medication has been taken, check it off. This informs both the aide and the client that the medicine has been taken. Refer to the schedule and remind the client when medicine is due. Your nurse or pharmacist may prepare your client's medication in special containers that have all the medication needed for a specific time.

3. Check with the client each time to make sure the medicine is the correct one listed on the schedule.

4. Make sure the correct method of taking the medication is followed. For example, some medicines are taken with juice or milk instead of water. Others are taken on an empty stomach, still others with food.

5. Certain medications such as nitroglycerin tablets must be within the client's reach at all times. When the client has chest pain, the client needs to place these tablets under the tongue immediately.

6. Be sure sleeping and pain medication bottles are kept in a safe place after each use. They should only be taken as often as the doctor ordered.

7. Review the times with the client when the prescribed medicines are to be taken. Leave the medication within easy reach of the client. Remind the client to take the nighttime dose in a well-lit room.

8. If the client has questions about the medications, encourage the client to ask the pharmacist, nurse, or health care provider. The client should be knowledgeable about medications that he or she is taking.

9. As a home health aide, you are not allowed to pour the client's medication from the bottle; the client needs to do this himself or herself.

Preventing the Spread of Infectious Disease

Unit 9
Principles of Infection Control

Principles of Infection Control

INFECTIOUS DISEASE

An infection is the invasion of body tissue by disease-producing organisms. An infectious disease is one that is readily communicable or easily passed on to others (contagious). Signs of a client having an infection are fever and chills, fatigue, loss of appetite, discharge from infected area, redness, pain or tenderness, nausea and vomiting, diarrhea, or a skin rash. An inflammation of a body part may have similar signs, but an inflammation does not have a pathogen (germ) in the area. An example of an inflammation would be a person who sprains an ankle. The ankle will be swollen, reddish, painful, and warm to the touch. These are called the classic signs of an inflammation. Infectious diseases can be spread through various routes: airborne, animal and insect carried, contact or human carried, prenatal, food, or soil and water carried.

The Chain of Infection

The first step in the chain of infection is that there is a source such as a pathogen or germ. The second step in the chain is that the germ must have a place to live and thrive—this is called the reservoir. The next step is for the germ to leave the reservoir and be transmitted to another host. In order for this to occur, the germ must have a portal of entry such as a break in the skin, through the urinary tract or respiratory secretions, or through the blood (such as HIV). The germ has a better chance of multiplying and surviving if the client (host) is weak. Instead of the term, weak, the term susceptible host is used. An example of a susceptible host would be a client in the later stages of cancer who suddenly develops a condition called herpes zoster (shingles). The primary sign of shingles is a painful itching rash that occurs over the body. The rash follows the nerves of the body. The virus that causes shingles is quite common, but a normal, healthy individual is able to resist the virus from entering and multiplying in the body.

If a client develops an infection while being hospitalized, this type of infection is called a nosocomial infection. There is less chance for this type of infection to occur if a client is discharged early from the hospital.

CAUSES OF PHYSICAL ILLNESSES

Microorganisms are so small that they can be seen only under a high-powered microscope. There are good microorganisms and microorganisms that can cause disease. The microorganisms that are capable of causing disease are called germs or pathogens. The time between the entry of germs into the body and the appearance of the first sign of disease is called the incubation period. Strong, healthy people are more able to fight off pathogens than weak or unhealthy people.

There are many different types of microorganisms. Bacteria are microscopic organisms that multiply rapidly. Protozoa are tiny one-cell microorganisms. Bacteria and protozoa can live for a long time and continue to multiply in air and water. Many types of bacteria and protozoa exist, but only a few cause diseases. Viruses are microorganisms that can live only by feeding on living cells. Most viruses are capable of causing infections. Diseases caused by viruses are flu, colds, human immunodeficiency virus (HIV) and hepatitis. Fungi include two groups of organisms—yeast and molds—that live normally in the body. Under certain conditions they can cause diseases such as athlete's foot (tinea pedis), ringworm (tinea capitis), thrush, or vaginitis (*Candida albicans*). Another example of a microorganism that can cause a disease and lives on lice, ticks, fleas, mites, and other insects is called rickettsiae.

Most germs grow and reproduce very rapidly. They spread disease from one part of the body to another. They also may spread disease from one person to another. This is called spreading germs by direct contact.

Practicing good infection control techniques is the best defense against the spread of germs. If there is a possibility of the presence of germs (pathogens) on an article, the article is considered contaminated. Articles that are free of all living organisms are sterile. The process of sterilization completely destroys microorganisms on objects. Aseptic techniques are used to prevent the spread of germs. Many sterile supplies such as gauze dressings, applicators, and instruments come prepackaged in paper for convenience. They must be opened, handled, and used in a special way so that they will not become contaminated. Disinfection is the process of destroying disease-producing organisms by using chemicals. For example, if a home health aide uses a stethoscope on one client, the diaphragm of the stethoscope must be disinfected or wiped with an alcohol sponge before using it on another client. This will prevent the spread of germs from one client to another.

Tuberculosis

Tuberculosis (TB) is an airborne disease, which means that it is spread by droplets in the air released from deep within the lungs when a TB sufferer coughs. Anyone sharing a poorly ventilated room with an individual with TB can contract the disease. The incidence of TB is on the rise. Individuals who live in crowded spaces, have poor nutrition, are substance abusers, are under a high amount of stress, or lack medical care are good candidates for this disease.

When an aide is assigned to care for a client with TB, the aide will need to use standard precautions, especially when handling the client's sputum and nasal secretions. Another important aspect of care is making sure to remind the client to take medication as prescribed. *The medication must be taken on schedule, otherwise the effects of the drugs will be decreased.* TB can be cured if caught in the early stages and if the client takes the medication as ordered usually for 6 months.

CONTROLLING THE SPREAD OF ILLNESS

Most everyone practices aseptic techniques for infection control in daily living. Some of the most common practices are:
- Handwashing
- Bathing, brushing teeth, shampooing hair
- Changing clothing regularly
- Cleaning bathroom sink, tub, bowl, and floor
- Cleaning kitchen, washing dishes
- Vacuuming and mopping floors
- Laundering clothing and linens
- Cleaning from the cleanest area to the dirtiest area
- Covering your nose when coughing or sneezing
- Flushing the toilet after each use
- Using separate towel and washcloth for each person in the household, if wet let it air-dry
- Keeping table and countertops clean and dry

When illness is present, added care must be taken to prevent the spread of germs. An ill person's body is producing germs. At the same time, the person is weak and cannot resist other germs. The person's body is so busy fighting one illness that it cannot fight off other germs.

Germs can enter the body in many ways. For example, if the germ that causes a cold enters the respiratory system (the nose, the lungs, etc.) the person would develop a cold because the respiratory system provides just the right climate for the cold germ to grow.

Germs can be spread when others touch contaminated objects or surfaces. This is called spreading germs

by indirect contact. Tissues used by the client should be placed in a paper bag at the client's bedside. Dressings or bandages from open cuts or wounds must be double-bagged in plastic and then discarded. Careful cleaning of the client's room is important in stopping indirect spread of germs.

Agency Requirements

Two government agencies are very involved in preventing the spread of infections and diseases while delivering care. Guidelines for working with clients with infectious diseases are issued from U.S. Centers for Disease Control and Prevention (CDC) and Occupational Safety and Health Administration (OSHA). In order to be accredited, a home health care agency must follow these guidelines. A few of the guidelines that affect the home health aide directly are:

1. The employer must provide the home health aide with training on working with protective care equipment (e.g., gloves, goggles, mask).
2. The employer must provide the home health aide with necessary protective equipment when caring for a client who has an infectious disease.
3. The employer must provide immunization against hepatitis B with no cost to the home health aide.
4. The employer must provide tuberculosis testing yearly with no cost to the home health aide.
5. The employer must provide training in biohazardous waste and what to do if the possibility of exposure exists.

These guidelines also state that if the home health aide accidentally pricks a finger by a needle or other sharp instrument that is contaminated, this must be reported to his or her agency immediately. The home health aide is also required to fill out an incident report. On this report the home health aide states (1) how the accident happened, (2) where it happened, (3) details about the injury or accident, (4) if there were any witnesses, and (5) date and time it happened.

Guidelines from these two government agencies are constantly being updated. It is the responsibility of the home health care agency to keep home health aides aware of changes that affect how they need to care for their clients. There are new diseases occurring all the time, for example, in the year 2003 there was a Severe Acute Respiratory Syndrome (SARS) epidemic. In the past 30 years, there have been 35 new infectious diseases worldwide. The U.S. death rate from infectious diseases, which dropped in the first half of the 20th century and then stabilized, is now double what it was in 1980.

INFECTION CONTROL MEASURES

A home health aide has a duty to protect clients from unnecessary harm. In addition to keeping the home environment clean and following everyday aseptic practices, the aide also should be in good physical health. An aide who is ill risks carrying germs into the client's environment.

The home health aide's hands are the most common means of carrying infection. To control the spread of germs and to protect the aide and client, the aide's hands must be washed frequently. Refer to Procedure 6 Handwashing. Just a quick rinse will not do it. The aide should use plenty of warm water and soap, rub hands to generate friction, and wash for 15 seconds. To dry the hands, the use of disposable paper towels is best. Cloth towels can spread germs when reused. If the hands are dry and chapped, lotion may be used after washing. Hands should be washed:

- On arrival at the client's home
- Before and after each client contact
- Before preparing food
- Before and after each meal
- After blowing the nose or sneezing
- After using the bathroom
- After handling soiled items such as linens, clothing, or garbage
- Before putting on gloves and after using gloves
- After contact with items contaminated with blood, feces, or other body fluids

The aide should keep in mind that handwashing is the most important procedure involved in controlling the spread of disease.

6   Procedure

Handwashing

Purpose
- To prevent the transfer of disease-producing organisms from person to person or place to place

Procedure
1. Collect the items needed for handwashing and bring them to the bathroom or kitchen sink.

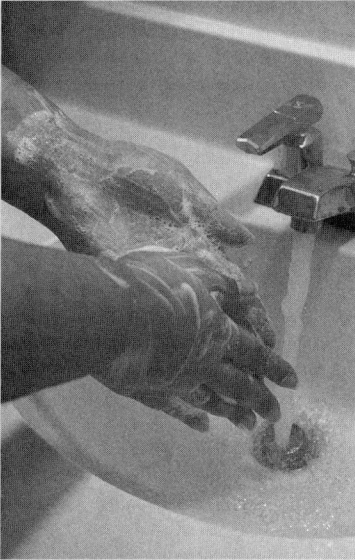

Figure 9-1 Wet hands, apply soap, and rub hands to cause lather. Keep hands pointed down so that water does not run up arms.

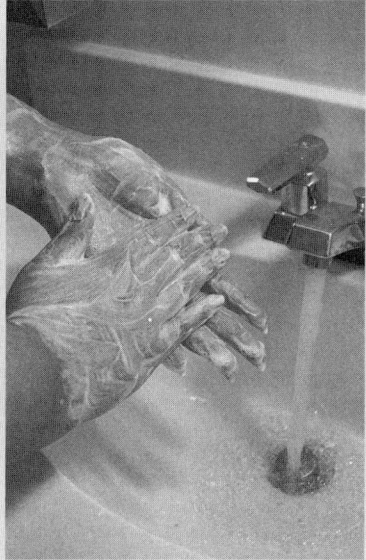

Figure 9-2 Use friction between hands to clean well.

soap (bar or liquid)
soap dish
towel (paper towels preferred)
2. Use a clean paper towel to turn on water and adjust temperature. Wet hands with fingertips pointing down (Figure 9-1).
3. Apply soap—either liquid or bar.
4. With fingertips pointing down, lather well. Rub your hands together in a circular motion to generate friction (Figure 9-2). Wash carefully between your fingers, palms, and back of hands, and rub fingernails against the palm of the other hand to force soap under the nails. Keep washing for 15 seconds. Be sure to clean under fingernails (Figure 9-3).
5. With fingertips still pointing down, rinse all the soap off. Be

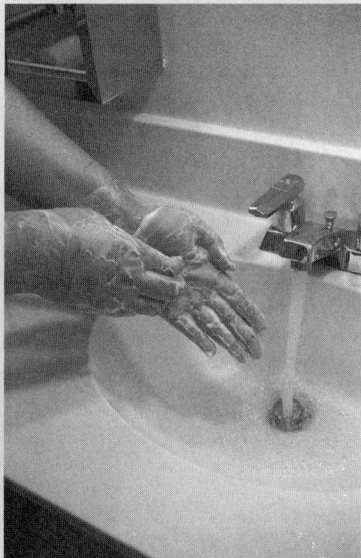

Figure 9-3 Always clean your fingernails.

careful not to lean against the side of the sink or touch the inside of the sink because germs are there.

6. With clean paper towel or clean hand towel, dry hands. Use a clean paper towel and turn off faucet (Figure 9-4). Do not turn off faucet with clean hands because the faucet handles are contaminated.

7. Discard the paper towel in the wastebasket.

8. Apply hand lotion if hands are dry or chapped.

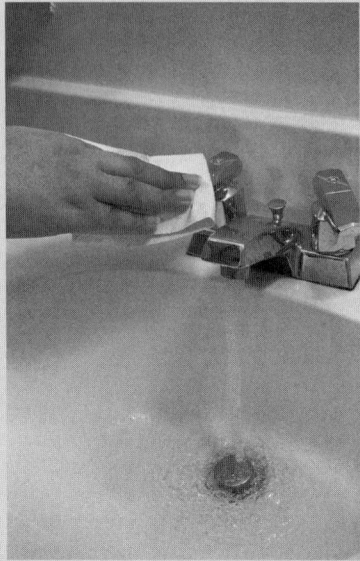

Figure 9-4 Turn off faucet with dry paper towel.

STANDARD PRECAUTIONS

We cannot tell if people have an infectious disease just from looking at them. Therefore, certain measures must be taken to prevent the spread of infection. These measures are called standard precautions and must be used at all times for all clients. Standard precautions are designed to protect the home health aide and the client. Standard precautions provide guidelines for handwashing, personal protective equipment (PPE) use (gloves, gowns, masks, goggles), client care equipment, environmental care, linen handling, and safe needle use. See Figure 9-5 for specific guidelines.

Although the use of special or standard precautions is important to prevent the spread of infection to, or from, a client, keep in mind how odd it must feel to a client to be cared for by a person wearing barriers. Most of us are used to health professionals and paraprofessionals using gloves, gowns, or masks. However, to a person who is feeling isolated or depressed, these protective barriers may increase their feelings of loneliness and sadness. Your tone of voice, what you say, and the gentleness of your touch become even more important.

TRANSMISSION-BASED PRECAUTIONS

Transmission-based precautions are precautions taken in addition to standard precautions. They are used when the pathogen that is causing the infection is highly contagious. There are three types of transmission-based precautions depending on

Standard Precautions for Infection Control

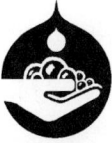

Wash Hands (Plain soap)
Wash after touching **blood, body fluids, secretions, excretions,** and **contaminated items.** Wash immediately **after gloves are removed** and before applying gloves.

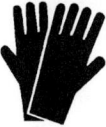

Wear Gloves
Wear when touching **blood, body fluids, secretions, excretions,** and **contaminated items.** Put on **clean** gloves just **before touching mucous membranes** and **nonintact skin.** Change gloves between tasks and procedures on the same client after contact with material that may contain high concentrations of microorganisms. Remove gloves promptly after use, before touching noncontaminated items and environmental surfaces.

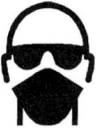

Wear Mask and Eye Protection or Face Shield
Protect mucous membranes of the eyes, nose, and mouth during procedures and client care activities that are likely to generate **splashes** or **sprays** of **blood, body fluids, secretions,** or **excretions.**

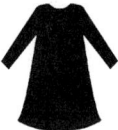

Wear Gown
Protect skin and prevent soiling of clothing during procedures that are likely to generate **splashes** or **sprays of blood, body fluids, secretions,** or **excretions.** Remove a soiled gown as promptly as possible and wash hands to avoid transfer of microorganisms to other clients or environments.

Client Care Equipment
Handle used client care equipment soiled with **blood, body fluids, secretions** or **excretions** in a manner that prevents skin and mucous membrane exposures and contamination of clothing.

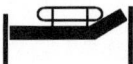

Environmental Control
Follow procedures for routine care, cleaning, and disinfection of environmental surfaces, beds, bedside equipment, and other frequently touched surfaces. Double-bag soiled disposable items (e.g., adult briefs). If blood gets on the floor or other surfaces, wash the area with a solution of 1 part bleach to 10 parts water.

(continues)

Figure 9-5   Standard precautions guidelines

Standard Precautions for Infection Control—continued

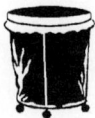

Linens

Handle, transport, and process used linens soiled with **blood, body fluids, secretions,** or **excretions** in a manner that prevents exposures and contamination of clothing. A large plastic bag or garbage bag can be used to discard soiled linens.

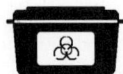

Biohazards

Prevent injuries when using needles, scalpels, and other sharp instruments or devices; when handling sharp instruments after procedures; when cleaning used instruments; and when disposing of used needles.

Do not remove used needles from disposable syringes by hand, and do not bend, break, or otherwise manipulate used needles by hand. Place used disposable syringes and needles, scalpel blades, and other sharp items in puncture-resistant sharps containers located as close as practical to the area in which the items were used, and place reusable syringes and needles in a puncture-resistant container. When the container is full, return it to your agency, do not throw it in the regular trash or garbage can.

Figure 9-5   Standard precautions guidelines—continued

how the organism is spread from one person to another. The first type is airborne, which is used when caring for a client with tuberculosis, chickenpox, or measles. The reasoning behind the extra precautions is that the organism is very small and can stay in the air for a longer period. Thus, the extra precautions deal with how the air is handled in the client's room and with the ventilation system. It is the responsibility of the home health care agency to deal with the home ventilation and air exchange system. The second type is called droplet precautions. These extra precautions are used when caring for a client who has an infectious disease such as influenza and the microorganism can spread by coughing, sneezing, or talking. The home health aide must wear a mask when caring for the client and when taking the client out of the home, the client must also wear a mask. Contact precautions are special measures that need to be taken if the client has an infection such as conjunctivitis (pinkeye), impetigo, or a staphylococcal wound infection. These diseases are highly contagious. Extra measures that need to be taken are (1) wear gloves at all times, (2) wash hands with antimicrobial soap (special soap that will kill microorganisms) before and after applying gloves, (3) wear a gown or apron when entering room and doing direct client care, (4) limit client's contact with others, and (5) take special care when disposing of all equipment and supplies that come in contact with the client. Contaminated items such as bloody dressings must be placed in a specially marked red bag with the biohazard symbol.

Antibiotic-Resistant Organisms

The most popular method used to treat an infection is with an antibiotic. Occasionally, a pathogen or microorganism is not killed by an antibiotic, which is called being antibiotic-resistant. Two organisms that are seen in home health care that are resistant to antibiotics are methicillin-resistant *Staphylococcus aureus* (MRSA) and vancomycin-resistant enterococcus (VRE). Although standard precautions are the same for hepatitis and HIV, there are extra precautions that should be taken for MRSA and VRE clients.

When caring for clients with VRE, the home health aide should use antimicrobial soap, as regular soap is relatively ineffective in removing VRE from the hands. Also, gloves should be worn whenever providing any personal care to these clients, not just when expecting to come into contact with bodily substances. This is primarily for preventing transmission from client to client, not necessarily from client to aide. If the client is incontinent, caregivers should wear gowns and aprons during catheter care, when bathing the client, or changing bed linens.

The client with a communicable disease may be placed in isolation. This means that the client is kept away from others in the household. Isolation helps prevent family members and the home health aide from getting the client's germs. In such cases home health aides will have to be especially careful in maintaining aseptic conditions. Gloves should be worn for most personal care procedures. Refer to Procedure 7 Gloving.

7 Procedure

Gloving

Purpose

• To prevent the spread of infections

NOTE: Gloves come in various sizes. Be sure you use the correct size gloves, because if the glove is too small, it will break or tear easily and if the glove is too large, germs can enter easily. Gloves are made from different materials. At one time, most gloves were made of latex, but because of so many allergies from latex the common material

used today is vinyl. If a home health aide is allergic to both materials, hypoallergenic gloves can be used.

Procedure

1. Wash your hands.
2. With your dominant hand pull out one glove and slide it onto your other hand.
3. With the gloved hand, pull out another glove and slide your dominant hand into it.

4. Interlace your fingers to make the gloves comfortable and adjust the top of the gloves to stay flat.

Removal of Contaminated Gloves

1. Use your dominant hand to grasp the opposite glove on the palm side, about 1 inch below the wrist (Figure 9-6).
2. Pull the glove down and off so that it is removed inside out and keep hold of that glove with the fingertips of the gloved hand (Figure 9-7).
3. Using your ungloved hand, insert the fingers into the inside of the remaining glove and pull it down and off, inside out, so that the glove you are holding with your fingertips is now inside the glove that you are taking off (Figure 9-8).
4. Drop both soiled gloves together into waste receptacle (Figure 9-9).
5. Wash your hands.

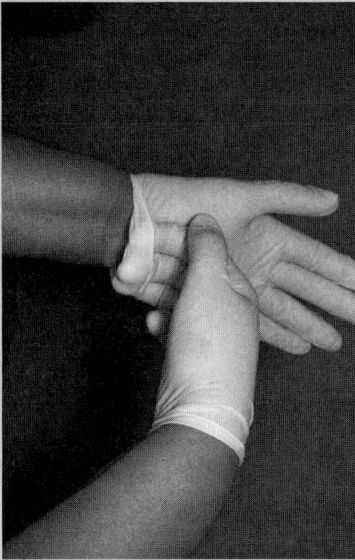

Figure 9-6 To remove gloves, grasp glove on the palm side.

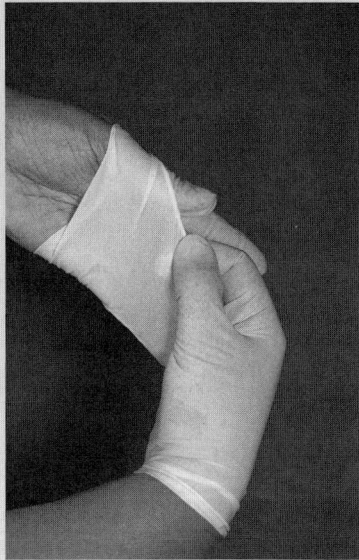

Figure 9-7 Pull glove down and off, inside out.

Standard precautions provide guidelines for wearing personal protective equipment such as gowns and masks. Wearing gowns and masks prevents the spread of germs and prevents the contamination of the aide's clothing. Refer to Procedure 8 Putting On and Removing Personal Protective Equipment.

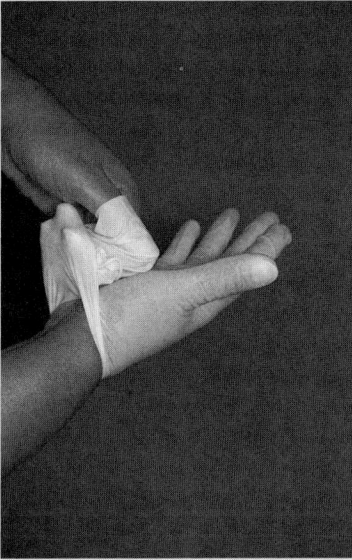

Figure 9-8 Use your ungloved hand, insert fingers into inside of remaining glove, turn inside out so glove you are holding is inside glove you're removing.

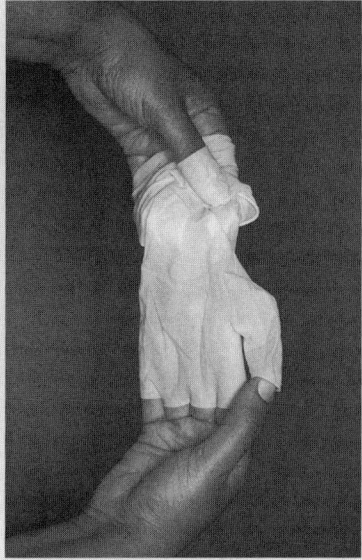

Figure 9-9 Drop gloves into proper waste container.

8 Procedure

Putting On and Removing Personal Protective Equipment

Purpose

- To prevent contaminating the aide's clothing
- To prevent the spread of germs through the respiratory tract

Procedure

1. Assemble personal protective equipment (Figure 9-10).
2. Wash your hands.
3. The first piece of equipment to apply is the mask.

4. Adjust the mask over your nose and mouth. Tie the top strings first and then the bottom strings. Your mask must always be dry, so that droplets are not absorbed into the paper of the mask. If the mask becomes wet, you must replace it.
5. Unfold and open the gown so that you can slide your arms into the sleeves and your hands come right through. Slip the fingers of

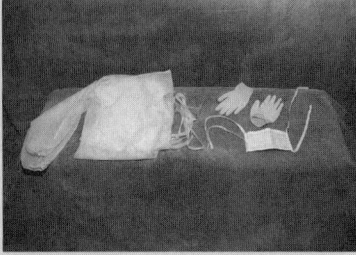

Figure 9-10 Protective barriers used in standard precautions: gloves, disposable gown, goggles, and disposable mask

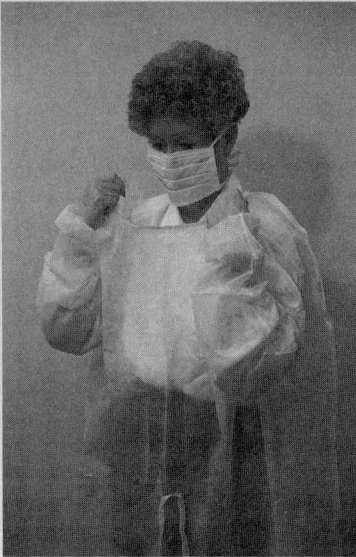

Figure 9-12 Tie waist ties in back.

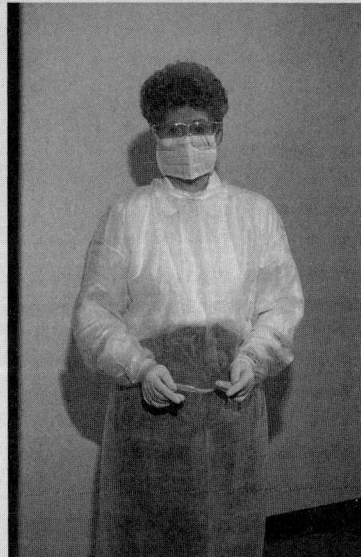

Figure 9-11 Putting on gown

both hands inside the neckband of the gown and grasp the two strings at the back and tie into a bow, not a knot, so that they can be undone easily after the procedure is completed (Figure 9-11). Reach behind you, overlap the two edges of the gown so that

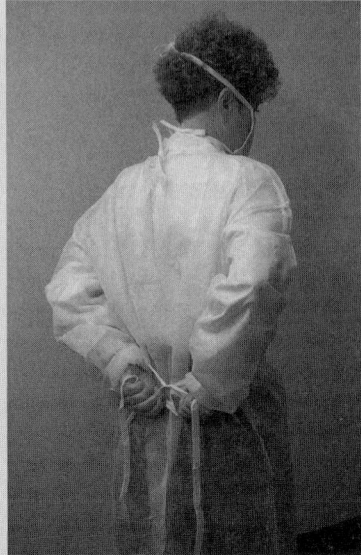

Figure 9-13 Properly masked, gloved, and gowned aide

your uniform is completely covered, and then secure the waist ties (Figures 9–12 and 9–13).

6. **REMEMBER:** Your moisture-resistant gown is only worn once and is then discarded in a container for contaminated waste.

Removing Contaminated Gown and Mask

1. Undo the waist ties of your gown.
2. Remove gloves.
3. Wash hands.
4. Undo your mask, bottom ties first, then top ties. Holding top ties, drop mask in appropriate waste container.
5. Undo neckties and loosen gown at shoulder.
6. Slip finger of right hand inside left cuff without touching outside of gown and pull gown over left hand. With your gown-covered left hand, pull gown down over right hand and then right arm.
7. Fold gown with contaminated side inward and dispose of it into the appropriate waste container.
8. Wash hands.

Isolation is more difficult to arrange in the home than it is in a hospital. Ideally, isolated clients should have a bathroom that only they may use. However, when this is not possible, the home health aide will have to clean the sink and toilet area each time the client uses it. The aide's hands and the client's hands should be washed often. Handwashing destroys many germs. Disposable dishes, equipment, or tissues should be used whenever possible. The client should use a separate set of dishes and utensils than is used by the family. Combs, brushes, toilet articles, towels, and washcloths used by the client should not be used by others. Keeping these items separate helps prevent indirect spread of infection.

Aides should wear a bib apron or smock over the uniform while in the client's room. Before leaving the room, the cover garment should be placed into a waste container or hung inside the door of the client's room. When changing the bed linens, the soiled linens should be held away from the aide's garment. Disposable gloves should be used to pick up soiled linens and place them into a waste container.

If blood is spilled on the floor, a preparation of 1 part bleach and 10 parts water must be used to clean it up.

All contaminated materials from the client's room must be discarded by placing them in a double plastic bag or placing in a covered garbage container. The client's linens and clothing must be washed separately from other family laundry. The client's dishes must be washed separately in hot, soapy water, rinsed, and air-dried. After the isolation period is ended, any items used by the client should be sterilized or disinfected completely. It is important to destroy all germs on the items used before returning to general family use.

Hepatitis

Hepatitis is a viral infection that mainly affects the liver. Classic signs and symptoms of this liver disease are jaundice (yellowing of the skin and white of the eye), fatigue, abdominal pain, loss of appetite, and nausea. There are many different types of hepatitis, depending on the name of the virus causing the infection. The three main types are Hepatitis A, B, and C.

Hepatitis A. The cause of this mild type is the hepatitis A virus (HAV). It is usually spread from person to person by putting something in the mouth that has been contaminated with the stool of a person who has hepatitis A. Signs are the usual signs plus the client may have a fever. Vaccine A is the best protection for this type of hepatitis. This disease is self-limiting.

Hepatitis B. This is a more serious type of hepatitis and could lead to complications that may cause liver cancer or cirrhosis of the liver. These complications may be fatal to the client. The virus that causes this condition is called hepatitis B virus (HBV). This virus may be found in the blood and body fluids including urine, tears, semen, vaginal secretions, and breast milk. The disease is spread through sexual contact, contamination by needle sticks, and using contaminated personal care items (e.g., razors, nail clippers, or toothbrush). Many individuals who are infected with the virus may not know it because the signs at first are silent. The only way one might know is through a blood test. The infected person can pass it on without knowing it. The primary signs of the infection are flu-like symptoms.

The home health aide may get vaccinated to prevent acquiring the virus. This vaccine is divided into three injections over a 6-month period. The Engerix-B Vaccine is recommended for health workers. The home health aide who is hypersensitive to yeast should discuss this with his or her health care provider prior to getting the vaccination.

Hepatitis C. Hepatitis C is caused by hepatitis C virus (HCV). This is a chronic disease that remains in the bloodstream, eventually destroying the person's liver. This disease is the leading cause for liver transplants in the United States. The disease occurs when blood and body fluids from an infected person enter the body of a person who is not infected. The virus is spread through shared needles of intravenous drug users, needle-stick injuries at work, or an infant can contract the infection while in utero, if the mother is infected.

Collecting a Specimen From a Client on Transmission-Based Precautions

To collect a specimen from a client on transmission-based precautions, it is important to also remember to use standard precautions. Both precautions need to be used because standard precautions alone will not always protect the client and home health aide. For example, if a client is on airborne precautions and you need to collect a urine sample, you must wear gloves (standard precautions) and a mask. Refer to Procedure 9 Collection Specimen from Client on Transmission-Based Precautions.

9 ——————————— **Procedure**

Collecting Specimen from Client on Transmission-Based Precautions

Purpose
- To obtain and send specimen to laboratory without spreading germs from the client's home

Procedure
1. Assemble equipment:
   clean specimen container, cover, label
   paper towels
   gloves
   plastic transport bag
2. Fill in label with client's name, date, time, and type of specimen.
3. Remove cover from the container and place all the equipment on the clean paper towel.
4. Wash your hands and put on gloves.
5. With gloved hands, pick up the specimen and place it in the container so that you do not contaminate any part of the container (Figure 9-14). Replace cover.
6. Remove gloves and wash hands.
7. Using the paper towel, pick up the container without touching it with your bare hands.

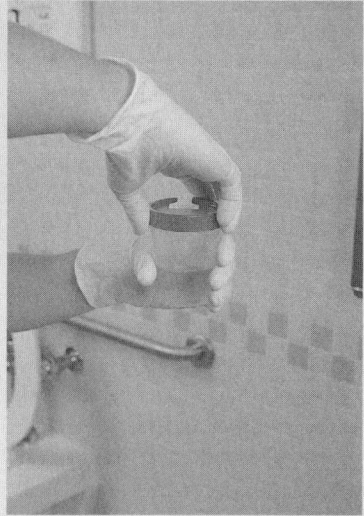

Figure 9-14   Collecting a specimen in isolation

8. Place the container in the plastic bag and seal it. Also label the outside of the bag.
9. Send specimen to the laboratory per instruction of your case manager.

AIDS

Acquired immunodeficiency syndrome (AIDS) is a severe immunologic disorder caused by the human immunodeficiency virus (HIV). In this disease, the body's immune system becomes severely depressed and unable to fight any type of infection. The HIV virus lives in the infected person's blood, semen, and other body fluids. It can be transmitted by intimate contact—oral, vaginal, rectal—or by direct contact with body fluids or blood. In most cases, AIDS is transferred by sexual contact and drug users sharing needles. AIDS can also be transmitted to newborn babies during delivery or through the mother's milk. A new mother infected with the virus can pass the disease by breast-feeding her infant. Prior to 1985, AIDS was also transmitted through contaminated blood transfusions. Contaminated blood is no longer a concern because the American Red Cross now tests all blood donations for HIV. HIV infection comes in three stages: acute infection, chronic infection, and AIDS. The acute infection phase is the shortest stage of HIV infection. The first signs are flu-like illness 3 to 6 weeks after being infected with the virus. Then for 7 to 10 years the symptoms disappear. The immune system during this time gradually becomes weaker. This is called the chronic stage. A blood test called the CD4 count is done to monitor the progress of the disease. A normal person would have a cell count of 450 to 1,200. Once the CD4 cell count is less than 200, the diagnosis of AIDS is given.

A diagnosis of HIV is made through a blood test. Today there is a test called OraQuick, which individuals who think they might have been infected with the virus can do at home. One can also obtain testing at a public health laboratory under complete secrecy, or see one's own health care provider for testing.

Each care plan will need to be individualized to meet the client's physical and emotional needs.

Children with AIDS need special attention and care. Often the scenario is that one or maybe both parents are HIV positive and will eventually die. The child is then left without any parental care. When caring for a child with HIV, be very observant for signs that may indicate an infection such as fever, vomiting, and diarrhea. It is better that the child has plastic or washable toys, as stuffed toys can hold dirt and hide germs that can make a child sick. Try to keep the child away from sandboxes and animals. Do the utmost to keep the child from contracting any type of infectious disease, as this could kill the child, as their immune system is very depressed.

As more information has come to light about AIDS, the public is more aware of what is and what is not true. According to Dr. C. Everett Koop, former Surgeon General of the United States, we must come to terms with the fact that we are fighting a disease, not the people who have AIDS. He also said that those who are already afflicted need to be cared for like any other sick individual. It is hoped that soon there will be a vaccine to protect a person against HIV.

HOW TO PROTECT AGAINST AIDS

At this time there is no vaccine to prevent AIDS and there is no cure for AIDS. The only way to lessen the impact of the AIDS virus is to avoid situations that are dangerous and take precautions, for example, practicing safe sex by using condoms, practicing abstinence, not "shooting" drugs intravenously, not using "dirty" needles (best of all, not getting involved in drug use of any kind), and using precautions when caring for an AIDS client.

The Surgeon General states that quarantine has no role in the management of AIDS because AIDS is not spread by casual contact, unless the AIDS victim deliberately exposes others by sexual contact and sharing drug equipment.

CARING FOR THE AIDS CLIENT

AIDS is a debilitating disease with no cure. Dealing with the effects of AIDS can be difficult for the client and family alike. AIDS often afflicts young adults at their most productive time of life, making it especially difficult for the client and their loved ones to face death. The emotional and physical support of caregivers, family, and friends is crucial in helping those with AIDS lead as normal a life as possible, for as long as possible.

What an Aide Can and Should Do

When working with an AIDS client it is important to know that many misconceptions about the disease exist. The home health aide should learn the facts about AIDS and remain nonjudgmental of the client, regardless of how the disease was contracted. A home health aide must never reveal to friends, neighbors, or anyone else the nature of a client's illness. That is considered an invasion of privacy and the client can file a complaint with the State Department of Human Rights if such information is revealed by the agency or the aide.

The home health aide should create a comfortable and pleasant environment for the client. Personal hygiene is crucial to maintain the client's comfort and to promote health. Regular bathing will be necessary if the client suffers from night sweats.

Understanding Health

Unit 10
From Wellness
to Illness

Unit 11
Mental Health

UNIT 10

From Wellness to Illness

Bodies come in all shapes and sizes. There are records of men who have been as tall as 9 feet and as short as 26 1/2 inches. These statistics are interesting because they show the tremendous contrasts possible within the human body. Just as there are contrasts in size, there are other individual differences. Heredity is the passing of traits from parents to their children. Heredity can determine height, weight, general appearance, skin color, talents and abilities, basic physical wellness, and many other things. All children get half of their heredity from each parent. However, some traits are more dominant than others. This explains why some children are more like one parent then the other.

Another factor that helps determine body size, shape, and wellness is environment. Environment is the sum total of the circumstances, conditions, and surroundings affecting the development of an organism. Some environmental factors that may affect growth are nutrition, financial conditions, climate, number of children in the family, and the parents' ages and occupations. The child who is born healthy with good hereditary characteristics is likely to start life as a well person.

THE REMARKABLE BODY

The human body is remarkable because it can continue to work when some of its parts break down. Damaged brain cells cannot be "repaired," but there are so many brain cells that new ones can be trained to take over. Many body structures are in "pairs." A body has two arms, two legs, two kidneys, two eyes. In the well body all of the parts work together.

What happens when one of a pair becomes diseased? In the case of kidneys, one can be removed surgically and the other will take over the work. The person with only one kidney must be more careful with diet and generally take more health precautions than the average person, yet a person can return to a state of wellness with even one kidney. The human body and mind are able to adapt. The home health aide's efforts are important in helping a client adapt physically, mentally, and emotionally. Human beings have often been compared to machines. When functioning perfectly, the body operates as

103

smoothly as a well-oiled machine. The human body, however, is much more efficient than any machine. Unlike a machine, the human body often can repair itself, for example, new skin can grow over a wound. When the body functions at its peak efficiency with all of its parts working like a finely tuned engine, it is in a state of wellness.

The body is a complex organism. It is made up of millions of cells, which are the smallest structural units of the body. Many cells make up a tissue and tissues make up organs (Figure 10-1). Organs act together in making the total body function. All of these separate units interact within the body in systems. There are nine body systems, each one performing a necessary function in the body (Figure 10-2).

INTERNAL HEALTH

Wellness is the normal state of the human body. Illness occurs when the body machinery is not working properly. This may be caused by external factors or it may result from an internal disorder (abnormality). Internal problems occur when some part of the body is not working correctly. Accidents and environmental hazards are examples of external causes of illness.

Illness, an accidental injury, a birth defect, or the normal sensory losses of aging may be the cause of a disability. A disability may involve impaired mental or emotional functioning or involve an impaired body function, such as eyesight or ambulation (walking). The Americans with Disabilities Act (a national law protecting the rights of people with disabilities) defines a person with a disability as someone who:

- Has a physical or mental impairment that substantially limits one or more major life activities

- Has a record of such an impairment
- Is regarded as having such an impairment

Because the home health aide will be caring for clients who are ill or disabled or who are recovering from an illness, it is important for the aide to understand the basic principles and terms related to disorders and diseases and to their treatment.

Internal Disorders

Internal disorders may happen at any age. However, they are more likely to occur as the body grows older and becomes more prone to breaking down. Usually young people recover more quickly from accidents and diseases because their body tissues and cells repair and grow at a faster rate. It takes longer for recovery in older persons because the growth rate of new cells is slower. The circulatory system often becomes less efficient as people age. Heart disease, stroke, diabetes, and hypertension are major physical disorders of the older adult.

Emotional Disorders

An internal disorder that can happen at any age is an emotional breakdown. Some mental disorders are so severe that the client must be hospitalized. Many times, a person who normally functions well suffers an emotional breakdown when external stress becomes too great. Depression is a normal response to illness. Illness, pain, and physical trauma put stress on the body and the person's emotions. On the other hand, physical care such as proper nutrition, exercise, companionship, and relief from pain can do much toward lifting depression and relieving mental stress.

Emotional and physical health depend on one another. Emotional ill-

LEVEL	EXAMPLES

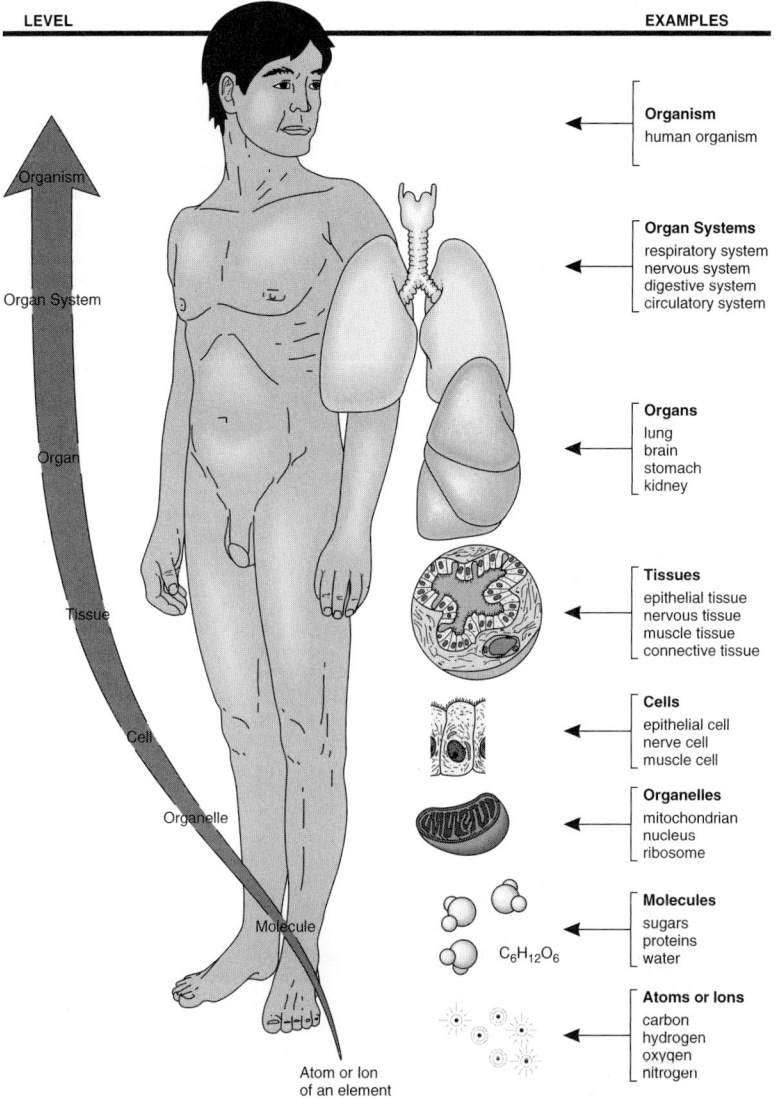

Organism
human organism

Organ Systems
respiratory system
nervous system
digestive system
circulatory system

Organs
lung
brain
stomach
kidney

Tissues
epithelial tissue
nervous tissue
muscle tissue
connective tissue

Cells
epithelial cell
nerve cell
muscle cell

Organelles
mitochondrian
nucleus
ribosome

Molecules
sugars
proteins
water

$C_6H_{12}O_6$

Atoms or Ions
carbon
hydrogen
oxygen
nitrogen

Atom or Ion
of an element

Figure 10-1   The human body is highly organized from the single cell to the total organism.

ness may sometimes cause a physical illness. Physical illness can bring on emotional problems, too. Some clients seem more able to cope with illness than others. A person who is ill or suffering from a disability caused by an accident, illness, or aging has to cope with an increase in physical and emotional pain as well as many losses. The individual who is ill experiences a decrease in physical and emotional energy, an

Body Systems	Major Organs		Functions
Integumentary system	Skin Sweat Glands Hair Oil Glands Nails Mucous membranes		Maintains temperature control Protects body areas Covers body framework
Musculoskeletal system	Muscles Bones Joints		Protects internal organs; makes movement possible
Nervous system	Brain Nerves Spinal cord Ganglia		Sends messages throughout the body
Circulatory system	Heart Lymph nodes Blood vessels Spleen Lymphatic vessels		Pumps blood carrying food and oxygen through body
Respiratory system	Nose Trachea Pharynx Bronchi Larynx Lungs		Provides oxygen to body Discharges waste gases
Digestive system	Mouth Stomach – Teeth Intestines – Tongue Liver – Salivary glands Gallbladder Pharynx Pancreas Esophagus		Prepares food for use throughout body, eliminates solid wastes
Urinary system	Kidneys Urinary bladder Ureters Urethra		Maintains body liquid balance; removes waste liquids from body
Reproductive system	**Male** Testes Epididymis Vas Deferens Seminal vesicles Ejaculatory ducts Urethra Prostate gland Bulbourethral glands Scrotum Penis Seminiferous tubules	**Female** Ovaries Fallopian tubes Uterus Vagina Bartholin glands Vulva Mammary glands	Provides for the growth and development of offspring
Endocrine system	Pituitary gland Adrenal glands Thyroid gland Islets of Langerhans Parathyroid glands Sex glands (ovaries, testes)		Secretes hormones and helps regulate various body functions

Figure 10-2   The body systems and their major organs and functions

	Oral	Axillary	Rectal/Tympanic
Average Temperature	98.6°F/37°C	97.6°F/36.5°C	99.6°F/37.5°C
Range	97.6–99.6°F (36.5–37.5°C)	96.6–98.6°F (36–37°C)	98.6–100.6°F (37–38.1°C)

Figure 10-3   Temperature variations in the same person

increase in physical discomfort, and perhaps chronic pain. Medications may cause drowsiness or confusion.

VITAL SIGNS

Vital signs are signs obtained by use of an instrument; they indicate the status of a person's life functions. They include temperature, pulse, respiratory rate, and blood pressure. Vital signs must be measured accurately and regularly. Changes outside the normal range must be reported to the nurse. The home health aide will be given exact instructions as to when to take these measurements for each assigned client.

Temperature

The difference between the heat produced and the heat lost is the body temperature. Temperature is measured with a thermometer. The most popular method of measuring body temperature is using either a tympanic/ear or digital thermometer. Refer to Procedure 10, Taking a Tympanic (Ear) Temperature.

Body temperature varies from person to person. When a person's body temperature is above normal, that is, over 100°F orally, the client is said to have a fever. Another term for fever is febrile. If a person's temperature is in the normal range, the term afebrile is used. Fever is a sign of a disease, not a disease in itself. When a person or child does have a fever, this indicates that the body is reacting to an infection. Fever can cause the immune system to start fighting the infection and producing more white blood cells. A normal healthy person can tolerate a fever for a short period without any complications.

A person's body temperature varies throughout the day. It is lower in the morning and higher in the afternoon, when the body has been more active. Certain factors can raise a person's temperature such as exercising, being outside in warm weather, or wearing too many clothes. Figure 10-3 shows the normal body temperatures taken by various methods.

10 Procedure

Taking a Tympanic (Ear) Temperature

Purpose
- To measure the client's body temperature in the most appropriate way
- To routinely check the temperature to note any significant change

Procedure
1. Gather the equipment needed:
   - ear thermometer and disposable probe
   - paper and pen
   - disposable gloves

2. Wash your hands thoroughly and put on gloves.
3. Tell the client that you plan to take a tympanic temperature.
4. With thermometer in hand, place a new probe on the thermometer (Figure 10-4).
5. Turn the thermometer on (Figure 10-5).
6. For an adult, pull top of ear up and back (Figure 10-6); for a child under 2, pull earlobe down and back (Figure 10-7) and gently insert probe into ear (Figure 10-8).

7. Press the top button as you insert probe into ear.
8. Listen for a beep, which will only take a few seconds, then remove probe from the ear.
9. Read the temperature indicated on the thermometer screen (Figure 10-9).

10. Remove the probe.
11. Record the temperature immediately.
12. Remove gloves and wash your hands.

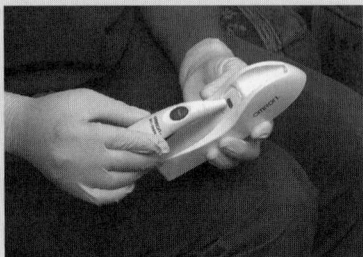

Figure 10-4 Applying a clean probe to the tympanic thermometer

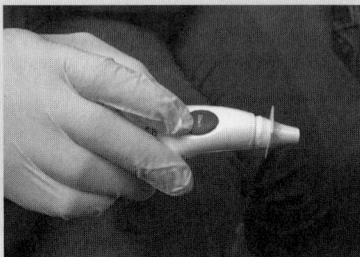

Figure 10-5 Press the button to turn thermometer on.

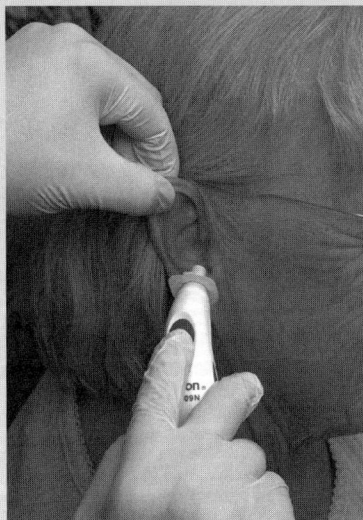

Figure 10-6 For adult, pull top of ear up and back.

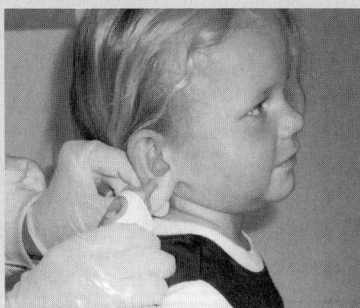

Figure 10-7 For a child under 2, pull earlobe down and back.

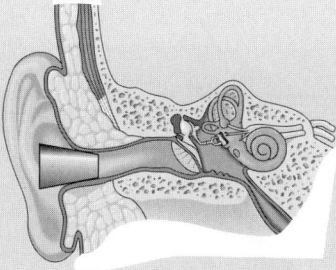

Figure 10-8   Inserting probe into ear

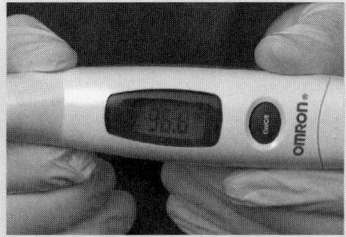

Figure 10-9   Screen showing temperature of client

Temperatures can be measured by mouth (oral), axillary (armpit), or rectally using a digital thermometer. Refer to Procedures 11, 12, and 13. A digital thermometer is easy to use, inexpensive, and offers a more accurate temperature reading. The tympanic or ear thermometer measures the temperature by inserting an electronic probe into a person's ear. The advantages of using this type of thermometer are that the ear has a large blood supply and a temperature can be taken quickly with little chance of error and little discomfort for the client.

11 Procedure

Taking an Oral Temperature (Digital Thermometer)

Purpose

- To obtain accurate reading of client's temperature
- To routinely check the temperature to note any significant change

Procedure

1. Gather the equipment needed:
   - thermometer and probe cover
   - paper and pen
   - disposable gloves
2. Wash your hands thoroughly and put on gloves.
3. Apply probe or sheath cover over end of the thermometer (Figure 10-10).
4. Insert the probe tip well under the client's tongue. Turn the thermometer on. Place the tip of the thermometer sublingually into a heat pocket (Figure 10-11).
5. Ask the client to close the mouth and wait 10 to 20 seconds.
6. Listen for the beeps and remove the thermometer.
7. Remove the plastic probe cover and discard it in the wastebasket.
8. Turn the thermometer off.
9. Record the temperature.
10. Remove gloves and wash your hands.

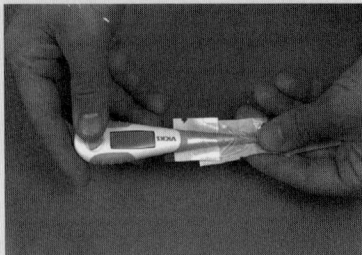

Figure 10-10 Apply plastic sheath over tip of thermometer.

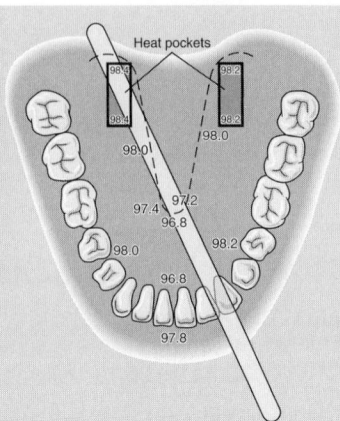

Figure 10-11 Place tip of thermometer sublingually into a heat pocket. (Courtesy 3M Health Care.)

12 Procedure

Taking an Axillary Temperature

Purpose

- To obtain the client's temperature reading when oral is not possible

NOTE: This method can be done for infants and young children, as they are unable to hold a thermometer in their mouths.

Procedure

1. Gather the equipment needed:
   - thermometer with probe cover
   - gloves and small towel
   - paper and pen
2. Wash your hands thoroughly and put on gloves.
3. Cover the thermometer with the probe cover.
4. Wipe the client's underarm area with a towel.
5. Place the probe tip in the center of the client's armpit so the tip is touching the skin. Position the client's arm close to the body (Figure 10-12).
6. Listen for beeps, which will take a few seconds longer than an oral temperature.
7. Remove the thermometer and read the temperature indicated.
8. Discard the probe in the wastebasket. (Optional: clean the probe tip with alcohol before using on another client.)
9. Record the temperature.
10. Remove gloves and wash your hands.

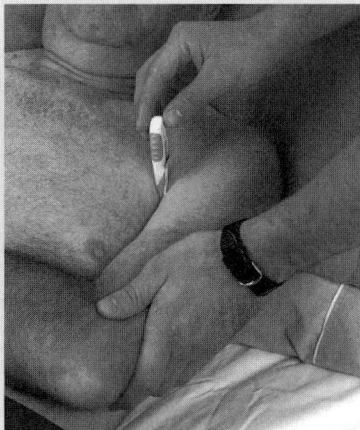

Figure 10-12 Place thermometer so the tip is touching the skin.

13
Procedure

Taking a Rectal Temperature (Digital Thermometer)

Purpose

- To obtain accurate reading of client's temperature
- To obtain the temperature of a client when an oral or ear is not possible

Procedure

1. Gather the equipment needed:
   - lubricant and alcohol wipe
   - disposable gloves
   - thermometer and probe cover
2. Wash your hands thoroughly and put on gloves.
3. Tell the client that you plan to take a rectal temperature.
4. Cover the thermometer with the probe cover and lubricate the probe tip with water-soluble jelly—not petroleum jelly.
5. Position the client on their side if an adult; an infant can be placed on their abdomen. Do not expose the client unnecessarily.
6. Gently insert the tip into the client's rectum, no more than 1/2 inch. Hold the thermometer in place and wait for the beep (Figure 10-13).
7. Remove the thermometer and discard the disposable probe and wipe the tip with alcohol.
8. Read the thermometer.
9. Remove gloves and wash your hands.
10. Record the temperature—remember this method produces a temperature 1°F higher than an oral temperature.

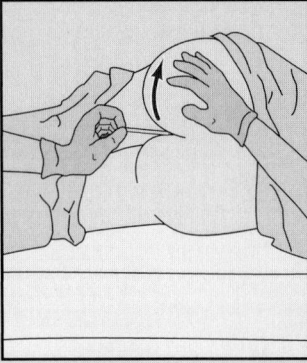

Figure 10-13 Hold thermometer in rectum and wait for a beep.

When recording a client's temperature, you need to indicate whether it was rectal, 99.6°F (R) or axillary, 98.6°F (Ax). A person's temperature can be measured using the **Celsius** or Centigrade scale (0°C for freezing and 100°C for boiling), or the Fahrenheit scale (32°F for freezing and 212°F for boiling).

Pulse and Respiratory Rates

Two other vital signs that a home health aide is required to take and record are the pulse and respiratory rates. These two readings are usually taken one after the other. After taking the pulse, the client's arm is held in the same position and the respirations are counted. It is better if the client does not realize that respirations are being counted. The results are more accurate if the client thinks that only the pulse rate is being checked.

Pulse. The pulse is the force of the blood pushing against the artery walls. Movement of the blood through the arteries is initiated by the heart's contraction. Thus, the pulse rate should be the same as the heart rate. The pulse may be felt at any of the sites shown in Figure 10-14. The most common site for checking the pulse is the radial artery, which can be felt inside the wrist on the thumb side. Procedure 14 demonstrates how to take a radial pulse. Procedure 15 demonstrates how to take an apical pulse. Pulse rates differ depending on age, sex, size, and physical condition of the client (Figure 10-15) A slow heartbeat is called bradycardia. A fast heartbeat is called tachycardia. Pulse readings show the rate, rhythm, and volume of blood pulsing through the artery. Rate is the times per minute. Rhythm is the evenness or regularity of the beat. An irregular pulse may indicate skipped heartbeats or changing rhythm patterns. Volume is the fullness of the beat. It can be described as strong, full, or weak; if it is very weak, the term *thready* is used.

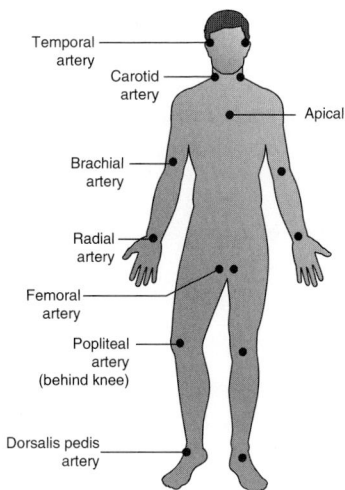

Figure 10-14   The pulse may be felt at any of the places shown.

Adults	60–100 beats per minute
Children over 6	70–110 beats per minute
Children under 6	80–120 beats per minute
Infants	100–140 beats per minute

Figure 10-15   Average pulse rate.

14   Procedure

Taking a Radial Pulse

Purpose

- To measure, record, and observe the character and rate of the client's pulse
- To report changes to the nurse

Procedure for Determining Pulse Rate

1. Gather the equipment needed: wristwatch with a second hand notepad and pen or pencil
2. Wash your hands before beginning the procedure.
3. Tell the client that you are going to check the pulse rate. Ask the client to help by remaining quiet and still while you are counting.
4. Have the client sit in a comfortable chair or lie in bed with arms resting gently on the chest.
5. Place the tips of your first two fingers lightly on the pulse site. The radial pulse on the inner wrist is most often used (Figure 10-16). **CAUTION:** Do not use your thumb to feel the client's artery. Using the thumb can result in an inaccurate reading.
6. Count the pulse beats for 1 full minute.
7. Record the pulse rate, regularity, and strength. Also record the time the pulse was taken.

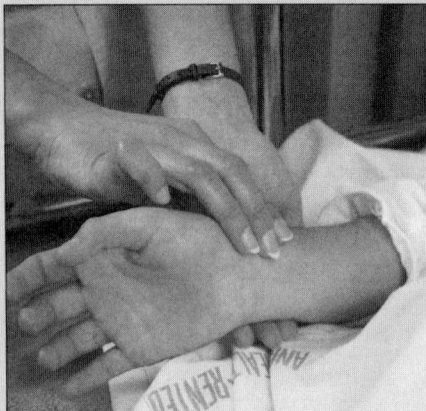

Figure 10-16 Locate the pulse on the thumb side of the wrist with the tips of your fingers.

15 — Procedure

Taking an Apical Pulse

Purpose

- To obtain accurate pulse rate
- To determine regularity and strength of pulse

Procedure

1. Gather the equipment needed:
   - stethoscope
   - wristwatch with a second hand
   - alcohol wipes
2. Explain the procedure to the client.
3. Clean stethoscope diaphragm and earpieces. Note: If you are using a stethoscope you used on a previous client, you will need to clean the diaphragm of the stethoscope.

If you, the home health aide, have your own stethoscope, you do not need to clean the earpieces each time.

4. Place the stethoscope earpieces in your ears.
5. Place the stethoscope diaphragm (Figure 10-17A) over the apex of the client's heart, 2 to 3 inches to the left of the breastbone, below the left nipple (Figure 10-17B).
6. Listen carefully for the heartbeat. It will sound like "lub-dub."
7. Count the louder sound (lub) for 1 complete minute and record. If you have a quiet environment, it will help you to hear the beats.
8. Record the pulse.

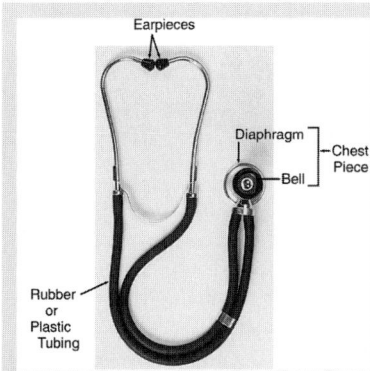

Figure 10-17A   Diagram of a stethoscope

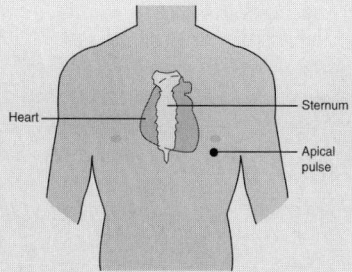

Figure 10-17B   Place diaphragm of stethoscope over apex of heart.

Apical-Radial Pulse

Taking the radial and apical pulse rates at the same time is done to see if one is the same as the other. For optimal comparisons you need two people for this procedure. A family member or client's friend may be recruited to assist the home health aide with the procedure.

1. Same beginning and ending procedures as in Procedures 14 and 15.
2. One person palpates (feels) the radial pulse and the other person counts the apical pulse at the same time. One aide is usually the timer and says "start," and then after 60 seconds, the aide says "end."
3. Compare the results and record the numbers on a notepad.
4. Document both pulse rates, e.g.,

   Apical pulse = 100 @ 10:00 AM

   Radial pulse = 92

   Pulse deficit: 8 (100 − 92 = 8)

Respiration.   Respiration is the sum total of processes that exchange oxygen and carbon dioxide in the body. However, respiration is most commonly known as breathing. The act of inhaling and exhaling once is counted as one respiration. The character of respirations is described as regular or irregular; labored, difficult, shallow, or deep; and noisy or quiet. Respirations that sound like snoring are called stertorous. Difficult or labored breathing is called dyspnea. Sometimes respirations stop for a few moments. This absence of breathing is called apnea. The bubbling sound may be heard when fluid or mucus gets caught in the air passages. This condition is called rales, and can often be heard in clients with pneumonia or emphysema. The normal rate of respirations for adults is 16 to 20 per minute. In adults, respiration rates of 25 or more are called accelerated. Weak respirations, which are characterized by only slight chest movements, are described as being shallow. Breathing characterized by many large breaths is described as being deep. Cheyne-Stokes is a term used to describe respirations that are very rapid and then stop and then start again. This type of breathing pattern occurs prior to the client's death. Procedure 16 demonstrates how to count respirations.

16   Procedure

Counting Respirations

Purpose

- To count the rate and observe the character of respirations

Procedure

1. Gather equipment needed.
   - wristwatch with a second hand
   - notepad and pen or pencil
2. After client's pulse has been taken, leave the fingers in position on the wrist. By doing this, the client is not aware that you are counting respirations.
3. One rise and fall of the chest counts as one respiration. Count the number of respirations during a full 1-minute period.
4. Note how deeply the client breathes. Also check the regularity of the rhythm pattern. Note the sound of the breathing.
5. Record the number of respirations occurring in 1 minute. Record the character of the client's breathing.
6. Report changes from the client's usual way of breathing. Report any difficulty in breathing to the nurse.
7. Wash your hands.

Blood Pressure.   Blood pressure is measured in two parts—systolic and diastolic—by using an instrument called a sphygmomanometer. Blood pressure is the amount of force the blood exerts against the walls of the arteries as it flows through them. It is expressed in numbers, with the higher number (systolic) representing the pressure while the heart is beating, and the lower number (diastolic) representing the pressure when the heart is resting between beats. The systolic number is always stated first and the diastolic second; for example: 134/72 (134 over 72); systolic = 134, diastolic = 72. Refer to Procedure 17. Normal blood pressure for an adult is 120/80, although it may vary depending on age, sex, emotional state, fitness, and weight. Blood pressure at or above 140 mm Hg systolic and 90 mm Hg diastolic is considered high blood pressure.

17   Procedure

Taking Blood Pressure

Purpose

- To take blood pressure correctly
- To accurately report blood pressure readings to the nurse

Procedure

1. Gather equipment needed:
   - sphygmomanometer
   - stethoscope

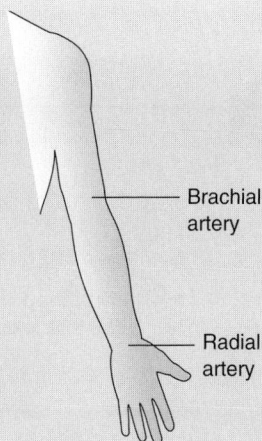

Figure 10-18   Location of brachial and radial arteries

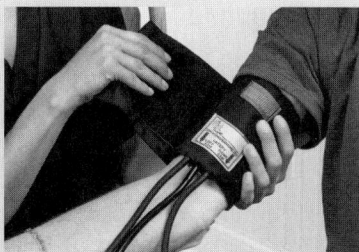

Figure 10-19   Apply cuff snugly to area at least 1 inch above the elbow.

- alcohol sponges
2. Wash your hands.
3. Explain to the client what you plan to do. Have the client sit or lie in a comfortable position with one arm extended at the same level as the heart. The palm should be upward. The arm should be in resting position. The arm should not be dangling by the hip because you may get an inaccurate reading. Locate brachial pulse (Figure 10-18).
4. Pick up the stethoscope. Wipe the earpieces. Place the stethoscope around your neck.
5. Place the cuff on the client's arm, at least 1 inch above the elbow (Figure 10-19). Make sure the cuff is evenly positioned around the arm and then tighten it so it fits snugly. If the cuff is marked with an arrow, place cuff so that the arrow points over the brachial artery.
6. Attach the dial gauge to the top of the cuff so you can read it (Figures 10–20A and B).

7. Palpate the radial pulse.
8. Explain to the client that as the cuff inflates, she or he will feel tightness in the arm that may be slightly uncomfortable. Begin to inflate the cuff by pumping the cuff with one hand while using the fingers of the other hand to feel for the radial pulse. Notice when you no longer feel the radial pulse. Deflate the cuff and wait 15 seconds.
9. Place the earpieces of the stethoscope in your ears and place the diaphragm over the brachial artery (Figure 10-21).
10. Inflate the cuff 30 mm Hg beyond the point at which you last felt the pulse.
11. Deflate the cuff at an even rate of 2 to 4 mm Hg per second. Turn the valve counterclockwise to deflate the cuff.
12. Note the point on the scale where you heard the first sound. This is the systolic reading. You should hear this sound near the point where the radial pulse disappeared.
13. Continue to deflate the cuff. Note the point where the sound disappears or becomes muffled, remember this number. This is the diastolic reading.
14. Deflate the cuff completely and record the blood pressure.

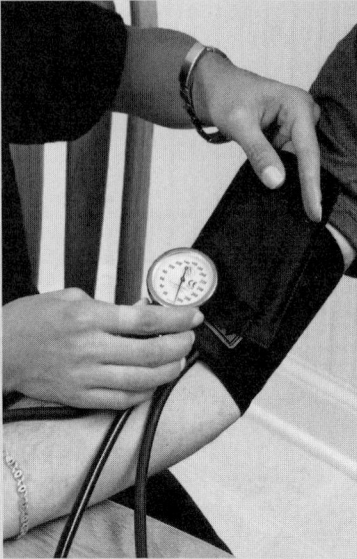

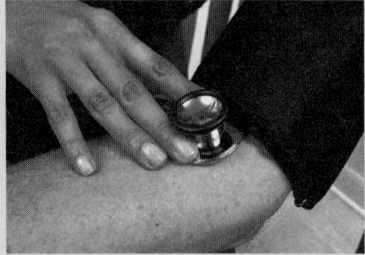

Figure 10-21   Notice placement of fingers over diaphragm to ensure firm fit to the skin.

Figure 10-20A   Attach gauge to top of cuff.

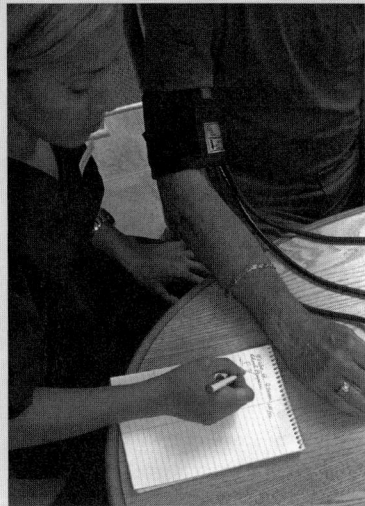

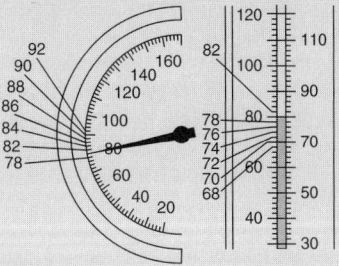

Figure 10-20B   The aneroid gauge (*left*) and the mercury gravity gauge (*right*). Take a reading at the closest line.

Figure 10-22   Record your reading right away. If repeat procedure is necessary, wait at least 1 minute.

15. Record the reading in even numbers, e.g., 134/78 or 102/64 (Figure 10-22).
16. If you are unsuccessful in obtaining a blood pressure reading after the first attempt, move to the client's other arm and try again, repeating the same procedure. (A second reading taken immediately, in the same arm, would probably be inaccurate and the client would become uncomfortable.) Never guess. If a blood pressure is hard to take

or you are not sure, tell the nurse. Record reading.

17. Wash your hands.

Precautions

- If you are taking the blood pressure of a stroke client or a client who has had a mastectomy, use the unaffected arm only.

- If your client is having home dialysis (as part of a kidney treatment), or is receiving intravenous (IV) fluids, take the blood pressure on the unaffected arm.
- Do not inflate cuff unnecessarily high.

Blood pressure is taken by the use of a sphygmomanometer (an instrument with a cuff, rubber bulb, and dial gauge for recording pressures) and a stethoscope (listening device that magnifies sound). The cuff should be the right size for the client's arm; otherwise an incorrect reading may be obtained. Cuffs come in various sizes: child, normal adult, and extra large.

When a person has a blood pressure that is higher than normal range, the person has hypertension; when it is below normal range, the person has hypotension. Blood pressure is lower among women than men. It is usually low in childhood, becoming higher with advancing age. African Americans and Native Americans have a greater incidence of high blood pressure than Caucasians. Several factors can cause an increase in blood pressure, including stress, obesity, and heavy alcohol use, lack of exercise, high salt diet, smoking, and aging. It is sometimes called the "silent killer" because a person can have high blood pressure and not know it. Hypertension is treated with diet, exercise, reduction of stress, and medications.

Occasionally, you may need to measure a client's blood pressure when the client is lying down, and again when the client is sitting up. The health care provider may order you to do it this way because the client may have a condition called orthostatic hypotension. When the person changes position, the person's blood pressure falls rapidly.

Height and Weight.   Occasionally it is necessary to obtain a client's height. You will need a tape measure to do this. You have the client stand to do it. Be sure the client is standing as straight as possible and that the client is not wearing shoes. Another task that may need to be done monthly, weekly, or daily is weighing a client. Refer to Procedure 18. Weight changes can make a difference in medical prescriptions, and often you may need to report daily to the nurse any change in the client's weight. For instance, some medication amounts are determined by the weight of a client, and a sudden weight loss would require a lesser dose.

18   Procedure

Measuring Weight and Height

Purpose

- To determine if unusual weight gain or loss has occurred
- To routinely check height

Procedure for Weight

If the client is bedridden and cannot stand to be weighed, the agency can bring a chair scale into the house. If the client is mobile, weight can be checked daily or weekly on a bathroom scale (Figure 10-23). Guidelines to follow:

1. Client should be weighed at the same time of day.
2. Client should be wearing the same amount of clothing each time.
3. Scale should be checked to see if it is balanced correctly.
4. Record and document weight.

NOTE: Height is not a common measurement for the elderly. As individuals age, there is some "settling" and a loss of height of perhaps an inch or two. If you need to take the height of an immobile client, you need a tape measure and a pad and pencil.

Procedure for Height

1. Have client positioned in bed flat on his or her back with arms and legs straight.
2. Make a small pencil mark at the top of the client's head on the sheet.
3. Make a second pencil mark even with the bottom of the heels.

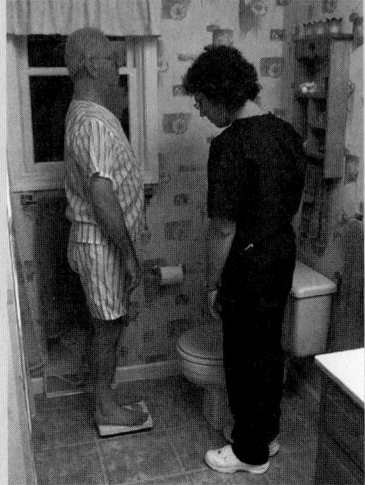

Figure 10-23   Weighing client using a portable bathroom scale

4. Using the tape measure, measure the distance between the two marks.
5. Record the height on the paper and record in client's record.
6. If client can stand, have the client stand with his or her back to the wall. Mark the wall with a small pencil mark on top of client's head. Client should not wear shoes.
7. Measure from floor to small pencil mark with tape measure.
8. Record on paper and then on client's chart.

Alert	The client is aware of the environment and responds promptly and appropriately to verbal, auditory, and visual stimuli.
Drowsiness	Client can answer questions but is confused and fades in and out of sleep.
Stupor	Client is restless and can only be aroused by continuous stimulation. Responds to bright lights, loud sounds, and can locate painful site.
Coma	Responds only to painful stimuli, if at all. In a deep coma, all responses are lost. Must be turned and repositioned or will remain in one position. Client is incontinent.

Figure 10-24   Levels of consciousness

LEVELS OF CONSCIOUSNESS

In most cases, a home health aide will be assigned to care for clients who are conscious. Consciousness is the normal state of awareness. Conscious people are responsive and know who and where they are. Normal consciousness varies in intensity throughout the day.

Have you had the experience of going to look for an item only to forget what it was when you got into the room? Have you ever been talking to someone and at some point lost the purpose of the conversation? These examples show that different levels of consciousness exist. While doing routine work, thoughts may wander and daydreaming may occur. At other times, a person may be extremely aware and sensitive of surroundings and events (Figure 10-24).

Sleep is a temporary state of unconsciousness. Other types of unconsciousness are due to a body malfunction or an injury. Fainting is an example of a temporary loss of consciousness. The blood supply to the brain is decreased; the person feels dizzy and may black out. When the head is lowered, the blood rushes back to the brain and the faintness disappears.

The deeply comatose client is totally helpless and the home health aide must follow a nurse's instructions carefully. The client's bed should be comfortable and kept clean and dry. The client should also be given frequent mouth care. Two of the greatest potential problems for a comatose client are pressure sores and contractures. Contracture is the abnormal shortening of muscle tissue. When contractures occur, the muscles become inelastic and fixed. Exercising the client's limbs can help prevent contractures. Exercises done to prevent contractures and the loss of motion in the joints are called range of motion exercises.

A comatose client must have special care. Figure 10-25 indicates the special needs of the unconscious client and how to meet those needs.

DANGERS OF EXTREME BODY TEMPERATURE

Hyperthermia (heatstroke) and hypothermia (abnormally low internal

Care Required	Frequency	What to Do
Mouth care	Every 2 hours	Wipe tongue, lips, gums, and teeth with gauze pad or lemon-glycerine swab. Lubricate and moisten mouth tissues with glycerine or vegetable oil. Wipe away saliva as it dribbles from the mouth.
	When client vomits	Turn client to side at first sign of vomiting. Catch vomitus in a bowl or basin held to the side of the mouth. Wipe mouth with gauze pads or clean damp cloth.
Eye care	Wipe clean in AM and PM	Cover eyelids with soft cloth moistened in water. (Prevents eye cavity from becoming dry because eyes may not close or blink.)
Repositioning	At least every 2 hours	Turn from back to side, and side to front, etc. (This prevents pressure sores from forming.)
Range of motion (ROM) exercises	As ordered	Exercise all client's body parts if permitted. (Keeps blood circulating, prevents contractures, and prevents loss of motion in joints.)
Body massage with lotion	At least daily	Rub skin firmly but gently. Rub in a circular motion around bony prominences.
Care of bowel and bladder drainage	At least every 2 hours	Check perineal area and bed linens to see if they are clean and dry. If client has not voided for 8 hours, report it to the nurse. If client has not had bowel movement for 2 days, report it to the nurse.

(continues)

Figure 10-25   Meeting the special needs of the unconscious client

Accident prevention	At all times	Put up guardrails or place chairs beside bed to prevent falls. Observe for signs of vomiting and keep saliva wiped away; client may choke or inhale fluids into the lungs. Keep blankets and pillows away from the client's nose and mouth to avoid smothering.
Room ventilation	Open windows or vent daily	Keep temperature between 66–70°, keep drafts from client. Open windows or vents to circulate air.
Tender loving care (TLC)	At all times	Talk to the client as if the client were conscious. Client may be able to hear and understand. (Communication gives client link with reality.) Use gentle touch often; if time allows, hold the client's hands and run fingers across forehead.

Figure 10-25   continued

body temperature) are two conditions that may occur when the environmental conditions are extreme and the person's skin is unable to regulate body temperature, a situation not uncommon among the elderly and children.

Hyperthermia

Older people are more likely to die from heat-related causes than younger persons. Chances of experiencing heatstroke are increased by a weak or damaged heart, hypertension, circulatory problems, diabetes, being overweight, infection or fever, drinking alcohol, or a previous stroke.

Hyperthermia Signs and Symptoms

1. Lack of energy
2. Mild discomfort
3. Lack of appetite
4. Dizziness
5. Muscle cramps
6. Diarrhea, nausea
7. Chest pain
8. Excessive weakness
9. Severe mental changes
10. Breathing problems
11. Vomiting
12. Dry skin (no sweating)

An older person may be reluctant to run an air conditioner or a fan because of the cost. He or she may not want to keep open a window due to fear of crime, or may be unable to manage opening a window that is stuck or painted shut. For the client's and your own safety try to gently convince the client to open a window while you are there. If the client is afraid, be sure to close it again before you leave. Be sure to encourage your client to drink plenty of fluids on very hot days.

If any client, older or younger, shows many of the above symptoms and has an elevated body temperature due to heat, take the following steps:

1. Loosen clothing.
2. Place the client in a semi-sitting position, the head slightly elevated to the body.
3. Bathe the head and body in cool water to lower the body temperature.
4. Give drinks of cool water or ice chips to suck on.
5. Call for medical assistance whenever you suspect a person is suffering from hyperthermia.

Hypothermia

Hypothermia is a condition marked by an abnormally low internal body temperature, usually 95°F (35°C) or under. This decrease in body temperature is due to exposure to a cold environment. Infants are at risk because of immature temperature control. The risk factors to the elderly are increased due to chronic illness, poverty, and some medications. Antidepressants, sedatives, tranquilizers, and cardiovascular medications can increase the risk of hypothermia.

Hypothermia Signs and Symptoms

1. A change in appearance or behavior during cold weather
2. Uncontrollable shivering or lack of shivering

3. Slow and sometimes irregular heartbeat, shallow or very slow breathing
4. Weak pulse, low blood pressure
5. Confusion, disorientation, or drowsiness
6. Pain in the extremities
7. Slurred speech
8. Lack of coordination, sluggishness
9. Stiff muscles
10. Low indoor temperatures and other signs that the person has been in a cool or cold room

You may visit a home that has little or no heat due to a lack of money for gas or oil, a lack of wood for a wood-burning stove, or no heating appliances in the home. If the client is experiencing money problems that have caused the heat to be turned off be sure to let your case manager know. Most states have emergency money available for utilities that can be given to individuals or families in need.

If your client's primary source of heat is a wood-burning, oil, or kerosene stove, you may find that bringing in the wood or filling the stove with oil is a part of the care plan.

Be cautious about the use and placement of electric space heaters. Never place a space heater near loose bed covers, clothing, or tablecloths. **NEVER** turn on an oven with the door open to heat a room. The danger of breathing in gas fumes or starting a fire is too great.

To warm a person whom you suspect of having hypothermia take the following steps:

1. Take the person's temperature. If it is below 95°F (35°C) call for help.
2. Wrap the person in a warm blanket, quilt, towels, or extra clothes.

Make sure that you cover the head and neck.

3. Use hot water bottles or electric heating pads on the person's abdomen (never on a high setting or with water too hot). Do not place hot water bottles on the feet. Do not rewarm extremities and the core (trunk of body) at the same time.

4. If the person is alert give small quantities of warm (not hot) food or a sweet, warm drink—but nothing alcoholic.
5. Do not rub the person's limbs.
6. Call for medical assistance whenever you suspect the person is suffering from hypothermia.

UNIT 11

Mental Health

UNDERSTANDING EMOTIONS

Stages of Personality Development

The stages in the development of one's personality are determined over an individual's life span. There are critical time frames when cognitive (being able to reason and make judgments), functioning, and motor skills are being developed that allow one to feel a sense of achievement or failure. According to Erikson, social and cultural influences are significant during an individual's growth and development phase. A person must successfully master each period in order to develop a positive image. If a person does not successfully master each phase then negative feelings occur (see Figure 11-1).

Emotions are common to all people and are neither good nor bad. An emotion is a strong, generalized feeling. The way a person shows emotion may be healthy or unhealthy. There is a wide range of acceptable levels of emotional behavior. Well-adjusted people most often use emotions in a healthy way to serve their purposes; they can control emotions so as not to harm themselves or others. There are a wide range of emotions that are regarded as normal, including fear, anger, grief, and others. Whether emotional behavior is healthy depends on whether a person can express these emotions in a manner that is socially acceptable.

Emotions may cause physical reactions. Anger and fear sometimes cause the heart to beat faster, respirations to increase, and chemical changes to occur within the body. The mouth may become dry; the person may become pale and may start to shake. Such physical changes are common and usually of short duration. Emotions can trigger the release of hormones and produce unusual results. For example, it is not unusual for those experiencing a shocking or traumatic event to find that they are physically capable of functioning at unusually high levels of strength and energy.

Individuals develop a pattern of emotional response. This may be a hereditary characteristic although environment also can influence mental health. Some babies, for instance, seem calmer and happier than others. The social environment of a family can influence whether a baby's early experiences are pleasant or unpleas-

Physical Stage	Year of Occurrence	Tasks to be Mastered
Oral-sensory	Birth to 18 months	To learn to trust—Trust vs. Mistrust
Muscular-anal	18 months–3 years	To recognize self as an independent being from mother—Autonomy vs. Shame and Doubt
Locomotor	3–6 years	To recognize self as a family member—Initiative vs. Guilt
Latency	6–12 years	To demonstrate physical and mental skills—Industry vs. Inferiority
Adolescence	12–20 years	To develop a sense of individuality as a sexual human being—Identity vs. Role Confusion
Young Adulthood	20–35 years	To establish intimate personal relationships with a mate—Intimacy vs. Isolation
Adulthood	35–50 years	To live a satisfying and productive life—Generativity vs. Stagnation
Maturity	50 plus	To review life's events and examine how they have influenced the development of a unique individual—Ego Integrity vs. Despair

Figure 11-1   Tasks of personality development according to the stages defined by Erikson

ant. As years pass, the child's successes and failures in daily life influence the child's emotional patterns. The child who is healthy and who is given tender, loving attention from birth has a good chance of growing up to be well adjusted.

The type of emotion (pleasant or unpleasant) that a person feels most of the time is referred to as his or her disposition. A disposition is the usual mood of an individual. An optimist probably feels more pleasant emotions and, therefore, has a brighter outlook than a pessimist. The aide who has a cheerful outlook may transfer this pleasant mood to the client. Words, tone of voice, actions, and facial expression show how a person looks at life. This often exposes the person's inner feelings. Pessimists may be just as well adjusted as optimists but their viewpoints differ. Pessimists tend to take a negative view of situations. A classic example showing the difference between an optimist and a pessimist is to consider a glass filled half-way with water. An optimist would be more likely to regard the glass as half full, whereas the pessimist may regard the glass as half empty.

Mentally healthy people learn to make their emotions work for them. One can deal with negative emotions in a positive way. When a home health aide feels angry with a client, the aide cannot have a tantrum. Strong outbursts of emotion are not acceptable while on duty. Sometimes anger must be expressed, but it should be done in a way that is constructive. A home health aide must not only deal with her own emotional needs, but must also be aware of the emotional needs and reactions of the client. This requires a great deal of self-control and self-discipline. The home health aide must be sensitive to the emotions of the client. Clients are often frightened and worried about their health. The home health aide must be kind and understanding and think of the client's needs first. Illness can cause temporary changes in the client's personality. This often requires the client to make many adjustments. It takes time to accept the physical changes caused by a disease. The home health aide must be willing to allow clients to express their emotions. The well-adjusted aide will be able to endure the client's strong emotional feelings without becoming a part of them.

STRESS

Stress is defined as a mentally or emotionally disruptive influence or upsetting condition that occurs in re-

sponse to adverse external stimuli. Stress may be seen as anger, depression, silence, outbursts, crying, sadness, jealousy, and frustration, to name a few of the symptoms. If stress occurs too fast and too often, even normal individuals have a problem dealing with it. The home health aide must realize that the client and family members are undergoing great stress at the time of illness.

Handling stress effectively is an important component of mental health and is essential for avoiding both physical and mental illness. Stress can make the body more vulnerable to physical illnesses such as colds, ulcers, headaches, and high blood pressure. In severe and prolonged cases, stress can lead to emotional illness.

Although no one can avoid stress all the time, steps should be taken to either eliminate the stressor or to diminish its negative effects. Regular exercise and adequate sleep will help to strengthen the body's resistance to stress. Relaxation is another useful technique to diminish stress and may include participation in hobbies, quiet meditation, or some other activity that an individual enjoys. It is often helpful to talk about stressful situations with a trusted friend. If these measures are not enough, it may be necessary to consult with a professional.

MENTAL DISORDERS

Emotions play an important role throughout our lifetime. Although there is a broad range of feelings that are considered normal reactions to everyday life, other feelings or behaviors may signal a problem that requires medical attention. A person is said to have a mental disorder if he or she is having difficulty functioning satisfactorily in society as a result of changes in thoughts, behavior, personality, or emotion. A mental disorder can be temporary or permanent and can affect people of all backgrounds and economic levels. Mental disorders can be caused by physical or chemical changes in the brain, genetics, and social and psychological factors. There are different kinds of mental disorders. A few of the more common ones are anxiety disorders, post-traumatic stress disorder, delirium, obsessive-compulsive disorder, schizophrenia, and bipolar disorder.

Anxiety Disorders

Individuals with anxiety disorder can live a fairly normal life, but they are always worrying. They are constantly worrying about their marriage, their job performance, their past mistakes, and future problems. This disorder can cause tension, irritability, and difficulty sleeping. It is not uncommon for this type of individual to be prone to panic attacks. During a panic attack, this person may display shortness of breath, pounding heart, and light-headedness. These individuals do have insight into their problem, but are unable to quit worrying.

Post-traumatic stress disorder is a form of mental disorder. This condition develops after a traumatic event, and is seen often in soldiers returning home from war or in rape victims. These individuals repeatedly relive the event either by remembering details about the event or through recurrent nightmares. If not treated, the individuals eventually become more violent and less interested in things they once enjoyed.

Obsessive-Compulsive Disorder

Obsessive-compulsive disorder is characterized by recurrent obsessions and compulsions that are time consuming and causes noticeable distress in the person. Obsessions are thoughts, images, or ideas that repeatedly go through a person's mind. Compulsions are acts that correspond with these obsessions. An example of an obsession would be fear of germs and the compulsion would be repetitive handwashing or cleaning one's home. Other common obsessions are the need for perfection and exactness or fear of harming someone close. Common compulsions are the need to rearrange items in a certain way, such as newspapers or dishes, and saving things that no longer have any need. The home health aide may walk into a home full of old newspapers and magazines with little space for the client to move around. The first thought might be to toss them away and make space for the client. This would be the logical thing to do, but a client with this disorder will not allow this to happen. The client would be extremely upset and distressed if this were to happen.

Delirium

Delirium is a disturbance of consciousness, making it difficult for a person to focus or shift his or her attention. A person who is delirious often looks confused or intoxicated. Delirium is a disorder of brain functioning often seen in patients with multiple diseases and is regarded as the final stage of a severe disease process.

Mood Disorders or Bipolar Disorders

Mood disorders are the most common mental disorders for people of all ages. Mood disorders include depression, and its opposite, mania (extreme happiness and hyperactivity). Depression is a term that is used to describe a range of emotions from blue feelings to a severe clinical condition.

The new term given to mood disorder is bipolar disorder. A person with bipolar disorder can alternate from being excessively depressed to very elated and back again, with little reason for these mood swings.

Depression. People who are depressed show signs of feeling extremely sad, worthless, or hopeless. They may become forgetful or seem unfocused. They can become angry easily or are constantly irritable. Anxiety is another sign of depression. Also, depressed people often express feelings of guilt.

People suffering from clinical depression are unable to enjoy any aspect of their lives and have great difficulty focusing or paying attention. Although a person may not complain about feeling depressed, he or she does frequently complain about things that can add up to depression. For example, many older adults have physical problems, but people who are preoccupied with their physical illnesses may be depressed. They may say things like "I don't know what's the matter with me. I just don't feel right." These complaints may be covering up their depression.

Depression can also affect the way a person thinks. Depressed people can have false beliefs about themselves. They often believe they are worthless and that nothing they do is right. Depressed people can be irritable, disagreeable, and at odds with everything.

People with depression think nothing will ever get better, and they are overwhelmed by guilt. They put themselves down and cannot see anything good about themselves. A depressed person may have difficulty paying attention and also may be forgetful. Encourage the client to seek help for his or her depression. Many home health agencies can provide mental health services by a licensed professional, so be sure to alert your case manager if you believe that your client is depressed.

Psychotic Disorders

Psychosis is a serious condition in which the thinking process is distorted by hallucinations, delusions, or both. The most common form of psychotic disorder is schizophrenia.

Schizophrenia. Schizophrenia is a serious mental disorder producing various degrees of chronic mental dysfunction and varying degrees of mental impairment. There are different forms of this disease and each form has its own specific signs and symptoms. Common symptoms of this disorder are disorganized thoughts, bizarre behaviors, attention deficits, and withdrawal. When talking, the person with schizophrenia will switch from one topic to another with no correlation; if asked a question, the person will give an irrelevant answer. These individuals often carry on a conversation with themselves and often suffer from delusions (false beliefs) and hallucinations (hearing voices or seeing objects that are not really there). Common delusions with this disorder involve themes of grandeur, persecution, or religion. The client might tell a home health aide that he or she is the pope or the president. The client may also tell you that "the CIA or the FBI is out to get them." This person may also display bizarre posture and movements. She or he may sit in one position for hours and then suddenly get up and start pacing for hours using the same path over and over again. Individuals with schizophrenia do not realize they are not acting normal and have no control over their actions. If you are caring for a client with schizophrenia, be sure the client takes his or her medications as ordered. Do not try to reason with the client, as this will make the client more upset and more difficult to manage.

Generally, people with severe psychotic episodes will be treated in a hospital to ensure their safety. In less severe cases, antipsychotic medications are prescribed to decrease excitement and agitation and to improve the thought processes. Supportive psychotherapy may also be helpful for those with psychotic disorders to improve functioning in everyday life.

EFFECTS OF EMOTIONS ON HEALTH

Sometimes a physical illness can aggravate a mental illness; but a person's emotional health may also affect his physical health. Wellness means different things to different people; people feel better on some days than on others. Temporary discomforts are not necessarily a health hazard or danger. After a very hard day at work, an argument with a close friend, or the death of a loved one, people may feel unwell. A tension headache caused by an emotional crisis can make a person feel ill for a short time. When the upset is resolved, the person forgets the pain and feels well again. Persons who are acutely or chronically ill also have

good and bad days. To a great extent these changes are related to their emotional outlooks. When routines have gone smoothly or when a special friend has called or visited, a person may feel very well despite physical problems. On a day when the home health aide comes late and is in a bad mood, the client may complain of feeling much worse than the physical condition warrants.

No two people react the same to external stimuli. The stress situation causing one person to feel unwell may have no effect on another person. People react to personal crises in their own ways. It has been proven that an emotionally depressed person is more likely to catch a cold or develop a physical disorder. Wellness may be described as freedom from discomfort—both physical and mental. Emotional health may strongly influence a person's state of wellness.

The home health aide can help the client by being aware of the client's mental health status and responding to the client in a supportive and nonjudgmental way. The aide should be aware of the signs of depression, and report any changes to a supervisor. *An aide must take all suicidal threats expressed by the client seriously and report these immediately to the case manager.* In addition, the home health aide must pay close attention to his or her own stress level and find constructive ways to cope with stressful situations on the job.

Body Systems and Common Disorders

SECTION 5

UNIT 12

Digestion and Nutrition

DIGESTIVE SYSTEM

Food is the fuel burned by the digestive system to provide energy for the entire body. The process of burning this fuel is called metabolism.

Metabolism depends on the proper functioning of each organ of digestion (Figure 12-1).

COMMON DISORDERS OF THE DIGESTIVE SYSTEM

Ulcers, hiatal hernia, and heartburn are common disorders of the digestive tract.

Ulcers

Ulcers occur when there is a break in the protective mucous membrane of the stomach or the duodenum. The client may complain of heartburn or a feeling of fullness after eating. If left untreated, ulcers can start to bleed. Treatment consists of medications, change in diet, and adjustment in lifestyle.

Hiatal Hernia

Hiatal hernia occurs when the upper part of the stomach protrudes through the esophageal opening of the di-

aphragm into the lung cavity. It is very common in older adults. It is treated primarily by eating small amounts of food at a time and sleeping with the head of the bed elevated with blocks. Sleeping with the head of the bed slightly elevated will prevent backflow of stomach juices.

Heartburn/Reflux

So-called heartburn results from a backflow of the digestive juices into the lower portion of the esophagus, which is called reflux. These juices, because of their high acid content, cause irritation of the lining of the esophagus. Those affected experience a burning sensation, frequently occurring at night. The client will experience belching that can cause vomitus to go into the mouth. Other symptoms might be a burning sensation in the chest and mouth. A coughing spell often follows one of these attacks.

Tips to prevent reflux are:
- Avoid high-fat foods
- Avoid spicy foods
- Decrease alcohol and caffeine intake
- Do not lie down after eating

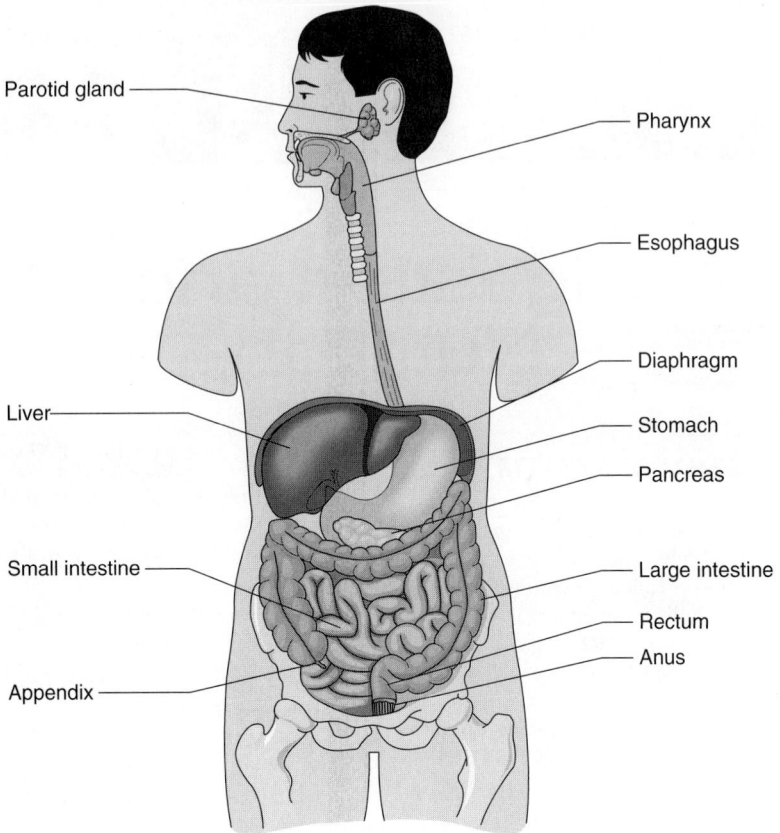

Figure 12-1 The digestive system

- Do not eat at bedtime
- Eat food in small amounts

FOOD GUIDE PYRAMID

The foods recommended in the food pyramid are the fruit group; vegetable group; milk, yogurt, and cheese group; bread, cereal, and rice group; meat, poultry, and fish group; and the fats, oils, and sweets group. Each individual needs the nutrients that can only come from a proper balance of the food guide pyramid (Figure 12-2).

GENERAL GUIDELINES FOR MEAL PLANNING

There are some general rules to follow when planning nutritious meals for clients. The home health aide should consider the ethnic and regional preferences of the client when planning a menu.

If the client is on a special diet, the dietician will prescribe a sample diet to follow. There will also be a list of foods allowed on this special diet. The sample diet and list of foods are a great resource in planning menus for a week.

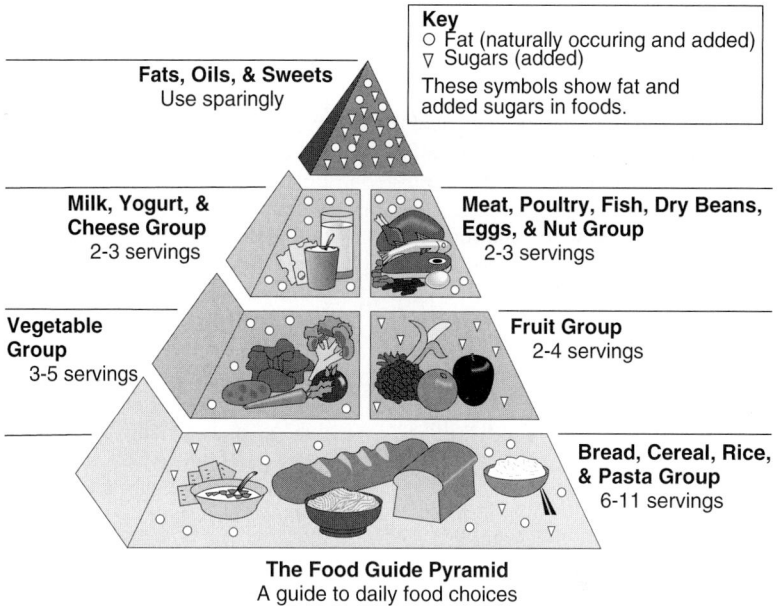

Key
○ Fat (naturally occuring and added)
▽ Sugars (added)
These symbols show fat and
added sugars in foods.

Fats, Oils, & Sweets
Use sparingly

**Milk, Yogurt, &
Cheese Group**
2-3 servings

**Meat, Poultry, Fish, Dry Beans,
Eggs, & Nut Group**
2-3 servings

**Vegetable
Group**
3-5 servings

Fruit Group
2-4 servings

**Bread, Cereal, Rice,
& Pasta Group**
6-11 servings

The Food Guide Pyramid
A guide to daily food choices

Figure 12-2   Food guide pyramid—a guide to daily food choices

Eating Patterns

Generally, people expect to have three meals a day—breakfast, lunch (dinner), dinner (supper). The midday and evening meals are a cultural choice.

Some older adults find that eating the main meal in the evening makes them uncomfortable. They find that they feel better having their main meal at midday and then eating a light meal in the evening. This relieves the feeling of heaviness and discomfort when they go to bed.

SHOPPING AND MEAL PREPARATION

Shopping and meal preparation require time and use of special skills. Planning nutritious meals and buying foods the family can afford require knowledge and use of judgment. Storing foods properly is also important.

Menus and Shopping Lists

Most meal planning is done for an entire week. Weekly planning saves the home health aide from making frequent trips to the market. The following steps are helpful planning guides.

• Sit down with the client or client's family and ask what foods and menus they want. This could be an important activity for the client because it may foster the client's feelings of being useful and in charge of the care.

• Plan menus for a full week. Make sure that the menu follows any specific guidelines provided by the dietician.

• Be sure all staple items, such as spices and seasonings that are needed for each planned meal, are on hand.

• Make a shopping list and include all items needed in the household.

Shopping time can be reduced by organizing the shopping list so that all items of one type are under one heading.

- Look in the newspaper and check the prices of products advertised. Cut out any coupons of items on the shopping list.
- Plan to use only the amount of money budgeted for food and supplies.

Purchasing Food

Planning done in the home saves the home health aide time in the store. Shopping should be done at a time when the client can be safely left alone or has a visitor.

Practical guidelines for shopping are presented in the following list.

1. If there is time, walk through the store with the shopping list in hand. Compare prices and decide on the best buys for the budget. If the allowed money will not cover all the items, make substitutions. For example, if beef prices are very high, buy ground beef instead of cube steak. If the quality of fresh produce is poor, buy frozen or canned vegetables.

2. Select the needed foods by starting at one side of the store and moving from aisle to aisle. Compare the prices of brand names and store brands. Read labels. Buy the size best suited to the needs of the client or family. Large quantities are not practical if they cannot be stored, handled, or used before the expiration date.

3. Do not buy sale items unless the client normally uses the products and has storage space for them. A bargain the client cannot use is no bargain at all.

4. If the client needs to prepare food when you are not there, you may need to purchase nutritious convenience foods such as frozen entrees that the client can prepare with little assistance. You will need to check food labels if the client has diet restrictions.

5. Be aware of how much area is available for storage of food. Use this space wisely and purchase items that are going to be needed within the month only.

6. If the client just wants a small quantity, it may be wise to purchase a small serving of this in the delicatessen rather than preparing a large amount and throwing it away in a few days.

7. If only one person is living in the home, it may be wise to put the bread in the freezer and remove when needed.

8. Fresh fruits and vegetables are less expensive during their growing season. Compare fresh vegetable prices with canned and frozen vegetable prices while vegetables are in season. Out-of-season produce is quite costly.

9. Eggs have the same food value whether they are jumbo, extra large, large, or small. Brown- or white-shelled eggs are equally tasty and nutritious.

10. When buying meat, consider how the meat will be prepared. Most meat cuts have the same food value. Cheaper cuts can be just as tasty when prepared with imagination and care. When comparing the price per pound, consider the waste due to bones and fat. Figure the number of servings needed and the cost per serving.

11. When selecting poultry, buying the whole bird is the best choice. Buying separate parts such as the breast, legs, or thighs is more expensive.

12. If there is enough freezer space in the home, meats can be purchased in bulk; there is a considerable saving in the cost per pound. At home, meat can be rewrapped for the freezer in the smaller meal-size portions. However, do not buy more than can be used. Waste occurs from overstocking the freezer. Most meats can be safely frozen for up to 6 months. Some meats lose flavor and food value when stored longer. Foods not properly wrapped can be ruined by freezer burn. Be sure to label and date each item put in the freezer.

13. Make sure meats purchased are fresh. If they do not smell, look, or feel right, do not buy them. Fresh meat will regain its shape when poked with a finger. If the meat feels slimy, slick, or soft, do not bury it. If the color is off, the meat may be spoiled already.

14. Do not buy damaged cans, no matter how low the price. Cans with bulging tops, dents, or rust may contain spoiled food.

15. Purchase perishable foods last. These include foods that spoil easily, such as milk, meats, and frozen foods.

16. Cheese can be frozen and used in smaller quantities.

Storing Food

After returning from the store, the aide should put foods and supplies away. This should be done before any other major task is begun.

- Always refrigerate perishable foods immediately.
- Frozen fruits and vegetables should be placed in the freezer as soon as possible. Do not overstock on frozen foods.
- Wash and clean poultry before refrigerating. If poultry is not planned

for a meal within 2 days, wrap, date, label, and freeze it.
- Dried and packaged foods should be stored in airtight containers.
- Canned goods store easily and keep very well.

Meal Preparation

When preparing meals, the home health aide must check to see if the client has a special diet ordered or if the client has allergies to any foods. Occasionally the client may be taking medications that cannot be taken with certain types of foods.

Cooking in a Microwave. Microwave ovens have been in general use for a few years, and are now a standard appliance in all homes.

Never place anything metal (including twist ties, labels with metal content, or dishes with metal trim) in the microwave. It will ruin the oven and probably the metal also. Special microwave utensils, plates, and dishes can be used, as well as glass, china, and paperware. Most microwave owners will have a simple manual with instructions for proper use.

DIET THERAPY

Certain medical conditions require special diets. The home health aide must carefully follow directions in preparing special diets.

Special Diets

Special diets may be ordered by the dietician to meet a client's specific health needs. A description of some special diets follows. Figure 12-3 lists recommended foods and foods to avoid for these special diets and why these diets are ordered.

Vegetarian Diet. A vegetarian diet is one that generally does not contain animal products. A lacto-ovo-vegetarian

Diet	General Use	Foods Allowed	Foods to Limit/or Avoid
Low-calorie	Overweight	Skim milk, fresh fruits, lean meat or fish, vegetables, sugarless gelatin	Fried foods, rich gravies and sauces, jams, jellies, rich desserts
High-calorie	Underweight	Peanut butter, eggnog, jellies, ice cream, desserts, frequent snacks, milk shakes	None
Bland	Stomach or intestinal precaution; ulcers	All food groups	Highly seasoned, fried foods, raw vegetables and fruit, whole grains and cereals, spices such as chili peppers or powder, black pepper, red pepper, caffeinated and alcoholic beverages. Decaffeinated coffee or tea will be served according to individual tolerance.
Diabetic	Diabetes	Canned fruits in natural juices, fresh fruits, meat, vegetables, bread, sugarless gelatin, custards	Foods containing sugar, alcoholic beverages, gravy, sauces, chocolate; sweetened carbonated beverages

(continues)

Figure 12-3   Special diets that are ordered for clients with specific medical conditions

Carbohydrate-controlled diet	Use exchange list for appropriate amount		
Low-sodium	Fluid retention; heart problems; high blood pressure	Foods cooked without salt, regular meat, vegetables, fruits, salt substitute	Smoked, cured, canned fish and meats, cold cuts, cheese, potato chips, pretzels, pickles, bouillon, mustard, catsup, salad dressings, soy sauce
Low-fat, low cholesterol	Heart disease; liver disease; gallbladder	Veal, poultry, fish, skim milk, buttermilk, yogurt, low-fat cottage cheese, fat-free soup broth, fresh fruits and vegetables, cereals, gelatin, angel cake, ices, carbonated beverages, coffee, tea, jams, jellies	Fatty meats, bacon, butter, whole milk, cheese, kidney, liver, heart, fried foods, rich desserts, sauces, eggs, sour cream
Clear-liquid	Preoperative or postoperative	Tea or black coffee with sugar, apple juice, plain gelatin (no fruit), clear broth or bouillon	Solid foods
Full-liquid	Gastrointestinal problems; chewing problems; cancer	All foods in clear-liquid diet, strained juices, milk, cream, buttermilk, eggnog, strained cream soups,	Solid foods

Figure 12-3   continues

Full-liquid (continued)		strained cereal, cocoa, carbonated beverages, ices, ice cream, gelatin, custard puddings, sherbets, milk shakes, bouillon, yogurt	
Soft	Gastrointestinal conditions; chewing problems When clients are weak or have no teeth to chew	All food groups but food needs to be chopped up finer	Fibrous meat, coarse cereals, fried foods, raw fruits and vegetables, rich pastries, highly seasoned food
Pureed	Difficulty or discomfort in swallowing	All semisolid foods, foods put through a blender, and liquids of a viscous nature such as nectars	Sticky foods such as peanut butter or melted cheese, thin liquids such as water
High-fiber	Constipation	Whole grain breads and cereals, raw and cooked vegetables, fruit juices, dried beans, bran or bran flakes, nuts, seeds, and dried fruits	

NOTE: This chart is a general guide to special diets. Always follow the dietitian's prescribed diet plan.

Figure 12-3   continued

will eat eggs and dairy products. A vegan is a vegetarian who omits all animal products from the diet. Vegetarian diets can be very healthy. However, it is important that the diet provides sufficient protein, iron, and vitamin B_{12}.

Lactose Intolerance Diet. Many people have a difficult time digesting dairy products and are considered lactose intolerant. Symptoms include nausea, stomach pain, diarrhea, and gas. There are milk and dairy substitutes such as lactaid, soymilk, soy yogurt, and soy cheeses available in most supermarkets today. Those foods should be eaten to ensure adequate calcium intake. Also, lactose-intolerant individuals can take lactose tablets to help them digest dairy products.

FEEDING THE CLIENT

On occasion, it may be necessary for the aide to assist with feeding the client to provide the proper nutrition for the client who is unable to feed himself or herself, or who needs assistance with feeding. Procedure 19 demonstrates the proper way to feed the client.

19 Procedure

Feeding the Client

Purpose
- To provide proper nutrition for clients who are unable to feed themselves or who need assistance in feeding
- To provide suitable food, based on client's condition, meeting dietary standards
- To provide a pleasurable experience for the client
- To encourage client to use adaptive devices for feeding

If the client needs to be fed, it is desirable that the client be sitting up in a chair. If this is not feasible, you can position the client up in bed with the use of a few pillows. The food will be digested better if the client is in a sitting position. It is recommended that the aide sit while feeding and be at the eye level of the client.

Most clients will prefer to feed themselves if possible. Many different feeding devices available today make this possible (Figure 12-4). The feeding device will need to be chosen according to the client's disability.

If your client chokes easily, it may be recommended to mix a com-

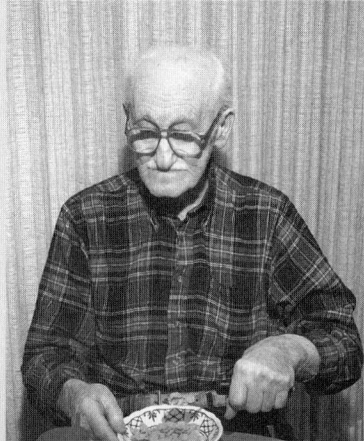

Figure 12-4 client feeds himself using special feeding devices.

mercial thickener in the liquid foods. This may prevent the client from aspirating (drawing by suction) liquids into the lungs. Clients do choke more readily on thinner liquids than thick liquids. If the client has a poor appetite and is becoming malnourished, it is advisable to offer high-calorie and high-protein drinks often throughout the day.

Some clients are fed through a feeding tube inserted through an opening in the abdominal wall. This tube is called a gastrostomy. A special control apparatus monitors the rate at which fluid nourishment is supplied to the client. It is the nurse's responsibility to teach the family how to administer and monitor a tube feeding.

Procedure

1. Wash your hands.
2. Prepare the client to eat. Check to see if the client's dentures are in. Wash the client's face and hands. Position client in sitting position in bed or sitting up in a chair. Make environment as pleasant as possible. If necessary, do mouth care before to increase the client's desire to eat. Place large napkin over client's chest.
3. Bring food to client. Tell client what foods you have prepared.
4. How you feed or assist your client depends on the handicap or physical problem the client has. If the client is blind, you need to tell the client where each food is on the plate in relation to a clock. If the client has use of only one hand, a suction plate or plate guard may be used. If the client cannot chew food, the food will need to be at the right consistency.
5. Ask the client which food is desired first. (Getting the client's cooperation and participation is important.)
6. If the client must be fed by the aide, remember:
   - Check to see if dentures are in place.
   - Feed slowly; let the client set the pace. Thermal bowls and cups will assist in keeping foods at proper temperature.
   - Feed small amounts of food at a time.
   - Make sure the consistency of the food is appropriate.
   - Do not use a syringe to feed the client. A child's feeder cup or plastic glass or plastic spoon works well in this situation.
   - If possible, have client hold finger foods or bread.
   - Do not mix food together. Feed each food item separately, identifying the food to the client.
   - Offer liquids between solid foods.
   - Do not eat client's food. Bring your own food to the client's home.
   - If you need to record food intake, do it in percentages such as 20% or 90%.

Total Parenteral Nutrition

Clients who cannot be nourished by being fed through the mouth or through a gastrostomy (tube inserted into the stomach through the abdomen) may receive nutrition intravenously. The client would have a small catheter (tube) inserted into the blood vessel by a health care provider. Through this line or catheter, the client may receive total parenteral nutrition (TPN). The fluid that goes through this line contains a high dextrose (sugar) solution that contains all the necessary nutrients. It is administered via a special pump to make sure the rate is consistent and to prevent fluid overload. The solution is hung by the nurse or family member. The home health aide will be given instructions on how to manage the client while the feeding is in progress, and how to troubleshoot the pump. Clients receiving TPN need daily weights obtained and urine checked with a Keto-Diastix for sugar in their urine.

Elimination

URINARY SYSTEM

The urinary system consists of the kidneys, ureters, bladder, and urethra (Figure 13-1).

Signs and symptoms of urinary problems may include:

- Dysuria—painful urination
- Hematuria—finding traces of blood in the urine
- Oliguria—voiding in small amounts
- Pyuria—having pus in urine
- Flank pain—pain in the area between the ribs and the hip bone in the person's back
- Change in stream of urine—urine is expelled slower or at different rates
- Color of urine—change to deep red, brown, or yellowish green
- Frequency—going to the bathroom more often than usual and only voiding a small amount of urine
- Hesitancy—delay in starting to void
- Retention—inability to void
- Urgency—having to void immediately

If you notice any of the above signs or symptoms when caring for a client, you need to report them. If a urinary tract disorder is treated early, the results of the treatment are better. It is also a good idea to be aware of the preceding terms and what they mean so that if these words are used on a client's chart, you will better understand the client's problems.

Prevention of Urinary Tract Infections

A goal of good health maintenance in caring for your client is to prevent urinary tract infections. Good rules to follow for your client are:

- Wipe perineal area from front to back after voiding or defecating (having a bowel movement)
- Drink an adequate amount of liquids throughout the day
- Avoid bath salts, oils, and vaginal sprays
- Drink cranberry juice, which will make the urine less odorous and is often ordered when a client has a urinary tract infection
- Empty the bladder completely when voiding
- Wear cotton underwear

COMMON DISORDERS OF THE URINARY SYSTEM

Incontinence, cystitis, renal failure, and kidney stones are four common disorders of the urinary system.

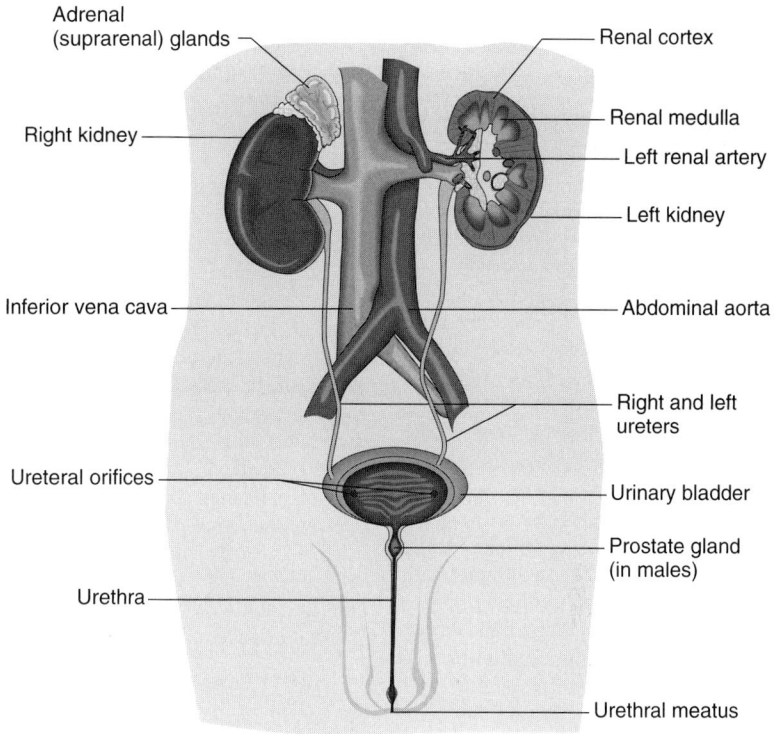

Adrenal
(suprarenal) glands

Renal cortex

Right kidney

Renal medulla

Left renal artery

Left kidney

Inferior vena cava

Abdominal aorta

Right and left
ureters

Ureteral orifices

Urinary bladder

Prostate gland
(in males)

Urethra

Urethral meatus

Figure 13-1   The urinary system

Incontinence

Some individuals have no voluntary control of their bladder muscles. This causes them to be incontinent, or to expel urine unexpectedly.

According to Newman and Jakovac-Smith:

Stress incontinence refers to the involuntary loss of small amounts of urine during activities that increase intra-abdominal pressure, such as coughing, running, laughing, or lifting heavy objects. Typically caused by weakened pelvic floor muscles or a weakened or damaged urethral sphincter, stress incontinence is most common in women but may affect men following prostate surgery.

A client with stress incontinence can be taught to do Kegel exercises (pelvic floor strengthener). The client is told to tighten the pelvic muscles, as though to stop the urine stream when voiding, and then release. The client should try to do this about 10 times each time when voiding and do it three or four times a day. Eventually, this will tighten the muscles around the meatus (opening where urine is expelled).

Urge incontinence refers to the involuntary loss of urine because of the inability to reach the bathroom in time. Most common in older adults, this type of incontinence usually is caused by weakened pelvic floor muscles, tumor, kidney or bladder stones, or diverticula. Detrusor instability (unstable bladder) is associated with disorders of the lower urinary tract or neurologic system, including multiple sclerosis and diabetes.

Overflow incontinence refers to the continuous or periodic dribbling of urine because of an atonic bladder (bladder that has lost tone), or an anatomic obstruction, such as an enlarged prostate or a urethral stricture. This type of incontinence accounts for 10% to 15% of all incontinent clients.

Functional incontinence refers to involuntary urination because of the inability to reach a bathroom due to a specific disability, such as a physical or cognitive impairment, an inaccessible toilet, inattentive or inaccessible caregivers, or an unwillingness to move. This type of incontinence, which accounts for 25% of all incontinent clients, is common after admission to an acute care hospital.

D. Newman and D. A. Jakovac-Smith, *Geriatric Care Plans* (Springhouse Corp., 1991), p. 128. Figure 13-2 provides an illustrative guide to help you understand and remember the causes of incontinence.

Cystitis

Cystitis occurs when the membrane lining of the urinary bladder becomes inflamed. It can be caused by bacterial infection or a kidney inflammation that has spread to the bladder. Signs and symptoms of cystitis are urinary frequency and urgency, dysuria, nausea, anorexia (loss of appetite), and fever. The health care provider will order a urine specimen to be collected on the client to find out what organism is causing the infection. If an organism is found in the urine, the common treatment consists of medication, avoiding carbonated beverages, and increasing fluid intake.

Kidney Stones

Kidney stones are usually caused by an excess of calcium. The urine becomes crystallized (hardened) and stones may block the ureters and cause painful urination. The stones can be of various sizes: some large, some very small. Signs and symptoms of renal colic are sudden severe pain in the flank area, hematuria (due to the stones trying to pass through the ureters), nausea, and fever. If the health care provider suspects that a client may have kidney stones, the client's urine will need to be strained through a strainer every time the client voids. If the stones are not passed, the health care provider may have to perform a special procedure to dissolve the stones through laser therapy. A new technique is available now for some clients, whereby the stones can be destroyed by sound waves rather than by surgery.

Renal (Kidney) Failure

When a client's kidneys no longer produce urine in the body, waste materials build up in the body, and if nothing is done, the client can die. Early signs of renal failure are weakness, fatigue, and lethargy. Eventually, signs like hypertension, edema, and fluid retention appear throughout the body. This condition can be treated by kidney dialysis or kidney transplant.

COMMON DISORDERS OF THE LOWER INTESTINES AND RECTUM

Cancer of the colon, diverticulitis and hemorrhoids are three common disorders of the lower intestines and rectum.

Diverticulitis

This condition occurs when the tiny sacs that are in the inside of the intestines become inflamed and irritate the intestines. Research shows that more than 50% of individuals over the age of 50 have some form of this disease. It is usually discovered when a client has a colonoscopy (exam of the colon). Signs are constipation or diarrhea, cramping pain in the abdomen, and increased rectal gas. Diverticulitis is treated with diet, and medication and if it becomes too severe, surgery may be indicated.

Hemorrhoids

Hemorrhoids are varicose veins that occur inside the rectum or around the outside of the rectum. They are caused by a weakness in this area, which can occur with straining on defecation or pregnancy. They can be very painful, itch, and can bleed if irritated. Treatment consists of the application of special cream, cold packs, and avoidance of constipation.

Cancer of the Colon

Cancer of the colon is the second most common cause of cancer deaths in the United States. It tends to occur in individuals over the age of 50. Signs and symptoms are silent at first, but as the tumor grows, the signs become more pronounced. Signs and symptoms are

pain, a palpable mass in the lower right side of the abdomen, vomiting, and dark red stools. The aim is to detect the tumor in the early stages of the disease, which is why a test for occult blood in the stool is done. Refer to Procedure 34 later in this unit.

CLIENT CARE PROCEDURES

The remainder of this unit addresses commonly performed client care procedures that are related to the elimination system. It is important that you check with your agency to clarify those procedures that will be your responsibility and those responsibilities that belong to other members of the team.

Measuring and Recording Fluids

Intake is a measure of all the fluids or semiliquids that a person drinks. Output is all the fluid that passes out of the body. The abbreviation for measuring fluid intake and output is I&O. Procedure 20 demonstrates the proper method for measuring and recording fluid intake and output.

20 Procedure

Measuring and Recording Fluid Intake and Output

Purpose

- To identify food items that need to be measured for fluid intake
- To measure and record fluid intake and output accurately

Fluids that should be included in the measurement of intake and output include:

Measure for Intake

ice	water
juices	pop
coffee	ice cream
yogurt	soup
jello	pudding

any other food that is liquid at room temperature

Measure for Output

vomitus (emesis)
liquid stools
urine
blood or drainage from wounds

Procedure

1. Assemble supplies:
   measuring cup or container for intake
   large measuring container for output
   disposable gloves
2. Wash hands and apply gloves if measuring output.
3. Measure and record all liquids taken by the client. This includes all fluids taken with meals and between meals: coffee, milk, fruit juices, beer, and water. Liquids are recorded in cubic centimeters,

abbreviated cc. You need to remember that 30 cc equals 1 ounce. (One cc equals one mL.) Example: If a client drank a can of pop that is 12 ounces, you need to multiply 12 by 30, which equals 360 cc.

4. Ask the client to use a urinal or bedpan for all voiding. If the client can use the toilet, a special plastic hat can be placed in the toilet to collect the urine. All urine must be collected so that it can be measured.
5. Pour urine from bedpan or urinal into a measuring device. Record the amount. Always record output in cc.
6. Be sure to explain to the client how to keep exact records. The client will need to record the fluids at times when the aide is off duty.
7. Clean equipment after each use.
8. Remove gloves and wash hands.

Giving and Emptying the Bedpan or Urinal

The bedpan is used for clients who are confined to bed. The bedpan should be given whenever the client requests it. The client may be undergoing retraining to establish bowel and bladder continence. The aide should follow a regular schedule of

offering the bedpan or urinal. If the client does not remember to ask, the home health aide should offer to bring the bedpan or urinal.

Procedures 21 and 22 demonstrate the proper way to give and empty a bedpan and urinal. Procedure 23 demonstrates the correct way to assist a client to use the portable commode.

21

Procedure

Giving and Emptying the Bedpan

Purpose

• To provide for routine elimination of bladder and bowels

• To observe or measure urinary or fecal output

Procedure

1. Assemble equipment and supplies needed:
   disposable gloves
   bedpan and bedpan cover
   toilet tissue
   moistened washcloth
2. Wash hands and apply gloves.
3. Tell client what you plan to do.
4. If a metal bedpan is used, first warm it by running hot water over the rim. Dry the rim and sprinkle it with powder if available. The powder prevents the client's buttocks from sticking to the bedpan.
5. Place bedpan near the bed. Put toilet tissue near the client's hand.
6. Fold top blanket and sheet at an angle. Remove the client's bottom clothing.
7. To raise the buttocks, have the client bend knees and push on the heels. As the client lifts, place your hand under the small of the client's back.
8. Lift gently and slowly with one hand. Slide the bedpan under the hips with the other hand. The client's buttocks should rest on the rounded shelf of the bedpan. The narrow end should face the foot of the bed. If the client cannot assist, turn the client to one side and position the bedpan over the buttocks. Roll the client onto the bedpan. The aide holds the bedpan in place when the client is lying on his or her backside and then turns the client. Make sure the client's head is elevated.

9. Pull sheet over the client for added privacy. Make sure the client is as comfortable as possible. An extra pillow under the head may be used.
10. While client is using the bedpan, the aide can be moistening the washcloth.
11. Remove the bedpan when the client is finished using it. Do not leave the client sitting on the bedpan for longer than 15 minutes. Remove the bedpan by having the client bend the knees and push on the heels. Place one hand under small of client's back and lift. Remove the bedpan with the other hand.
12. If possible, have client wipe him or herself. If client is not able to do this, the aide must wipe the client. Remember to wipe from front to back on a female client. Discard tissues in the bedpan.
13. Replace the client's clothing. Give client washcloth to wipe hands.
14. Take bedpan to toilet, observe contents and measure if necessary. Empty contents into toilet. Flush. Fill bedpan with cold water and empty. Clean bedpan by using warm soapy water or disinfectant and the toilet brush. Empty water into toilet and rinse bedpan. Dry well.
15. Return bedpan to proper storage area.
16. Remove gloves and wash hands.
17. Record color and amount of urine; color, amount, and consistency of stool.

22

Procedure

Giving and Emptying the Urinal

Purpose

- To provide for routine elimination of urine for a male client

Procedure

1. Wash your hands and apply gloves.
2. Lift the top bedcovers and place the urinal under the covers so that the client can grasp the handle. If he cannot do this, you must place the urinal in position and ensure that the penis is placed in the opening of the urinal. If possible assist the client to stand when using the urinal.
3. Remove gloves and dispose of them properly. Leave client alone if possible. You may give the client a bell to ring when he is done.
4. Put on gloves and remove urinal once client is done using it.
5. Take the urinal to the bathroom and observe contents. Measure if required. Empty the urinal. Rinse with cold water. Rinse with disinfectant or water; dry and store properly.
6. Remove gloves and wash hands.
7. Record amount and color of urine, if required.

23

Procedure

Assisting Client to Use the Portable Commode

Purpose

- To assist client to use a portable toilet who because of mobility problems cannot use a regular toilet

Procedure

1. Assemble equipment:
   commode and bucket
   toilet paper
   moistened washcloth with soap applied
   disposable gloves
2. Wash hands and apply gloves.
3. Bring commode to area closest to client. Detach bucket from commode, if you need to wipe the client. If you place water in the bucket, it will make it easier to empty.
4. Transfer client to commode and pull down the client's underwear.
5. If client is stable, leave the room to provide privacy.
6. After client is done, check to see if you need to wipe the client.
7. Remove gloves and assist client to chair or bed.

8. Return to commode and apply gloves. Empty bucket in toilet. Rinse with disinfectant and cold water. Return the bucket to commode. Store commode in designated area.
9. Remove gloves and wash hands.
10. Record amount of urine or stool.

Collecting a Urine Specimen

A clean-catch specimen is requested to obtain a urine sample that is as free of contamination as possible. This is required to provide a urine sample for a diagnostic test and to ensure that the test results are as accurate as possible. Procedure 24 demonstrates the correct way to collect a clean-catch urine specimen.

24 Procedure

Collecting a Clean-Catch Urine Specimen

Purpose
- To obtain and send specimen to laboratory for analysis

Procedure
1. Assemble supplies:
   disposable gloves
   sterile urine specimen container with completed label
   biohazard transportation bag
   clean bedpan or urinal
   antiseptic soaked wipes
2. Wash hands and apply gloves.
3. Inform client of what you plan to do.
4. Wash the client's genital area or have the client do so, if able. It is especially important for the urinary opening to be cleansed.
5. Give the client a labeled specimen container.
6. Explain the procedure to the client.
7. Have the client begin to void into the bedpan, urinal, or toilet.

After a small amount of urine has been voided, have the client catch some of the urine in midstream in the sterile specimen container. You will only need 2 ounces, or 60 cc. After the specimen has been collected, the client can resume voiding into the bedpan, urinal, or toilet.
8. Immediately place the sterile cap on the specimen container so the specimen will not become contaminated.
9. Remove bedpan and wipe client.
10. Place labeled specimen container inside a biohazard transportation bag.
11. Remove gloves and wash hands.
12. Store the specimen bag according to the nurse's instructions until time to take to local laboratory.
13. Document time of collection and type of specimen.

Caring for Catheters

A urinary catheter is a tube inserted into the bladder to drain urine. Germs can easily enter the bladder while the catheter is in place. Therefore, cleaning around the urinary opening is important. The catheter is inserted by the nurse. The catheter is replaced weekly or once a month. Procedure 25 demonstrates the proper way to care for a urinary catheter.

25 Procedure

Caring for a Urinary Catheter

Purpose

- To clean the area around where the catheter enters the body
- To prevent infection of the urinary tract
- To decrease odors and make the client comfortable
- To maintain closed drainage system

NOTE: The collection bag, tubing, and catheter are referred to as the *closed drainage system.* The system should never be disconnected except to reconnect it to a leg bag. The reason the system should not be disconnected is to prevent germs from entering the system. You should never raise the collection bag higher than the client's bladder. Always check to see if the tubing is lying in correct position and not kinked. Never pull on a catheter. If possible, cover bag with a cloth to prevent embarrassment of your client. Newer closed drainage systems have a stop valve in the tubing and in the bag, which will prevent backflow of urine.

Procedure

1. Assemble supplies:
   disposable gloves
   antiseptic wipes or
   moisten warm washcloth, and
   soap
   plastic bag for waste
2. Wash your hands and apply gloves.
3. Tell client what you plan to do.
4. Position client on his or her back. Expose only the small area where the catheter enters the body. Using moistened washcloth with soap or antiseptic wipes, wash area surrounding the catheter. Observe for any skin breakdown, signs of infection, crusting, leakage or bleeding, which should be reported to the nurse.
5. Using antiseptic wipes, or soap and moist washcloth, wipe the catheter tube. Make only one stroke with each wipe. Discard each wipe after one stroke. Start at the urinary opening and wipe *away* from it. Be careful not to dislodge the catheter. Clean the catheter down to the connection of the drainage tubing.
6. Remove gloves and discard into plastic bag.
7. Check to be sure tubing is coiled on bed and hanging straight down into the drainage container. Check level of urine in the

collection bag. Tubing should not be below the collection bag.

8. Cover client and discard wastes properly.
9. Wash hands.
10. Always remember to keep the collection bag below the level of the urinary bladder. This is to assist the gravity drainage and backflow of urine into the bladder.
11. Document procedure, your observations, and client's reaction.

The leg urinary collection bag is smaller than the closed urinary collection bag to provide a smaller collection bag for the client when out of bed. The leg bag is attached to the client's thigh (upper leg). Otherwise, a client can have an extension tube put on the leg bag and have it attached to the lower leg. The leg bag allows for greater mobility for the client, but must be emptied more frequently. A client may use the leg bag while in the wheelchair or ambulating, and it can be connected to the closed drainage bag when in bed for the night. The leg bag must be rinsed according to agency directions. A clean cap or stopper must be used at the end of the tubing while the closed urinary drainage bag is not in use. Refer to Procedures 26 and 27 for the proper ways to connect a leg bag, and to empty a drainage unit. Procedure 28 demonstrates the proper way to apply a condom (external) catheter.

26   Procedure

Connecting the Leg Bag

Purpose

- To connect a leg urinary drainage bag

Procedure

1. Assemble equipment:
   disposable gloves
   urinary leg bag with straps
   alcohol wipes
   paper towels
2. Wash your hands and apply gloves.
3. Tell client what you plan to do.
4. Place paper towel underneath catheter connection area.
5. Use alcohol wipes to disinfect area to be disconnected.
6. Disconnect catheter from tubing. Wipe end of catheter with alcohol wipe (Figure 13-2). Remove cap from end of leg bag and connect leg bag to catheter. Wipe end of closed drainage bag tubing with alcohol wipe. Place cap on end of closed drainage system.
7. Attach leg straps and bag to leg of client. Check to see if the part marked "top of bag" is in the correct position.

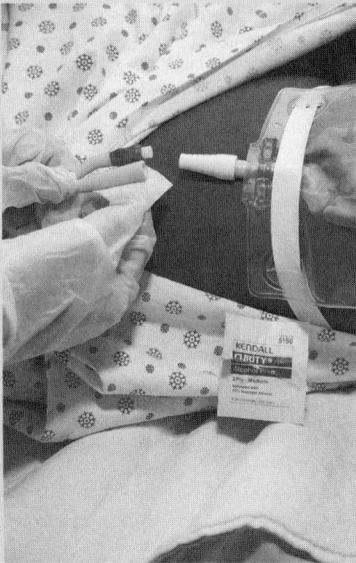

8. Empty and measure urine from closed drainage bag.
9. Clean and disinfect bag and store in designated area.
10. Remove gloves and wash hands.
11. Note: If the client wants the leg bag to be connected to the lower leg, an extension tube can be used.
12. Document procedure completed.

Figure 13-2   Wipe end of catheter with alcohol wipe before connecting leg bag.

27 Procedure

Emptying a Drainage Unit

Purpose
• To empty urinary drainage bag

Procedure
1. Assemble equipment:
   disposable gloves
   alcohol wipes
   measuring device
   paper towel
2. Wash hands and apply gloves.
3. Tell client what you plan to do.
4. Place paper towel underneath measuring device on floor below drainage bag.
5. Open drain or spout and allow the urine to drain into measuring device (Figure 13-3). Do not allow the tip of tubing to touch sides of the measuring device.
6. Close the drain and wipe it with the alcohol wipe. Replace it in the holder on the bag.
7. Note the amount and color of urine. Empty urine into toilet. Wash and rinse measuring device.
8. Remove gloves and wash hands.
9. Record amount.

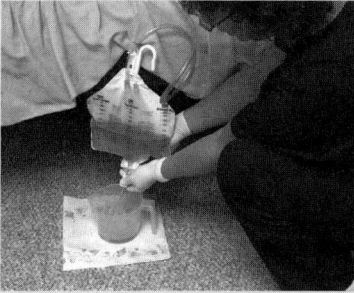

Figure 13-3 Open the drain on the bottom of the urinary drainage bag, be sure you place a paper towel underneath the container.

28

Procedure

Applying a Condom (External) Catheter

Purpose

- To drain urine from the urethra through a tube to a drainage bag

Procedure

1. Assemble equipment:
   disposable gloves
   condom catheter
   special wipes or moistened washcloth with soap applied
   special adhesive (optional)
   drainage bag
2. Wash hands and apply gloves.
3. Clean penis and dry if needed.
4. Place the tip of the penis into the condom.
5. Roll the condom over the penis.
6. If using a self-adhesive condom, it needs to be gently squeezed on top to seal it.
7. Special adhesive may come with the condom to apply after it is rolled to the top.
8. Connect to the urinary leg bag or bedside drainage bag.
9. Remove gloves and wash hands.

The condom catheter is used primarily on younger men who have no control over their urination. Problems with this type of catheter are that the urine is in constant contact with the skin, which can cause the tip of the penis to become reddened and sore; also leakage can occur because sometimes the fit is not the best. If leakage does occur, another brand of catheter may be indicated.

Retraining the Bladder

A home health aide may need to keep a record for a few days of how often and how much the client voids throughout the day and night. Once the client's voiding pattern is known, the nurse can analyze the client's voiding record and formulate a schedule for the aide to follow. The schedule developed by the nurse will include regularly scheduled times for the aide to have the client drink a measured amount of fluids, and then to toilet the client at regular intervals.

Procedure 29 discusses the proper method to retrain the bladder.

29 Procedure

Retraining the Bladder

Purpose

• To regain bladder control

Procedure

The schedule developed by the nurse will include regularly scheduled times for the aide to have the client drink a measured amount of fluid. After the client has drunk the liquid, the aide notes the time and then 30 minutes later the aide will toilet the client.

The aide will need to encourage the client to void each time the client is positioned on the commode or toilet. It is helpful at times to run water from the faucet to give the client an urge to void. Other methods of encouraging the client to void are to have the client apply light pressure to the bladder area to stimulate the urge to empty the bladder; to pour warm water over the genital area; or have the client lean forward on the toilet to stimulate emptying the bladder.

Remember that the client needs to be toileted at regular intervals to prevent accidents. The client will need consistent positive reinforcement to remain dry. At first it may be necessary to take the client to the bathroom every 2 hours; intervals may be lengthened as control is gained. A common cause of incontinence is delay in getting the client to the bathroom. It is of utmost importance to take the client to the bathroom on a *regular* time schedule.

The plan will also call for the aide to maintain the client's fluid intake at about 2500 cc/day, except for persons with fluid restriction (i.e., congestive heart failure or renal failure). The aide should encourage the client to wear regular underwear to enhance the client's self-esteem and to help the client from reverting back to the previous incontinence habit.

Bowel Movements

When a client has a bowel movement, this rids the body of waste products that have accumulated after the food has been digested. Everyone has a different pattern in frequency of bowel movements. For some clients having three bowel movements a day may be normal, whereas another client may have a bowel movement every three days. The medical term for having a bowel movement is defecation. When a client has a defecation, the stool or feces should be observed for: color—black, tarry, brown, tan; consistency—hard, form, liquid, pasty; amount—large, medium, or small. If a client has a bowel movement often and the stool is very runny, the client has diarrhea. When a client passes gas through the colon, the medical term for rectal gas is flatus.

Enemas and Rectal Suppositories

An enema is the technique of introducing fluid into the rectum to re-move feces and flatus (gas) from the rectum and colon. Procedures 30 and 31 demonstrate the proper way to give a commercial enema and a rectal suppository. Procedure 32 discusses regulating the bowels.

30 ━━━━━ Procedure

Giving a Commercial Enema

Purpose

• To help cleanse the bowel

NOTE: Because enemas distend or dilate the rectum, the client may experience a feeling of urgency in the bowel, that is, a very strong need to empty the bowel as soon as possible.

Enemas can only be given on a health care provider's orders.

The two commercially prepared enemas are the chemical (often referred to as Fleets) and oil-retention enemas. Oil-retention enemas are given to soften hard feces in the rectum and are usually followed by a soap solution enema.

Procedure

1. Assemble supplies:
   disposable gloves
   commercial prepackaged enema
   protective pad
   bedpan or commode
   toilet paper
   lubrication jelly
   water, washcloth, soap, towel
2. Wash hands and put on gloves.
3. Tell client what you plan to do.
4. Provide for the client's comfort and privacy.
5. Place protective pad underneath the client's buttocks.

6. Have client turn to the left side. Turn covers back to expose only the buttocks.
7. Remove cover on the tip of enema. Apply extra lubricant to tip to ensure easy insertion.
8. Separate the buttocks and insert the tip into rectum for at least 3 inches. Slowly squeeze the plastic container (Figure 13-4). This forces the solution to flow evenly into the rectum.
9. Remove enema tip while holding the client's buttocks together.
10. Instruct client to hold the enema for at least a few minutes.
11. Position client on bedpan, commode, or toilet.
12. After client has expelled feces and enema solution, assist the client in cleaning area around anus and buttocks.
13. Return client to comfortable position. It may be necessary to leave the protective pad in place until the effects of the enema are complete.
14. Remove gloves and wash hands.
15. Record results of enema—color, amount, consistency; for example: 10:00 AM, Fleets enema given, good results—large, brown, formed stool.

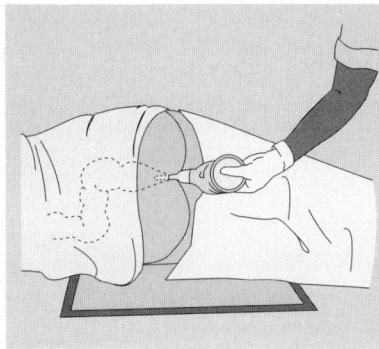

Figure 13-4 Squeeze the plastic container from the bottom until all the liquid has gone into the rectum.

31

Procedure

Giving a Rectal Suppository

Purpose

• To stimulate a bowel movement

NOTE: Suppositories are usually stored in the client's refrigerator and are wrapped in foil. The suppository will melt once inserted into the warm environment of the rectum and colon. It will take the suppository at least 5 to 10 minutes to melt. It is important that the aide inform the client to wait a few minutes after the suppository is inserted before trying to have a bowel movement.

Procedure

1. Assemble supplies:
   disposable gloves
   rectal suppository
   lubricant
   protective pad or paper towels
2. Wash hands and apply gloves.
3. Tell client what you plan to do and provide privacy.
4. Open foil-wrapped suppository.
5. Turn client to one side and place protective pad under buttocks.
6. Lubricate gloved finger well, insert gloved finger with suppository, tip end first, into rectum (Figure 13-5). Push the suppository along the lining of the rectum with your index finger as far as your finger allows. Be careful not to insert suppository into the feces. The suppository needs to be next to the lining of the rectum for it to be effective.
7. After 10 minutes have passed, assist the client to the toilet or commode.
8. After client has had a bowel movement, assist client back to bed or chair.
9. Remove gloves and wash hands.
10. Record results. Note color, consistency, and amount of stool.

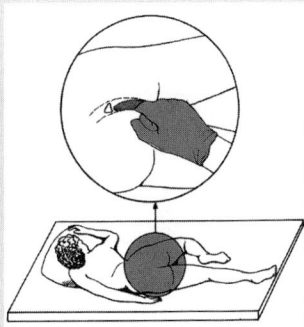

Figure 13-5 Carefully place the rectal suppository into the rectum about 3 inches for adults.

32   Procedure

Regulating the Bowels

Purpose

- To retrain a client to be continent of bowel movement
- To regulate a client to have regular bowel movement

NOTE: Among the elderly, constipation is often encountered. If a client is unable to exercise and move about regularly, bowel action becomes sluggish. Sometimes medications, especially painkillers, can cause constipation. If a client has hemorrhoids, there may be a fear of pain and so the client avoids trying to have a bowel movement. If a client does not have a bowel movement for three days, the client may develop a fecal impaction. An impaction is a large amount of hard stool in the lower colon or rectum that cannot be expelled normally. Signs of an impaction are pain in the lower abdomen and continuous liquid stools, which are caused by leaking around the hard stool. If a client does develop an impaction, the nurse will need to remove the stool manually.

Procedure

1. The health care provider assesses prior habits of client. If client always had a bowel movement early in the morning, this would be important to know in planning the client's bowel regulating program.
2. A plan is designed and implemented. Important elements of the plan are:
   - High intake of fiber foods
   - Adequate intake of liquids
   - Regular exercise
   - Toileting client at regular intervals
   - Praise by aide of slightest progress
   - Privacy for client for bowel movements

3. Follow bowel regulating program developed by the health care provider. If plan does appear to be working, note success of program. If plan does not work, re-

port. It is also important to give some suggestions to the health care provider of possible solutions for regulating the bowels.

Adult Briefs

The adult brief is used to keep the incontinent client dry and to minimize embarrassment to the client in the event of accidents. The adult brief

will also reduce odor and the chance of developing urinary infections and pressure sores, and save on laundry. Refer to Procedure 33.

33   Procedure

Applying Adult Briefs

The adult brief comes in various styles and sizes. One design may be an insert to go inside a specially designed brief. Another popular type is a "wraparound brief" fastened with Velcro-like tabs. It is important to have the correct size for your client to ensure their effectiveness. If an adult brief is too large, it will be ineffective and leakage will occur; if the brief is too small, the brief will also be ineffective and leak. It is a good idea to place a maximum absorbency brief on the client at night. It is also important to read the instructions on the package on how to apply each particular style of brief. Many briefs have a strip on them that changes color when the brief needs to be changed. The brief should be checked at regular intervals and changed as needed. Do not apply powder to the client's perineal area when adult briefs are used. Many of the briefs have specially treated wipes to use to clean

the client's perineal area (**perineum**) when changing the briefs. They are very reasonable in cost and are recommended over soap and water. If a certain brief does not appear to be working, report this to the nurse. There are many different types on the market, and some work better on some clients than others.

Purpose

• To confine urine or feces to one area when the client is incontinent

Procedure

1. Assemble supplies:
   adult brief
   cleansing wipe
   disposable gloves
   plastic bag
2. Wash hands and apply gloves.
3. Tell client what you plan to do and provide privacy.
4. Remove soiled brief and place in plastic bag.

5. Cleanse genital area with cleansing wipe and place in plastic bag.
6. Apply new brief underneath client's buttocks. Be sure to position brief correctly under buttocks. Bring lower end of brief through the client's perineal area. Fasten tabs on brief.
7. Remove gloves and wash hands.
8. Record output—urine or stool and approximate amount, if required.

Bowel Regulating Programs

There are several methods that can assist clients to evacuate. Each method is designed according to the client's specific need. For instance, if any medication is to be administered, or a digital exam is to be performed (lubricated finger is inserted into the rectum and irritates the rectum area for a minute) it needs to be part of the daily routine. A bowel regulating program is developed with the client to set up a designated time for a bowel movement. Consuming dietary foods that are high in fiber and bulk, drinking eight glasses of water a day, and exercising will help the client to achieve this goal. Medications such as Metamucil, stool softeners, suppositories, or enemas may be needed to supplement the program.

Collecting a Stool Specimen

On occasion it may be necessary to collect a stool sample for a diagnostic test. Procedure 34 demonstrates the proper method to collect a stool specimen.

34   Procedure

Collecting a Stool Specimen

Purpose
- To collect a stool sample for a diagnostic test

Procedure
1. Assemble supplies:
   disposable gloves
   bedpan or other collecting
     container
   specimen container or
     hemoccult
   slide packet with label completed
2. Inform client of need for specimen. Certain foods, such as organ meats, can change the color of stool and test positive or false. Many of the tests on the market will indicate which foods should be avoided for several days before testing.
3. After client has had a bowel movement in bedpan or toilet, apply gloves and with wood applicator remove stool (Figure 13-6A). If specimen is to be collected in specimen container, place small amount (approximately 1 tablespoon) of stool in

container (Figure 13-6B). If the test is for occult blood or guaiac, place small amount of stool on hemoccult blood card with the applicator stick included in the test (Figure 13-7).

4. Place specimen in proper storage place until it is sent to the laboratory.
5. Remove gloves and wash hands.
6. Document stool specimen collection.

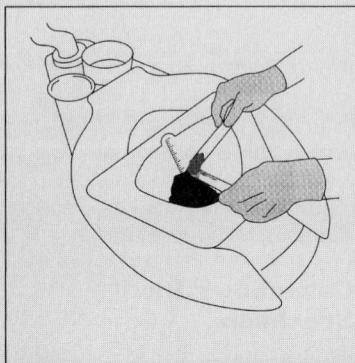

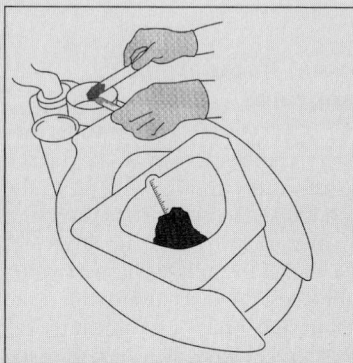

Figure 13-6 Using tongue blades to transfer the stool specimen from the collection container (A) to the specimen container (B).

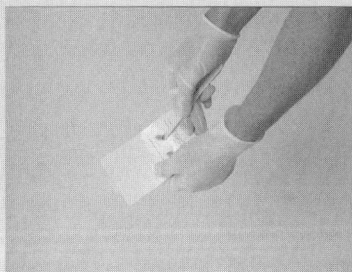

Figure 13-7 Open card and apply a small sample of stool on the designated area on the card for occult blood or guaiac test.

Caring for an Ostomy Bag

An ostomy bag is sometimes called a stoma bag. It is used for clients who have had a surgical operation called a colostomy or an ileostomy. Instructions for changing an ostomy bag are discussed in Procedure 35.

35   Procedure

Assisting With Changing an Ostomy Bag

Purpose

- To keep the client clean
- To prevent skin breakdown around the stoma
- To regulate and establish a daily routine for removing wastes

NOTE: An ostomy bag should be changed when it becomes one-third or one-half full. Once regulated the client can change it at about the same time each day. In some cases, the client may wear a gauze pad instead of a bag or pouch.

In addition to changing the bag, the client may need to irrigate the intestines. If the client needs to do this, the client would have been taught at the hospital or by the nurse how to irrigate (wash out) the intestine. An aide may assist the client with this procedure.

Until a client has adjusted to using the ostomy bag there may be strong feelings of embarrassment. The home health aide can help the client accept the inconvenience by being understanding. The aide should not show displeasure in assisting the client.

The bags and attachments come in many styles today. They are lighter, odor proof, and fit more tightly. Many types of bags and appliances are available; a few require a belt to attach the appliance, others do not require a belt. Colostomy bags can be in one-piece disposable pouches or two-piece disposable pouches. A popular method of attachment is with a synthetic preparation resembling real skin that is attached to the area around the stoma. On this artificial skin is a raised seal that the colostomy bag may attach to. This artificial skin protects the real skin from irritation and contamination with the client's feces and also serves as a place where the colostomy bag can be put on and taken off. Another popular method for attaching a colostomy bag is with a brown-colored, gum-type substance called karaya, which does not irritate the client's skin and prevents skin breakdown. The nurse or enterostomal therapist will give you special instructions on the type of skin attachment and bag the client is using.

Procedure

1. Assemble supplies:
   disposable gloves
   washcloth
   basin of warm water and soap
   clean ostomy bag
   plastic bag
   skin ointment (if ordered)
   toilet tissue
2. Wash your hands and apply gloves.
3. Tell client what you plan to do and provide privacy.
4. Gently remove soiled colostomy bag from the stoma. Place in plastic bag. In a few instances, the colostomy bag can be washed and reused.
5. If there is stool on the skin remove with toilet tissue. Wash area around the stoma with mild soap and water. Pat the area dry. Occasionally a special substance may

be applied to assist the new colostomy bag to adhere better.

6. Apply ointment if ordered. Observe area around the stoma for redness or open areas.

7. Apply client's pouch.
   - If one-piece pouch or bag is being used, remove self-stick backing from new ostomy appliance. Press the new bag to the area around the stoma, being sure to seal tightly.
   - If two-piece pouch is being used, be sure to cut opening to the correct size. (A few bags are premeasured and this step is not necessary.) Remove adhesive backing on face plate. Firmly apply face plate to client's skin around stoma, working from the stoma out-

ward. Then apply the bag to this face plate. Let your client assist you as much as possible. Be sure to follow any special manufacturer's instruction in application of appliance.

8. Assist the client to connect belt to appliance, if client is using this type of appliance.

9. Remove wastes. Observe stool for color, amount, and consistency. If necessary spray the room with deodorizer.

10. Remove gloves and wash hands.

11. The karaya seal should be changed every 5 to 7 days, unless leakage is occurring around the seal.

12. Document procedure and time, your observations, and client's reaction.

UNIT 14

Integumentary System

INTEGUMENTARY SYSTEM

The skin, hair, and nails make up the integumentary system. The skin is the largest organ of the body. It covers the entire outer surface of the body. Skin is made up of two layers of tissue. The outer layer is the epidermis and the inner layer is the dermis (Figure 14-1). Other parts of the integumentary system are the nails, hair, oil and sweat glands, and mucous membranes.

The integumentary system protects the body but also has other functions. It regulates body temperature and works with the nervous system to sense touch, pressure, pain, heat, and cold.

COMMON DISORDERS OF THE INTEGUMENTARY SYSTEM

Pressure Areas

The care given to the skin of a person confined to bed or a wheelchair is extremely important. When the body gets little exercise, the skin is one of the first areas to break down. Breakdown most often occurs where the

skin covers the bones. These places are called bony prominences.

The back of the head, buttocks, coccyx, elbow, knees, and heels are common places to watch for signs of skin breakdown. A pressure sore is a breakdown in the skin that covers a bony area. Some common causes of pressure sore development are injury to the skin due to leaving a client in one position too long, friction and shearing when turning or repositioning a client, poor skin cleansing, poor nutrition, and incontinence.

Signs and Symptoms of Pressure Sores. Pressure sores are characterized by stages, depending on the degree of severity.

Stage 1: A warm-looking reddened area. Within 18 to 24 hours the reddened area can become an open sore. If not treated it will soon develop into Stage 2.

Stage 2: A blister will form and there will be small breaks visible on the client's skin. If not treated it will soon progress to Stage 3.

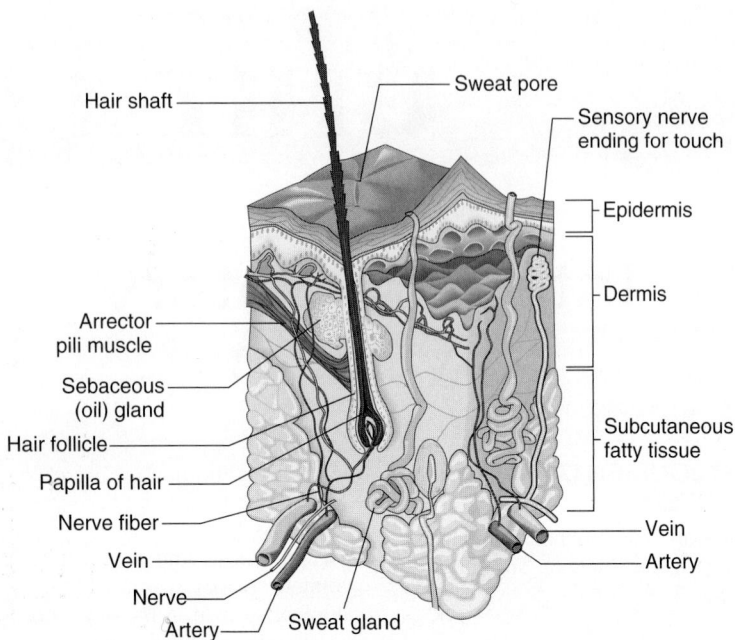

Figure 14-1 Cross section of the skin

Stage 3: The blister breaks open and there is a well-defined sore visible.

Stage 4: The open area extends to the muscle, bones, and underlying structures. These sores can vary in size and are places where infections can easily and quickly set in.

Preventing Pressure Sores. Certain medical conditions such as diabetes, stroke, and paralysis make the client more susceptible to skin breakdown. Clients with circulatory problems or clients who are obese or very thin are also more susceptible. Nursing care is aimed at prevention, as once a pressure sore occurs, more skilled nursing care is required. The home health aide must pay particular attention to the bony prominence areas on the client. Skin should be cleansed when necessary and at routine intervals. The aide should avoid hot water and use a mild cleansing agent that minimizes irritation and dryness of the skin. If soap is used on the skin it must be completely rinsed off, as soap has a drying effect on the skin. Care must be exerted to minimize the force or friction used on the skin as it is cleansed. If the skin gets dry, it is more vulnerable to the development of pressure sores. If the client is incontinent or has wound drainage that cannot be controlled, underpads or briefs that absorb moisture and present a quick-drying surface to the skin can be used. Topical ointments that act as barriers to moisture can be used with the briefs. A nutritious high-protein diet should be offered and, if need be, a nutritional supplement can be given to the client. Nutrition plays a big part in the development of pressure sores. Once an individual becomes malnourished, pressure sores can develop quickly if the client is bedridden. The client also needs to be kept as mobile as possible. It is important that the client's position be changed often and passive range-of-motion exercises be provided as part of a daily routine.

Many special devices are available to place on the bed or on the specific part of the body to aid in the prevention of pressure sores. Examples are alternating air pressure mattress, eggcrate mattress, gel foam cushion for wheelchairs, lamb's wool or sheepskin pad, bed cradle, elbow pad, heel pad, and ankle elevator.

An alternating air pressure mattress is a mattress filled with air. This works by continuously changing the pressure areas on the client's back. One can improvise an air mattress designed for camping instead of buying a medical air mattress. A water mattress is also effective in reducing pressure on the skin, but causes problems when transferring clients in and out of bed, because it is not as firm as a regular mattress.

An eggcrate mattress is a mattress made of foam rubber that is molded like an egg crate. They are inexpensive but effective in reducing pressure on the skin. A gel foam cushion is a special cushion filled with a solution or gel. This style of cushion is effective in the prevention of pressure sores for a client who sits in a wheelchair for long periods of time.

Sheepskin or lamb's wool pads prevent pressure sores by acting as a barrier between the client's skin and the sheets. A bed cradle is another device to keep linens off the client's legs and feet. In the home a client may substitute a box or other device to keep linens off the legs and feet.

These special devices can prevent the skin from rubbing against the bedclothes, but do not take the place of good skin care.

The home health aide should watch for skin irritation when applying braces and splints, and report the first sign of a reddened area to the nurse.

Applying Over-the-Counter (OTC) Ointments. There are numerous types of creams, salves, and ointments available today that can be applied to the skin. Some are used for infections, others for rashes, and some for relief of pain or just plain lubrication of the skin. Home health aides are allowed to apply these ointments to the unbroken skin areas. Be sure to read the directions on the care plan for each ointment that needs to be applied. Double-check to make sure you are applying them to the right area of the body. Always wear gloves when you are applying the ointments so as not to absorb them into your own body.

Applying Skin Dressings. Occasionally it may be necessary to apply a dressing for minor cuts and scrapes. Applying a clean dressing and ointment to broken skin helps to protect the area from contamination and irritation. Although most dressings will be changed by the nurse, occasionally the dressing change is done by the home health aide, with the approval of the nurse. In these cases, the aide should observe and record the color, amount, and consistency of the drainage, the progress of the healing, and the surrounding skin condition. Refer to Procedure 36.

36 Procedure

Applying Clean Dressing and Ointment to Broken Skin

Purpose

- To help skin heal and avoid infection.
- For relief of pain

Procedure

1. Assemble supplies:
   disposable gloves
   two or more 4 × 4 gauze pads prepackaged
   over-the-counter ointment (if ordered)
   receptacle for wastes (e.g., plastic bag)
   tape and scissors
2. Wash your hands and apply gloves.
3. Tell client what you plan to do.
4. Position client so area with dressing is accessible while maintaining client comfort.
5. Remove old dressing. If the dressing does not lift off easily, pour warm water over it to loosen it. Discard used dressing in open waste receptacle (plastic bag). Note color, amount of drainage, and condition of surrounding skin.
6. Open the package of gauze pads without touching the pads. Be careful not to have dressing touch bed linens or client's clothing. Cut tape. Apply medication in a thin layer to the affected area. Apply ointment if ordered. Apply dressing. Do not touch center of dressing. Hold

all dressings on the corners only. Apply tape correctly.

7. Position client comfortably.
8. Discard wastes and return supplies to storage. Be sure to follow standard precautions throughout this procedure.
9. Remove gloves and wash hands.
10. Record observations of the wound and skin condition. Report signs of redness, swelling, heat, foul odor, or amount of drainage. Document that dressing was changed. In addition, report client complaints of pain around the wound.

Topical Applications to Unbroken Skin

1. Obtain correct topical medication. Check label of medication with care plan.
2. Wash hands and apply gloves.
3. Position client so area is accessible, while maintaining client comfort.
4. Apply medication in a thin layer to affected area only. Note color and appearance of skin. Is the affected area larger or smaller? Is there drainage? Is the skin red?
5. Remove gloves and reposition client.
6. Wash hands.
7. Return medication to correct storage area.
8. Chart application [treatment] and appearance of skin.

HYGIENE

Good hygiene is an important part of the care a home health aide provides to a client. Practicing good hygiene is important to maintain skin integrity, prevent infection, as well as to refresh and clean the client. The home health aide may be responsible for providing bathing, oral care, and personal care to the client. It is important for the aide to be sensitive to cultural reactions of clients with regard to providing this type of care. A client's cultural ideas about health, illness, hygiene, and rules for behavior may be different from your own. It will be helpful for you to understand your client's customs, practices, and beliefs so you can provide the best care and be respectful of individual differences. If you are unsure of your client's cultural patterns with regard to personal hygiene, it is a good idea to talk with your case manager.

Bathing a Client

A tub bath or shower will clean and refresh the client, as well as stimulate the circulation in the skin. While bathing a client, the aide should check the client's skin for any signs of irritation. Procedure 37 demonstrates the proper procedure for assisting with a tub bath or shower.

37 Procedure

Assisting with Tub Bath or Shower

Purpose

- To clean and refresh the client
- To check client's skin for signs of skin breakdown
- To stimulate circulation in the skin

Procedure

1. If possible, plan the tub bath or shower for a time convenient for the client. A tub bath or shower should not take more than 15 minutes unless there is a special reason for a longer bath.
2. Assemble needed supplies and place in bathroom:
   clean clothing
   bath seat or stool
   2 washcloths and towels
   shampoo (if needed)
   plastic pitcher (if shampooing client's hair)
   hose attachment
   comb and brush
   skidproof bath mat
   soap
3. Wash hands.
4. Tell client what you plan to do.
5. Fill tub one-third full with warm water. **CAUTION:** Test the temperature with a thermometer or inside the wrist to be sure it will not burn the client. The water should be about 115°F (46°C). Place a skidproof bath mat in the bottom of the tub. If client is taking a shower, regulate the flow and be sure the temperature is correct.
6. Assist the client to sit on a chair or on the closed toilet seat. Help the client undress. Place soiled clothing in the hamper. Close the bathroom door so the client will not be chilled.

7. For a tub bath, help client to sit on the edge of the tub. If there is a safety bar, have client hold onto it. When client has gained balance, help the client to turn and lift both legs into the tub. Give assistance by supporting the client under the arms and helping the client to slowly sit down in the tub facing the faucets. If the client cannot sit in the tub, place a bath stool in the water. Help the client to sit on the stool.

8. If the client needs a shampoo, wet the hair, rub in shampoo, lather, and massage head. If possible, have the client tilt head back. Pour water over the head using the pitcher, or attach the hose to the faucet and use it to rinse the head. Repeat shampoo, massage, and rinse. Client may hold a washcloth over the eyes during the shampoo to prevent soap from entering the eyes.

9. Give the client a washcloth and soap. Allow the client to do as much bathing or washing as possible. Assist as necessary. If shower is running, make sure the flow is not too heavy; check water temperature often.

10. Remain beside the tub at all times during the bath or shower. CAUTION: Be ready to help the client at any moment. If the client should feel faint, empty water from the tub, cover the client with a towel to avoid unnecessary chilling, and lower the

client's head between the client's knees.

11. For a tub bath, help the client raise out of the water. Assist the client out of the water. Assist the client to sit on the edge of the tub. Bring client's legs over to outside and assist the client to stand. Allow the client to sit on the closed toilet seat or the chair.

12. Make certain that the client's body is thoroughly dry. Do not dry the client by rubbing with the towel, instead pat the area to be dried. Help dry difficult areas such as the back and shoulders. Be sure underarms are completely dry. Protect the skin from unwanted moisture with a moisture barrier lotion. Pay special attention to the feet. Dry soles of feet and between toes. Apply lotion to the client's skin as required.

13. For a shower, make sure the client is completely washed and rinsed and then turn off the shower. Towel dry and assist client out of the shower area.

14. Assist client to dress in clean clothes.

15. Help client back to bed, to a wheelchair, or to a chair.

16. Return to the bathroom and drain and clean tub or shower stall. Place dirty clothes and towels in the hamper. Put supplies away.

17. Wash hands.

18. Document procedure, any observations, and client's reaction.

Giving a Bed Bath

If the client is bedridden, the bath will need to be given in bed. Procedure 38 demonstrates the proper way to give a bed bath. A partial bath is given on days a complete bed bath is not given. A partial bath is given the same as a bed bath, except that the legs and feet are not washed. If the client is able, this type of bath can be given by the bathroom sink.

38 Procedure

Giving a Bed Bath

Purpose

- To clean and refresh the client
- To stimulate circulation
- To observe the client's skin for signs of skin breakdown

NOTE: The bed bath is usually given in the morning. This procedure is one of a series of procedures performed in the same time period. This will require the home health aide to organize and plan ahead. All materials and supplies needed can be gathered and placed conveniently so that each separate procedure can be completed easily.

- If client needs to use the bedpan, offer it before the bath.
- Gather supplies needed for making the bed and put them near at hand.
- Organize materials needed for oral hygiene, denture care, and nail care to move easily from one procedure to another as needed.

Procedure

1. Gather supplies for the complete series of procedures including:
   body wash and disposable gloves (optional)
   washcloths and towels
   fresh clothes
   body lotion and deodorant
   change of bed linens
   bath basin, two-thirds filled with water
2. Close windows to prevent a draft from blowing on the client. If there are other people in the home, ask not to be disturbed. Close the door for privacy.

3. Wash your hands.
4. Tell client what you plan to do.
5. Remove blankets, leaving the top sheet covering the client. Place one pillow under client's head.
6. Pull out bottom part of top sheet so it covers client loosely. Remove client's clothing.
7. Place a basin of water on the chair or dresser at the bedside.
8. Assist client in moving to side of bed nearest you. Apply gloves.
9. Moisten washcloth, squeeze out excess water. Form a mitt by folding a washcloth around one hand (Figure 14-2).
10. Using clear water only, wash the client's eyes first. Wipe from the inner corner to the outer corner of the eye. Using a mild soap, wash the face, ears, and neck. Pat dry with the face towel.
11. Lift client's farthest arm and lay a bath towel under the area to keep bed dry. Wash with body wash, rinse, and pat dry, making sure the arm, underarm, and hand are cleaned and thoroughly dry. Repeat for other arm. Apply underarm deodorant or bath powder if client desires.
12. Give nail care and clean under nails. Trim nails *if allowed*. Refer to Procedure 46 for a description of the proper method to give nail care.
13. Place towel over client's chest, then pull sheet down to waist. Working under the towel, wash with body wash, rinse, and dry

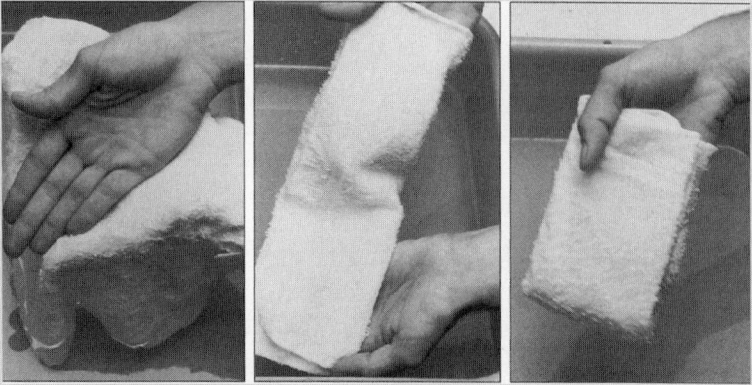

Figure 14-2 To make a bath mitt, wrap the washcloth around one hand, bringing the free-hanging end up over palm and tucking in the end.

chest. Rinse and dry area under a woman's breasts carefully to prevent skin irritation and redness. The abdomen is washed after the chest is washed. Replace sheet over chest.

14. Have client bend one knee. Fold sheet up from the foot of the bed. Expose the thigh, leg, and foot. Place a towel under the area, and put the basin on the towel, placing client's foot in basin. Wash and rinse foot. Remove the foot from the basin and dry it well.

15. Remove the basin from the bed. Follow the same procedure for the other leg and foot.

16. Lightly apply lotion on legs and feet if skin is dry (never massage legs).

17. Change the water in the basin before proceeding with the bath. If at any time during the bath the water becomes dirty or cool, change it.

18. Place bath towel lengthwise by the client's back and buttocks. Starting at the hairline use long, firm strokes while washing the back. Carefully wash the buttocks area.

19. Change the water at this point. Remember to wipe a female client from front to back. This method is highly recommended to reduce the spread of germs and prevent infection. Prepare washcloth with body wash and have client wash the genital area, if able. Rinse the cloth and have client wipe and dry the genitals, if capable. Remove gloves and wash hands.

20. Spread the towel under client's head and comb or brush hair.

21. Assist the client into clean clothes.

22. Remove the basin, dirty linens, and the other equipment away from the bed.

23. Change the bed linens using the procedure for making an occupied bed.

24. Leave the client in a comfortable position.

25. Wash your hands.

26. Document procedure and time, observations, and client's reaction.

A new type of bath introduced recently with much success is the bag bath. A commercial bag bath is very easy to use. Just put the package in the microwave for a few minutes and remove. The package contains five or six presoaked disposable washcloths. The aide bathes the client using one for the face, one for the arms and upper chest, one for the legs, another for the back, and the last one for the perineal area. The solution on the washcloth not only cleans the skin, but also gives the skin a pro-

tective coating so that it is less likely to break down. There is no need to dry the client because the solution is self-drying.

Back Rub

A back rub is helpful to increase the blood circulation to the back area, and to provide comfort and relaxation to the client. It is also a good opportunity for the aide to observe the skin for signs of skin breakdown. Procedure 39 demonstrates the proper way to give a back rub.

39 Procedure

Giving a Back Rub

Purpose
- To increase the blood circulation to the back area
- To give comfort to the client and provide relaxation
- To observe the skin for signs of skin breakdown

Procedure
1. Wash your hands.
2. Assemble supplies:
   small towel
   lotion
3. Provide privacy for the client.
4. Position client on back or side.
5. Place small amount of lotion on your hands. Rub together to warm the lotion.
6. Begin by starting at the base of the spine; rub toward the neck in the center of the back. Use both hands in one long stroke.
7. When reaching the neck, continue back down the sides of the back. When reaching the base of the spine, rub up the center again. Repeat several times.
8. If necessary, add more lotion and use a spiral motion for several minutes.
9. Remove excess lotion with small towel. Reposition client.
10. Wash hands and return supplies to proper place.
11. Record and report any sign of skin irritation.

Perineal Care

Part of good skin care includes keeping the perineum clean, which is the area from the genitals to the anus. Keeping the perineum clean is im-

portant to prevent infections, to prevent skin breakdown, and to reduce odor. Procedures 40 and 41 demonstrate the proper way to give female and male perineal care.

40
Procedure

Giving Female Perineal Care

Purpose

- To prevent infections
- To clean the genital and anal area
- To prevent skin breakdown
- To prevent odors

Procedure

1. Assemble supplies:
   disposable gloves
   soap or perineal wash
   basin
   water
   washcloths and towel
2. Wash your hands and apply gloves.
3. Tell client what you plan to do, and provide for privacy.
4. Position client on back and place sheet or thin cotton blanket over client.
5. Position towel under client's buttocks.
6. Wet washcloth with soap and water. Help the client flex her knees and spread her legs if able.
7. Separate the vulva. Clean downward from front to back with one stroke, first the inner labia, and then rinse. Repeat with outer labia. Repeat on other side. Dry with the towel.
8. Help the client lower her legs and turn onto her side away from you.
9. Apply soap or perineal wash to washcloth.
10. Clean the rectal area by cleaning from the vagina to the anus with one stroke. Rinse washcloth and repeat until area is clean.
11. Pat the area dry with towel.
12. Observe area for any unusual redness, open areas, or abnormal discharge.
13. Cover client and remove equipment.
14. Clean equipment and remove gloves.
15. Wash hands.
16. Document procedure completion and any abnormal observations.

41
Procedure

Giving Male Perineal Care

Purpose

- To prevent spread of infection
- To promote comfort
- To prevent odors
- To clean the genital and anal area

Procedure

1. Repeat steps 1 through 6 as for female perineal care.
2. Grasp penis gently with gloved hand. Clean the tip of the penis using gentle circular motion. You will need to pull back the foreskin if the man is uncircumcised. Start at the urinary meatus and work outward. Rinse the area well and dry. Return the foreskin to its original position.

3. Clean the remaining portion of the penis with firm downward strokes. Rinse well.
4. Wash the scrotum and pat dry.

5. Turn client to side and clean rectal area in the same way as for the female.
6. Follow steps 11 through 16 as for female perineal care.

Oral Care

Some clients will be unable to give themselves oral care. In these instances, the aide must assist the client with oral hygiene, including brushing teeth and caring for dentures. Procedures 42 and 43 demonstrate the proper ways to assist with routine oral hygiene and to care for dentures.

42   Procedure

Assisting with Routine Oral Hygiene

Purpose

• To keep client's teeth, tongue and gums healthy
• To refresh client's mouth and improve appetite

Procedure—Using Toothettes and Lemon Glycerine Swabs

1. Assemble equipment:
   disposable gloves
   toothettes or lemon glycerine swabs
   paper towels or small towel
   small container of water
   lip cream
2. Wash your hands and apply gloves. Tell the client what you plan to do.
3. Place small towels or paper towel under the client's head and turn head to one side.
4. Dip toothettes into water or mouthwash (optional). Lemon glycerine swabs can be placed directly from package into the client's mouth.

5. Insert into mouth and swab gums, teeth, and tongue. If need be, repeat with clean swab.
6. Apply pleasant-tasting lip lubricant to lips.
7. Place used swabs in paper towels.
8. Remove your gloves and add to paper towel for disposal.
9. Wash your hands.
10. Document procedure. **Note:** If a client is a mouth breather or is terminally ill, this procedure will need to be done at least every two hours.

Procedure—Routine Oral Care

1. Assemble needed equipment and supplies:
   disposable gloves
   toothbrush
   toothpaste
   glass of water
   towel
   small bowl or basin or emesis basin

mouthwash if available
tissues or moisten washcloth
2. Wash your hands and apply gloves.
3. Tell client what you plan to do and position the client in a sitting position (if allowed).
4. Place a towel over the client's chest and under the chin.
5. Moisten toothbrush and apply toothpaste.
6. Let client brush teeth, if able. If not, carefully brush the client's teeth (Figures 14-3A through D).
7. Client or aide should brush the teeth holding the brush at a right angle to the teeth, starting at the gumline and working upwards.
8. Give the client a glass of water; be sure client rinses mouth well. Hold the basin underneath the client's chin and have client return the fluid. If mouthwash is available, have client rinse mouth with the mouthwash.
9. Give the client a moistened washcloth to wipe mouth.
10. Reposition client.
11. Clean and replace equipment.
12. Remove gloves and wash hands.
13. Document procedure completed and time, any observations, and client's reaction.

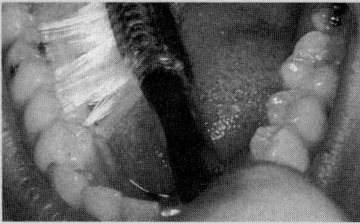

Figure 14-3A Hold soft, wet toothbrush at a 90° angle and brush back teeth.

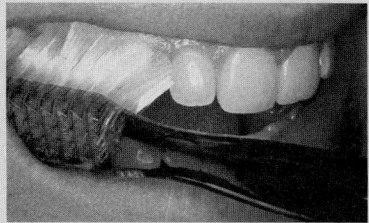

Figure 14-3B Brush top and bottom teeth thoroughly, including the gums.

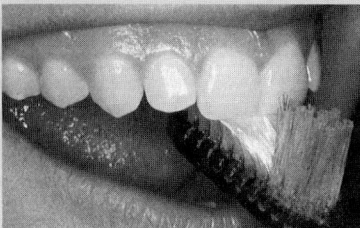

Figure 14-3C Be sure to brush behind the front teeth.

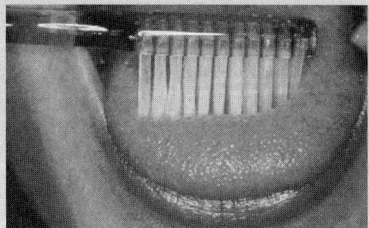

Figure 14-3D Brush tongue.

43   Procedure

Caring for Dentures

Purpose

- To clean dentures and refresh client's mouth
- To provide opportunity to observe client's gums for irritation or soreness
- To stimulate client's appetite

Procedure

1. Assemble the needed supplies:
   denture brush or toothbrush
   denture cleaner or toothpaste
   denture cleaning tablet (e.g., Efferdent)
   denture cup
   disposable gloves
   mouthwash and small cup
   emesis basin
   washcloth and small towel
2. Wash your hands and apply gloves.
3. Tell client what you plan to do.
4. Ask client to remove dentures (Figure 14-4A), helping if needed. Place dentures in padded container or denture cup. Be very careful in handling client's dentures. They may become slippery to hold.
5. Place approximately 2 to 3 inches of water and a washcloth in bottom of sink (Figure 14-4B). This will protect the dentures in case they are dropped. Turn on cold water and brush all surfaces of the upper and lower plate (Figure 14-4C). Rinse denture cup and fill with cold water. If the client is not going to wear the dentures, place denture cleaning tablets in the container. If the client is going to wear the dentures, take the clean dentures in the cup to the client.
6. Assist client to rinse mouth with mouthwash. Have client expel rinse into emesis basin.
7. Toothettes can be used to clean the gums and tongue (Figure 14-4D). This is a good time to observe the client's mouth for signs of irritation or sores.
8. Have client insert dentures in mouth, if able. Some clients may have denture adhesive applied to the area of the dentures that adheres to the gums. If you need to apply this paste, use it sparingly, as a little bit goes a long way.
9. Remove equipment and gloves.
10. Wash your hands.
11. Document procedure completed and any abnormal observations.

NOTE: If the client only wears the upper dentures and not the lower dentures, do store the lower dentures in a designated area in a container that is clearly marked. Occasionally, you will find clients whose dentures do not fit, and they most likely need to be relined by a dentist because they are very loose. Even though they are loose, please encourage the client to wear the dentures, as this will prevent the client's gums from receding more.

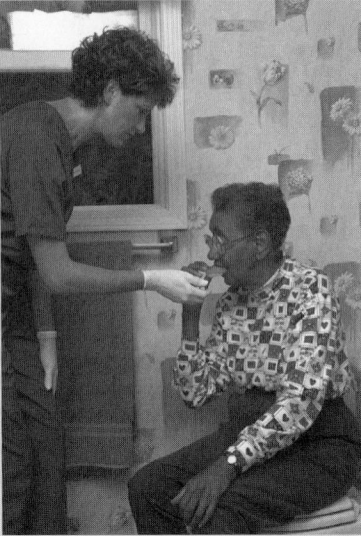

Figure 14-4A   Ask client to remove dentures.

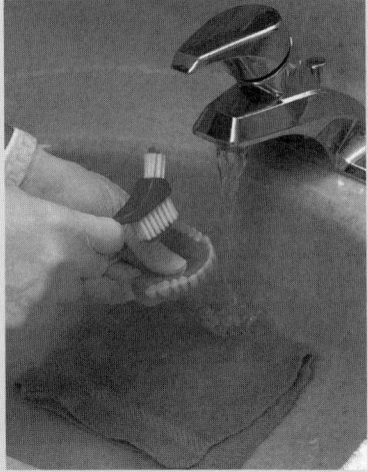

Figure 14-4B   When cleaning dentures, use cool running water and protect the dentures by placing washcloth in the bottom of the sink.

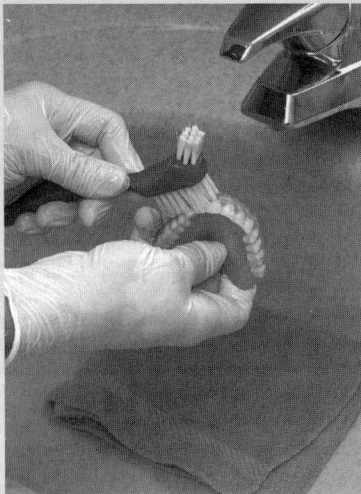

Figure 14-4C   Be sure to brush all surfaces of the dentures.

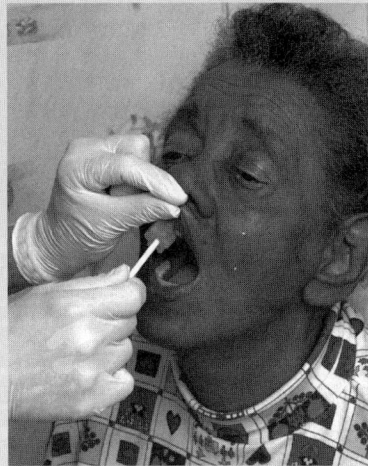

Figure 14-4D   Use toothette and clean inside of mouth. Remember to clean the tongue.

Personal Care and Grooming

The home health aide will be responsible for providing personal care to clients to keep clients well-groomed so that they look and feel good about themselves. Personal care will include shaving, nail care, and shampooing. Depending on the needs of your client, personal care may also include performing a warm foot soak. Procedures 44, 45, 46, and 47 demonstrate the proper ways to shave a male client, perform a warm foot soak, give nail care, and shampoo hair in bed.

44

Procedure

Shaving the Male Client

Purpose

• To remove unwanted facial hair

NOTE: Shaving can be planned for the same time that other daily hygiene tasks are done. If the client is taking a blood-thinning medication like warfarin, *always* use an electric razor. An ordinary razor may cause excessive bleeding from a cut in the facial area. For shaving, the electric razor is usually the easiest to use. However, it may be necessary to use a safety razor or disposable razor. In some instances, older women also may request to have facial hair shaved to improve cosmetic appearance. Remember standard precautions; wear gloves.

Procedure

1. Wash hands and apply gloves.
2. Ask client if he wants a shave.
3. Assemble needed supplies:
   disposable gloves
   razor and shaving cream
   basin of hot water
   washcloth and towel
   aftershave lotion (optional)
4. Position client in sitting position and place towel under chin and across his chest.

5. Apply shaving cream (Figure 14-5A). With one hand, pull the skin tight above area to be shaved. With razor in other hand, gently take short, even strokes. Shave in the direction the hair grows (Figures 14-5B through D). If client is able, let him do as much as possible. If feasible, have the client shave with a mirror in front of him.
6. Rinse the razor frequently. After shave is completed, rinse face and pat dry.
7. Apply aftershave lotion (optional).
8. Clean equipment and return to designated area.
9. Remove gloves and wash hands.
10. Document procedure completed and any abnormal observations.

NOTE: If using an electric razor, apply preelectric lotion before using the razor, as it will make the skin easier to shave. Hold the skin taut as you work the razor around the face. Clean inside of razor each time you use it. If cutting blades get dull, ask to have the blades replaced. It is almost impossible to shave an older man's wrinkled face with a dull electric razor.

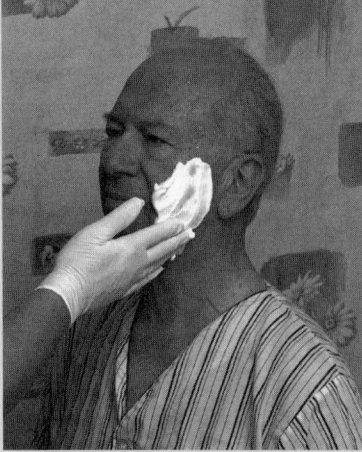

Figure 14-5A Apply shaving cream to face.

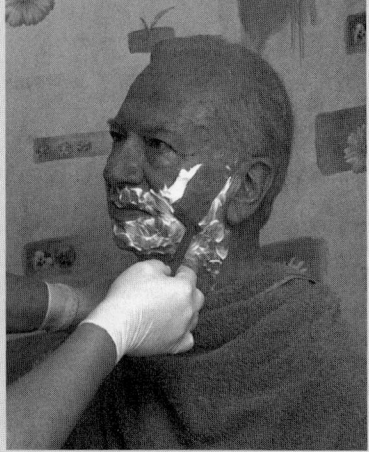

Figure 14-5B Shave in direction of hair growth.

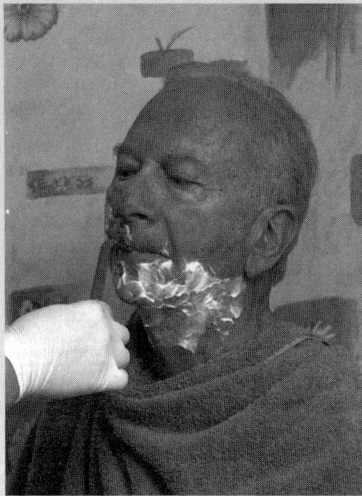

Figure 14-5C Be sure to shave area under nose and top of chin.

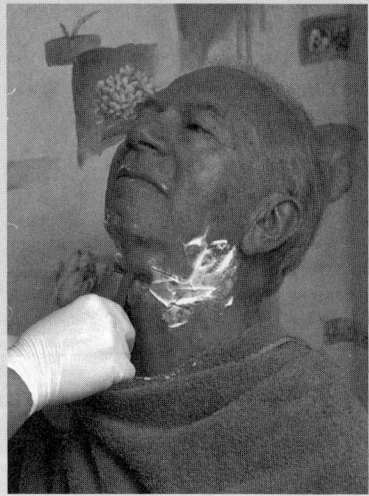

Figure 14-5D Shave area under the client's chin.

45

Procedure

Performing a Warm Foot Soak

Purpose

- To stimulate circulation in a client's feet
- To relieve pain or discomfort
- To soften the toenails to make them easier to cut

Procedure

1. Assemble equipment:
   disposable gloves
   large basin—plastic oblong dishpan
   warm water—100° to 110°F
   large plastic garbage bag or small rug
   small thin blanket
   2 towels
2. Wash hands and apply gloves.
3. Tell client what you plan to do.
4. Have client sit in comfortable chair if possible.
5. Place small rug on floor and place basin of water on top of rug.
6. Remove client's shoes and socks and slowly place client's feet in basin of warm water. Be sure to follow any special instructions for special soaps or solutions that might be ordered.
7. Place thin blanket over the client's legs and feet.
8. Replenish water as necessary to maintain proper temperature.
9. Soak feet for about 20 to 30 minutes.
10. Remove feet from the basin and pat dry. Be sure to dry the skin well in between toes. When feet are dry, massage lotion on both feet. Put socks and shoes on client's feet.
11. Clean up equipment and return to storage area.
12. Remove gloves and wash hands.
13. Record treatment and any abnormal observations such as swollen ankles or sores on feet.

46

Procedure

Giving Nail Care

Purpose

- To keep the client's nails clean and well groomed
- To observe for signs of irritation

NOTE: You are not allowed to cut the fingernails or toenails of clients who are diabetic or clients with poor circulation to their legs. Be aware if client is on a blood thinner medication. Cuts can produce excessive bleeding. Check with your supervisor about your agency's policy about cutting nails. Some agencies will allow a home health aide to cut nails whereas others will not allow home health aides to cut nails. Nail care is usually given at bath time or when there is a need because of a broken nail or hangnail. A manicure may be done to make the client feel more attractive. In the elderly, you might note very thick toenails, which require special clippers to cut; this usually is done by a podiatrist (health care provider who specializes in foot problems).

Procedure

1. Assemble supplies:
   soap, water, and basin
   nail brush
   towel and lotion, preferably lanolin lotion
   small scissors or clippers
   emery board or nail file
2. Wash your hands.
3. Tell client what you plan to do.
4. Soak toenails or fingernails in soap and water for 10 minutes.
5. Brush nails with nail brush. Clean under nails. Rinse well. Dry hands and nails.
6. Wear gloves if clipping nails/toenails.
7. If nails are too long, make a straight cut for toenails and a curve cut for fingernails. Check to make sure that you are allowed to cut nails. If you accidentally cut a client's skin while cutting nails, remember to use standard precautions. Report the cut to your nurse.
8. Use file or emery board and smooth edges of nails.
9. Massage lotion on the hands or feet.
10. Clean the basin, brush, and scissors or clippers. Return equipment to proper place.
11. Wash your hands.
12. Document procedure, any observations, and client's reaction.

47 Procedure

Shampooing Hair in Bed

Purpose

- To clean the hair and scalp
- To stimulate circulation in the scalp
- To make the client feel and look better
- To prevent accumulation of dandruff or formation of scalp crusts

NOTE: Dry shampoos can also be used if the client is too weak to tolerate a wet shampoo. Follow the directions on the package. If you need to shampoo a client's hair and the client is mobile, it is better to do it in the kitchen sink than the bathroom sink. It is easier to bend an older client's head forward rather than backward for the shampoo.

Procedure

1. Assemble equipment:
   shampoo and hair conditioner or rinse
   3 to 4 towels
   inflatable shampoo basin
   4 large empty garbage bags

large pitcher or empty gallon milk container
comb and brush
large empty bucket
disposable gloves

2. Wash your hands and apply gloves.
3. Tell client what you plan to do.
4. Prepare bed by applying plastic garbage bag under head with large towel on top of it.
5. Place bucket on floor with a plastic bag under the bucket. This allows the water to go from the basin into the bucket.
6. Place shampoo basin on top of large towel on bed and gently place client's head in basin (Figure 14-6A). Be sure to pad the client's neck area with a small towel.
7. Place one end of a plastic bag under end of basin and the other end in the plastic bucket.
8. Wet hair with warm water. The client can use a washcloth to cover the eyes for protection (Figure 14-6B).

9. Apply shampoo to the head, lather well, and massage scalp with your fingertips (Figure 14-6C). If a specific shampoo is ordered, follow any special instructions.
10. Rinse hair with water thoroughly, making sure to remove all traces of shampoo (Figure 14-6D).
11. If necessary, reapply shampoo, lather well, and rinse thoroughly.
12. Apply hair conditioner or rinse. Follow directions on the bottle.
13. Dry client's hair with large towel. Comb and brush hair. If female, you may need to set hair on rollers. If hair dryer is available, blow-dry hair. Remove and clean equipment. Return equipment to proper place.
14. Remove gloves and wash hands.
15. Observe scalp for buildup of dandruff or any other substance, sores or any break in the skin, or redness.
16. Record completion and any abnormal observations.

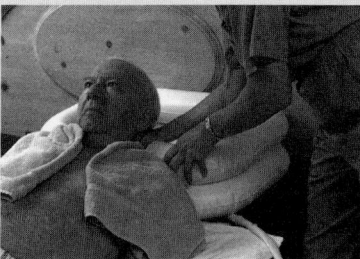

Figure 14-6A   Placing tray under client's head for bed shampoo.

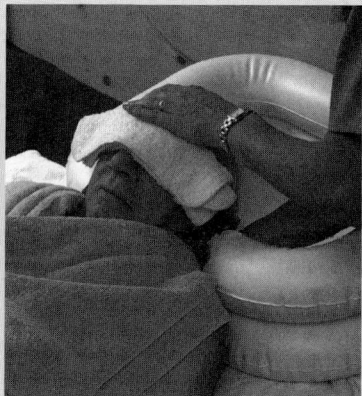

Figure 14-6B   Place washcloth or towel under client's neck and cover client's eyes with a washcloth.

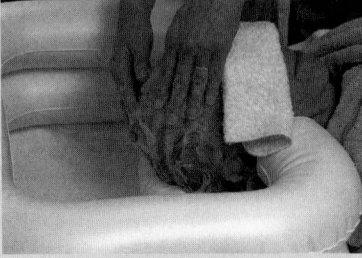

Figure 14-6C Wet hair and apply shampoo, using fingertips to massage scalp.

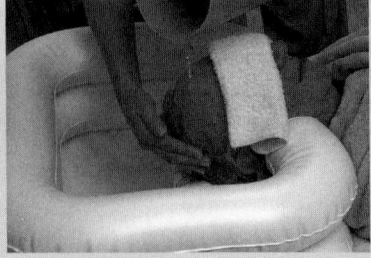

Figure 14-6D Rinse hair to remove all shampoo and apply hair conditioner.

UNIT 15

Musculoskeletal System: Arthritis, Body Mechanics, and Restorative Care

MUSCULOSKELETAL SYSTEM

The musculoskeletal system is made up of bones and muscles. It protects the internal body organs and makes body movement possible. The skull, for instance, forms a protective covering for the brain. The spinal column surrounds the spinal nerves leading from the brain.

There are more than 200 bones in the body (Figure 15-1A and B). Bones are joined together by tough elastic fibers called ligaments.

Joints allow the bones to be moved in certain ways. The elbows and knees have hinge joints, which move in only two directions like hinges on a door. The joints at the shoulder and pelvis are ball and socket joints. They provide circular movements. The wrist, ankles, and spinal column have gliding joints connecting the various bones. These allow only a limited sliding movement.

Skeletal muscles are attached to the bones by tendons and are stretched over joints. Certain muscles produce motion by pulling on the bone when they receive messages from the nervous system. These muscles are called voluntary muscles because their movement is controlled by the brain.

Other muscles, called involuntary muscles, form the walls of organs. They, too, receive messages through the nervous system but they work automatically, or without any conscious effort by the individual.

Common Disorders of the Musculoskeletal System

The musculoskeletal system can be invaded by disease-causing microorganisms. However, the most common

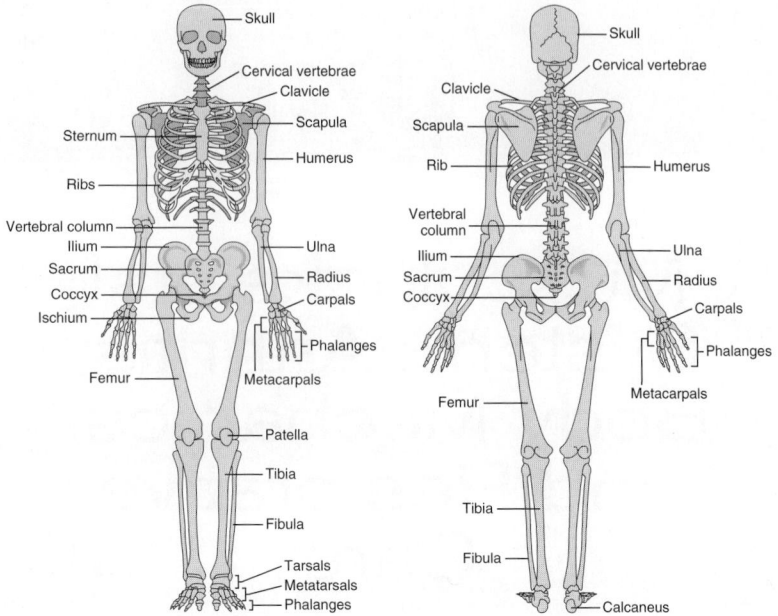

Figure 15-1   Bones of the skeleton. A. Anterior view B. Posterior view

problems are injuries that are caused by falls.

A sprain is a partial tear of a muscle, tendon, or ligament. Sprains usually involve damage to blood vessels and nerves. The site of the sprain may appear swollen and black and blue, with sharp intermittent pain that increases on movement. The cause of a sprain is usually due to trauma to a joint, such as falling down steps when wearing high heels or getting one's foot caught in a door. Treatment consists of immobilizing the joint with an elastic bandage, elevating the extremity, applying ice, and prescribing rest for the client. Depending on the severity of the sprain, it will generally take three to six weeks or longer to heal.

Bursitis is inflammation of a bursa, which is an enclosed sac containing fluid, which is found between muscles and tendons. The joints most affected with this disorder are the shoulder, elbow (sometimes referred to as tennis elbow), and the knee (sometimes referred to as housemaid's knee). The client may complain of tenderness, swelling, pain, and limitation of movement at the site. Treatment varies but generally consists of rest, painkillers, application of moist heat, and injection of steroids to the affected joint.

Fractures.   A fracture is a break in a bone. A closed fracture is a break in the bone but not in the skin. An open fracture is a break in the skin and the bone is fractured. With this type of break there is a high risk of infection due to the break in the skin where microorganisms can easily enter. Fractures are treated with surgery, cast application, and/or traction. Healing of the bones generally takes at least six weeks for a younger adult and a little longer for an older adult. Procedure 62, presented later in this unit, demonstrates the proper method of caring for casts.

DEFINITION OF ARTHRITIS

Arthritis means inflammation of a joint. Many people complain of rheumatism in relationship to their many aches and pains. The Arthritis Foundation states that arthritis is the number one crippler in the United States, affecting one in seven people. There are several types of arthritis. The two main ones are rheumatoid arthritis and osteoarthritis. Other types of arthritis are gout and ankylosing spondylitis. Arthritis affects 50% of persons over 65 years of age. Twice as many women as men are afflicted with the disease. The major warning signs of inflammatory arthritis are:

- Swelling in one or more joints
- Early morning stiffness
- Recurring pain or tenderness in any joint
- Inability to move a joint normally
- Obvious redness and warmth in a joint
- Unexplained weight loss, fever, or weakness
- Symptoms and signs of the above persisting for two weeks

Other infections such as gonorrhea, tuberculosis, syphilis, Lyme disease, and streptococcal infections can also cause arthritis. There is no cure for the disease. It can be managed with diet, medication, surgery, and exercise.

Rheumatoid Arthritis

Rheumatoid arthritis generally affects people between the ages of 20 and 45, but it is also seen in younger children and older adults. It affects more women than men. The cause of this condition is that the immune system that normally protects the body works the opposite way and fights the body. It is a disease that affects the entire body; the joints are affected the most. There is symmetrical swelling (both hands or both feet are affected, not just one side). It can occasionally cause problems with the muscles, skin, blood vessels, nerves, and eyes. The client may have a very mild case, which might cause mild discomfort, or a severe case where widespread joint deformities are present. For clients the morning is usually the most difficult part of the day or after a long period of inactivity, since at these times the pain increases and the stiffness is greater. The characteristic signs and symptoms of this disease are joint pain, stiffness and redness of the joints, and difficulty with range of motion. Other less common signs are mild fever, weight loss, and fatigue. As the disease progresses, joint problems increase in severity. These deformities of the joints are seen in the hips, knees, wrists, fingers, and ankles. This type of arthritis affects more than 2 million people in the United States.

Osteoarthritis

Another term for osteoarthritis is "wear and tear" arthritis. This type of arthritis affects the weight-bearing joints, such as the spine, hip, and knee. The affected joint or joints become enlarged and painful. If the finger joint is affected, the swelling occurs closest to the fingernail. The larger joints are the ones that cause the most pain and discomfort. It is most often seen in clients over 65 years of age. The cause of this type of arthritis is not clearly understood. A few of the possible causes might be attributed to the aging process, obesity, heredity, stress, trauma, unbalanced hormone levels, or overuse of the joint. This is the most common type of arthritis and it affects more than 20 million people in the United States.

Gout is a form of arthritis that affects mainly men over the age of 40. This type of arthritis is due to the presence of too much uric acid in the client's system. The first sign of this disease is a painful big toe. It can also affect other joints such as the foot, ankle, and wrist. These areas of the body have little out-pouches or protruding lesions called tophi that contain abnormal amounts of uric acid (see Figure 15–4B). The affected joint becomes extremely painful. This condition is treated with a low-purine diet, limiting the use of alcohol, and giving prescriptions drugs such as colchicine or allopurinol.

MANAGEMENT OF ARTHRITIS

Arthritis is a chronic degenerative (weakens and becomes abnormal) disease. It is generally managed with diet therapy, an exercise program, medication, and surgery. In some cases assistive devices can also be helpful.

Diet Therapy

The diet is individualized to meet the person's needs. Individuals crippled with arthritis may have a few of the following problems that interfere with their nutritional status.
- Pain may be a factor in lack of appetite.
- Decreased activity can cause weight gain, immobility, and pressure sore development.
- Impaired movement may cause lack of energy for preparing foods and grocery shopping.

As a home health aide, you will most likely be employed to work in the home to assist the client with cooking, cleaning, and laundry duties. The client will be able to assist you to do a few of these tasks but will tire easily. You need to encourage the client to do as much as possible. Be sure you do not overtire or rush the client. The client will need a longer time to accomplish a task.

Exercise

Another form of treatment for arthritis is exercise. Exercise can be passive (you do it for the client) or active (the client performs the exercise without assistance). The goals of the exercise program are to maintain complete joint movement and in some cases strengthen the muscles around the specific joint. The physical therapist will develop a care plan for your client.

Medication

The third method of treatment is through drug therapy. The specific drug used by clients will depend on many factors, such as:
- Severity of the arthritis
- Tolerance to the drug (aspirin may be the drug of choice, but many individuals with stomach problems cannot tolerate aspirin)
- Cost
- Type of arthritis (gout responds to certain drugs only)
- Client's response (some clients respond positively to a drug and others do not respond at all)
- Presence of other chronic diseases (if a client has a stomach ulcer, certain drugs cannot be prescribed)

Surgery

In the last 20 years, surgery has become successful in helping the arthritic client maintain independence. Surgeons can now replace arthritic knees and hips. Surgery can also be done on the client's spine, jaw, wrist, fingers, and shoulder. An aide may be employed to care for these clients on a temporary basis after they return home from the hospital. Clients will have their own individualized plan of care designed by a team consisting of the health care provider, nurse, physical therapist, occupational therapist, and case manager.

Nursing Care After Joint Replacement Surgery

Replacement of a joint is called an arthroplasty. The surgeon removes the damaged joint such as the knee or hip and replaces the joint with artificial parts, called prostheses. The client is hospitalized for about four to five days and then sent home. At home, this client will need assistance in dressing and walking. General guidelines for caring for a client who had total hip replacement or total knee replacement are:

- Have the client take sponge baths only. Do not shower or take a tub bath until staples are removed.
- Avoid movements that twist or cause pain, such as kneeling or strenuous exercises.
- Allow only the amount of weight on the affected hip or knee as instructed by the physical therapist.
- Walk often to keep the new hip or knee as mobile as possible.
- It is normal for the new hip or knee to be swollen and the client to have discomfort, especially on movement. Client can take painkiller as needed.
- Elevate the affected leg with a pillow in bed and when sitting in a chair.
- At first, the client will have a walker and gradually progress to the use of a cane as mobility of the knee increases.

- It is helpful for the client to have a long-handled gripper or picker-upper, elevated toilet seat, and long-handled shoehorn.
- The client may be sent home with an incentive spirometer, a device to help the client breathe more deeply.
- Ice packs may be ordered for 20 minutes to reduce swelling of the knee.
- Elastic stockings may used to help reduce the swelling in the affected joint.
- The site of the surgery will have a dressing applied and a nurse or health care provider will change this as needed. The home health aide should observe the site for an unusual amount of drainage or odorous drainage. Keep the area clean and dry.
- The aide may need to take the client to physical therapy sessions or, in some cases, the physical therapist may come to the client's home.

Assistive Devices

An aide employed in a home with a client with arthritis will need to take special care when moving or transferring a client. It is normal for the client to be able to do everything one day but the next day very little. Encourage the client to function at the highest level of wellness possible and to be as independent as possible.

PRINCIPLES OF GOOD BODY MECHANICS

The most common injuries for the home health aide involve the muscles, ligaments, and joints of the lower back. These injuries are caused by lifting, bending, pulling, twisting, and pushing incorrectly.

Much of your work as a home health aide requires physical effort. To avoid injury to yourself, use good techniques when you lift a client, transfer a client between bed and wheelchair, cook meals, do laundry, or even stand, sit, or walk. All require correct, careful, and efficient use of your muscles to prevent injury and reduce fatigue.

The way in which the body moves and keeps its balance through the use of all its parts is referred to as body mechanics. Use of body mechanics means that each part of the body works together.

Good body mechanics start with proper posture—the way you hold and position each part of your body. Correct posture means that there is a balance between your muscle groups and that the different parts of your body are in good alignment—in the correct position relative to each other.

Correct posture makes lifting, pulling, and pushing easier. Correct posture is important at all times—standing, sitting, walking, and lying. A good standing posture begins with having feet flat on the floor, separated by about 12 inches, knees slightly bent, arms at the sides, abdominal muscles tight.

Ten basic rules will help your body and muscles work well for you, prevent injury, and reduce fatigue.

1. Keep your back straight—do not twist or bend.
2. Keep your feet apart, to provide a good base of support.
3. Bend from the knees, particularly when lifting—do not bend from the waist or spine.
4. Use the weight of your body to help pull or push an object.
5. Use the strong muscles of your thighs and shoulders to do the work.
6. Hold objects close to your body. This allows your strong shoulder and thigh muscles to work most efficiently.
7. Avoid twisting your body as you work and bend. Pivot the whole body.
8. Push or pull, rather than lift.
9. Always get help if you feel you cannot do the lifting or moving on your own.
10. Synchronize movements with client or others; count 1 . . . 2 . . . 3 . . . and do the job together.

Remember, it is your body, they are your muscles, and you are responsible for the way you use them.

Applications of Good Body Mechanics to Client Care

Many client care procedures require moving and turning the client. To ensure the safety of the client and to avoid self-injury, the home health aide should apply the techniques of good body mechanics to the work situation. This means that the aide should do the following:

- Stand straight, rather than slouch. Keep the back and shoulder muscles in a straight line.
- Push, pull, slide, or roll the client whenever possible. Try to avoid lifting the client.
- When turning the client, try to make the movement smooth and fluid so that the entire body shifts at the same time.
- When repositioning the client in bed, turn the client toward you rather than away from you. This lessens the danger of the client falling out of bed and keeps your weight more evenly distributed.
- When walking with the client, remain on the client's weak side. Try to stay near chairs or a couch so you can quickly seat the client if the client tires.
- If the client becomes faint while walking, help the client to sit in a chair. If there is no chair nearby,

help the client slide slowly to the floor.

- When walking or transferring a client, remember to use a gait or transfer belt.

Procedure 48 demonstrates the proper method of using a transfer or gait belt. Procedure 49 demonstrates the proper method of dangling a client.

48 Procedure

Applying a Transfer or Gait Belt

Purpose

- Safely transfer a client or ambulate a client
- Prevent injury to client's shoulder while transferring

NOTE: There are various names for these belts (e.g., transfer, gait, or lift belt). When not using the belt on the client, the aide often wears the belt around the waist. If the aide needs it, it is right there and there will be no need to look for it. A transfer belt or gait belt is a wide canvas belt that is placed around the client's waist for the home health aide to hold onto when transferring or walking a client. The belts come in various styles and sizes.

Procedure

1. Assemble equipment: transfer belt
2. Tell the client what you plan to do.
3. Position client, to make application of belt possible. If the client is lying in bed, move the client up to a sitting position. If the client is sitting in a chair, ask the client to lean forward, so you can slide the belt around the client's waist.
4. Apply the belt around the client's waist over clothing, never over bare skin. It should be snug, but not too snug. The aide should be able to place two fingers in between the belt and the client's skin. Place the buckle side of the belt in the front.
5. When walking a client, place your hands under the belt in the back. Always walk the client holding on to the belt on the client's weak side.
6. If you are using the belt to transfer the client out of bed, place both hands under the belt and support the client to stand.
7. Remove the belt after you are done transferring or ambulating (walking) a client.

49 Procedure

Dangling a Client

Purpose

- To move the client's legs around to prevent blood clots
- To relieve pressure on client's back

NOTE: This procedure is usually done after surgery before a patient is allowed out of bed.

Procedure

1. Tell the client what you plan to do.
2. With hands supporting shoulder and back of client, sit client up in bed. Change position of hands and place hands under client's legs and slide legs over the side of the bed.
3. Once client is in sitting position with legs hanging loose over the outside of the bed (dangling), ask client to move legs around for a few minutes.
4. Check the pulse of the client to see if it is regular and strong. If client becomes faint, tip the client's head down for a few seconds.
5. After a few minutes, lay the client down in bed.
6. Record and document procedure and any abnormal signs.

POSITIONING

Often a home health aide will need to position a client with mobility impairments. Positioning can make the client more comfortable and assist the body to function more efficiently. The correct positioning can relieve pressure on body parts, aid in breathing, as well as preventing injury to the client. Some clients may need your assistance in positioning so that they can engage in activities such as eating, reading, watching television, or visiting. If the client is in the sitting position, you should check to make sure that the head is erect and the spine is in straight alignment. Body weight should be evenly distributed on the buttocks and thighs. Feet should be supported by the floor with ankles comfortably flexed. Forearms should be supported on an armrest, on the lap, or on a table positioned in front of the chair. For a side-lying position, pillows and other positioning supports should be correctly placed. The spinal column should be in correct alignment. Procedures 50 through 56 address many different positioning techniques and the proper procedures for each position.

50 Procedure

Turning the Client Toward You

Purpose

- To make the client more comfortable
- To change the client's position
- To improve circulation and reduce skin pressure

Procedure

1. Wash your hands.
2. Tell client what you are going to do.
3. Lift client's far leg and cross it over the leg that is nearest you.

4. Lift the far arm over the chest, bend the elbow, and bring the hand toward the client's shoulder. Position the nearest arm so you will not roll client on it when you turn him.

5. Place the hand nearest the head of the bed on the far shoulder and place your other hand on the client's hip on the far side.

6. Brace your one thigh against the side of the bed and smoothly roll client toward you. Make sure that the client's upper leg comes over and bend it at the knee to ensure that the new position is stable.

7. Go to opposite side of bed and place your hands over the client's shoulder and pull upper body to the center of the bed. Place your hands over client's hips and pull the rest of the client's body to the center of the bed and into good body alignment.

8. Place a pillow against the client's back and secure it by pushing part under the client's back. The client's upper arm also should be supported with a pillow.

9. Support the knee, ankle, and foot of the upper leg with a pillow, which also prevents the knees and ankles from rubbing against each other and causing skin irritation. Cover client.

10. Wash your hands.

11. Document procedure completion, time, and client's reaction.

51

Procedure

Moving the Client up in Bed Using the Drawsheet

Purpose

- To move client up in bed with minimum discomfort
- To relieve pressure on body parts

NOTE: Very often a client will slide down in the bed away from the headboard. This is uncomfortable for the client. The sheets become wrinkled and undue pressure may be placed on the bony prominences, allowing the formation of pressure sores. You will need a partner to accomplish moving the client.

Procedure

1. Wash your hands.

2. Tell client what you plan to do. Have your partner, either a friend or family member, stand on the opposite side of the bed to assist you.

3. Place pillow at the head of the bed to protect the client's head. Roll both sides of the drawsheet or flat sheet folded in fours toward the client. Place the client's feet 12 inches apart, so that they will not bump together as you move the client. Bend the client's knees, if possible.

4. With the hand nearest the client's feet, firmly grasp the rolled drawsheet or folded sheet. With the other hand, both of you cradle the client's head and shoulders and firmly grasp the top of the rolled drawsheet or folded sheet.

5. Turn your body and feet toward the head of the bed. Keep your feet about 12 inches apart and bend your knees slightly to

achieve good body mechanics as you lift the client.

6. Coordinate your lift—on the count of three, together lift the draw-sheet and the client up toward the head of the bed without dragging the client. Align the client's body and limbs so that the client is straight and comfortable.

7. Place the pillow back under the client's head, and tighten the drawsheet. Replace the covers and make the client comfortable.

8. Wash your hands.

9. Document completion of the procedure, time, and client's reaction.

52 Procedure

Log Rolling the Client

Purpose

- To ensure the spinal column is kept straight because of special medical conditions such as spinal injury and hip fractures

NOTE: You will need help to perform this procedure. It takes a minimum of two people to do this procedure.

Procedure

1. Wash your hands.
2. Tell the client what you plan to do.
3. With both you and your helper on the same side of the bed, remove the top covers.
4. Place your hand and arm under the client's head and shoulder to stabilize the neck. Your helper places her arms under the client's body and legs. On the count of three, lift the client toward you as a single unit.
5. Do not allow the client to bend and use good body mechanics yourselves by bending your knees and keeping your backs straight.
6. Place a pillow lengthwise between the client's thighs and legs and fold the client's arms over the chest.
7. Go over to the other side of the bed. You are in a position to keep the shoulders and upper body straight and your helper is positioned to keep the client's lower body, hips, and legs straight. Reach over the client and roll the drawsheet firmly against the client. On the count of three, the client is rolled toward you in a single movement, keeping the client's head, spine, and legs in a straight position.
8. To maintain the client's new position and alignment, place pillows against the spine and leave the pillow between the client's legs. Other small pillows or folded towels can be placed under the client's head and neck and under the arms for support.
9. Fold the drawsheet back over the pillows supporting the spine. Make sure the client's alignment is straight and that the client is

comfortable. Arrange covers for the client.
10. Wash your hands.

11. Record this repositioning, time, and any observations you made.

53   Procedure

Positioning the Client in Supine Position

Purpose

- To make client more comfortable
- To assist the body to function more efficiently
- To relieve pressure on body parts

Procedure

1. Wash your hands.
2. Tell client what you plan to do.
3. Place pillow under the client's head, so that the client's head is about 2 inches above the level of the bed. The pillow should extend slightly under the shoulders (Figure 15-2).
4. Have client's arms extended straight out with palms of the hands flat on the bed. The arms can be supported by pillows or covered foam pads placed under the forearms and extending from just above the elbows to the ends of the fingers.
5. Place a small pillow or rolled towel along the side of the client's thighs and tuck part of the sup-

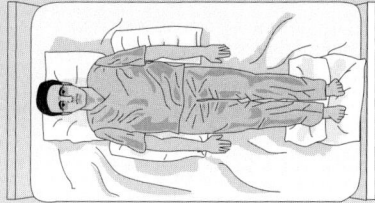

Figure 15-2   A client in supine position. The head of the bed may be elevated slightly with a pillow and the arms and hands may be elevated with a pillow.

port under the thigh, ensuring that the part under the thighs is smooth. This maintains alignment of the hips and thighs and helps prevent the hips from rotating outward or externally.
6. Place a small pillow or towel under the back of the ankle to relieve pressure on the heels.
7. Wash your hands.
8. Document the time, position change, and the client's reaction.

54   Procedure

Positioning the Client in Lateral/Side-lying Position

Purpose

- To provide for client comfort and change of position
- To relieve pressure on body parts

Procedure

1. Wash your hands.
2. Tell client what you plan to do.
3. Go to opposite side of bed from the direction you are planning to turn the client toward.
4. Cross the client's arms over the chest. Place your arm under the client's neck and shoulders. Place your other arm under the client's midback. Move the upper part of the client's body toward you.
5. Place one arm under the client's waist and the other under the thighs. Move the lower part of the client's body toward you.
6. Turn client to opposite side. Pull shoulder that is touching the bed slightly toward you. Pull buttock that is touching the bed slightly toward you. Place pillow under back and buttocks. Place bottom leg in extension and flex upper leg. Place small folded blanket or pillow between the upper and lower leg.

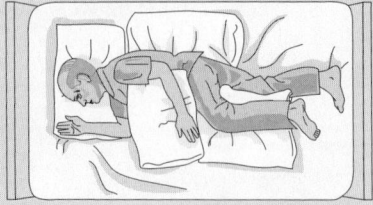

Figure 15-3   Lateral/side-lying position

7. Place pillow under client's head. Rotate the arm up to bring it up to the pillow with the palm facing up. Place the other arm on a pillow that extends from above the elbow to the fingers. Extend the fingers.
8. Check the client's position to see if the body is in good vertical alignment (Figure 15-3).
9. Wash your hands.
10. Document time, change of position, and client's reaction.

55   Procedure

Positioning the Client in Prone Position

Purpose

- To relieve pressure on body parts
- To provide for client comfort and position

NOTE: Most older adult clients are not able or do not like to be in this position for long because it is uncomfortable. In fact, it would be preferable to use frequent position changes from side to back (if possible), to side again, to increase client comfort and to reduce pressure points.

Before turning a dependent client in a prone position, make sure client's arms are straight down at sides to avoid injury while turning. Never leave an older client in this position more than 15 to 20 minutes.

Procedure

1. Wash your hands.

2. Tell client what you plan to do.
3. Turn client on abdomen. Check to see if spine is straight and face is turned to either side.
4. Client's legs are extended. Arms are flexed and brought up to either side of head.
5. A small pillow can be placed under the abdomen. (For women, this will reduce pressure against their breasts.) An alternate method is to roll a small towel and place it under shoulders to reduce pressure.

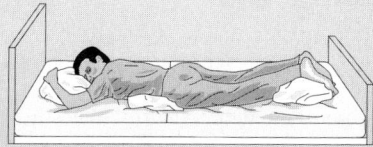

Figure 15-4   Prone position

6. Place another pillow under lower legs to prevent pressure on toes (Figure 15-4).
7. Wash your hands.
8. Document time, change of position, and client's reaction.

56 — Procedure

Positioning the Client in Fowler's Position

Purpose

• To provide client comfort
• To aid in breathing
• To position client so the client can engage in activities such as eating, reading, watching television, visiting

NOTE: If the client is weak or frail, the Fowler's position may be hard for the client to maintain. Supporting the client with pillows may help the client maintain the sitting position.

Procedure

1. Wash your hands.
2. Tell the client what you plan to do.
3. Check to see if the client's spine and legs are straight and in the middle of the bed.
4. Support client's head and neck with one, two, or three pillows. If

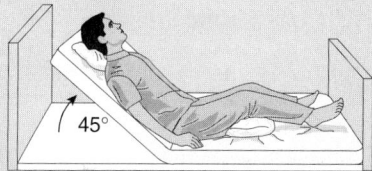

Figure 15-5   Fowler's position

   client has a hospital bed, raise bed to 45° angle.
5. Knees may be flexed and supported with small pillows (Figure 15-5).
6. Pillows may be placed under each arm from elbows to fingertips to support shoulders.
7. Place pillow or padded footboard against feet.
8. Wash your hands.
9. Document time, position change, and client's reaction.

TRANSFERS

Often an aide will be asked to transfer a client who is wheelchair bound. Using the proper transfer techniques will ensure that the client is moved safely from one location to another. Procedures 57 through 60 address various transfer techniques and the proper method for each. Procedure 61 demonstrates the proper method for using a stand lift.

57 — Procedure

Assisting the Client from Bed to Wheelchair

Purpose

- To move client from one location to another safely and without discomfort

NOTE: There should be a specific transfer procedure for each client who is not an independent, self-transfer.

Procedure

1. Wash your hands.
2. Tell the client what you plan to do.
3. Assemble needed equipment:
   wheelchair
   transfer belt
   client's shoes and socks
4. Place chair so client moves toward client's strongest side. Set chair at 45° angle to bed. Lock wheels. Move footrests out of the way.
5. Assist client to sit at edge of bed, as close to edge of bed as possible. Never pull on the client's arms or under the client's shoulders. Use verbal cues if necessary during transfer.
6. Wait a few seconds to allow the client to adjust to sitting position.

   Assist client to put on socks and shoes.
7. Apply transfer belt. Make sure the belt is not too tight or too loose.
8. Spread your feet apart and flex your hips and knees, aligning your knees with client's.
9. Grasp transfer belt from underneath. Rock the client up to standing on the count of three, while straightening your hips and legs, keeping knees slightly flexed.
10. If client has a weak leg, press your knee against it or block client's foot with yours to prevent weaker leg from sliding out from under the client.
11. Instruct client to use armrest on chair for support and be sure to flex your hips and knees while lowering client into chair. Remove transfer belt.
12. Check alignment of client in chair and make adjustments accordingly.
13. Wash your hands.
14. Document time, position change, and client's reaction.

58
Procedure

Assisting the Client from Wheelchair to Bed

Purpose

- To change client's position
- To transfer client safely from one location to another

Procedure

1. Wash your hands.
2. Tell client what you plan to do.
3. Position client with strong side toward bed with wheelchair at 45° angle. Lock wheels.
4. Apply transfer belt and place both hands on back of the belt. Have client slide forward in chair as far as possible; this will make it easier for the client to stand up. Instruct client, if able, to put feet flat on the floor and hands on the chair. On the count of three, have client push up to standing position. While standing, have the client pivot (turn) on strong leg toward the bed. Have the client lower himself or herself to the bed to a sitting position.
5. Assist the client to lying position. Position client in comfortable position and in good alignment. Remove shoes, socks, and transfer belt.
6. Wash hands.
7. Document time, change of position, and client's reaction.

59
Procedure

Transferring the Client from Wheelchair to Toilet/Commode

Purpose

- To enable client to sit on toilet for normal excretion of body wastes

NOTE: It is essential to have grab bars, preferably secured to the wall, but they can be attached to the toilet seat.

Procedure

1. Wash hands.
2. Tell client what you plan to do.
3. Have client in wheelchair with strong side nearer to the toilet or commode.
4. Lock the wheelchair. Apply transfer belt. Lift foot pieces out of way.
5. Loosen clothing on the client, but not too loose that the slacks fall while transferring.
6. Have client slide forward in chair and place feet apart. Place your hand on the back of the transfer belt. Have client place hands on armpiece and on the count of three push up.
7. Stand client up and have client place strong arm on grab bars. You continue to hold onto the transfer belt and slowly lower client onto the toilet or commode. Have client hold onto grab bar while you lower client's pants.

8. Remove belt and move wheelchair out of way.
9. Provide privacy for client. Check often to see if client is all right. Give client toilet paper.
10. Assist the client as needed, return to wheelchair, and assist back to prior activity.
11. Wash client's hands and your hands.

60   Procedure

Lifting the Client Using a Mechanical Lift

Purpose

- To transfer client from one place to another, usually from bed to chair
- To safely transfer a client who is heavy or has no weight-bearing ability

NOTE: Check slings, chains, and straps for frayed areas or defective hooks. Two types of slings are supplied with the Hoyer lift or other mechanical lifts: hammock style and two-piece canvas strips. The hammock type can be made out of mesh or canvas. This type of sling is better for clients who are weak and need support. The canvas strips can be used for clients with normal muscle tone.

Procedure

1. Wash your hands and assemble equipment.
2. Tell client what you plan to do.
3. Position chair near bed and allow adequate room to maneuver the lift. Be sure chair has adequate padding before transfer.
4. Roll client away from you.
5. Place hammock sling or canvas strips under client to form seat; with two canvas pieces, lower edge fits under client's knees (wide piece); upper edge goes under client's shoulders (narrow piece).
6. Go to opposite side of bed, roll client away from you and straighten hammock or strips through.
7. Roll client supine into canvas seat.
8. Place lift's horseshoe bar under side of bed (on side with chair). Have base of lift in maximum open position and lock.
9. Lower horizontal bar to sling level by releasing hydraulic valve. Lock valve.
10. Attach hooks or strap (chain) to holes in sling. Short chains/straps hook to top holes of sling; lower chains to bottom of sling. Point hooks to the outside when attaching.
11. Fold client's arm over the chest.
12. Pump handle until client is raised free of bed, but no higher than necessary.
13. Use steering handle to pull lift from bed and maneuver to chair.
14. Roll base around chair. Slowly release check valve and lower client into chair.
15. Check to see if client is positioned correctly. Unhook chains or straps and remove lift.
16. If straps are used, they can be removed. If the hammock sling is

used, sling will remain underneath client so it is in position for transfer back to bed.

17. Wash your hands.
18. Document transfer, time completed, and client's reaction.

---

61 Procedure

Using a Stand Lift

Purpose

- To safely transfer a client from bed to chair
- To safely ambulate a client

Procedure

1. Assemble equipment:
   watch with second hand
   stand lift
   belt that comes with lift
2. Bring stand lift to side of bed.
3. Tell client what you plan to do.
4. Assist client to sit on side of bed. Dress client and be sure the client is wearing a good pair of shoes with nonskid soles that will give support while walking or transferring.
5. Apply belt that comes with lift around client's waist.

6. Have client place hands on the bars on lift and gradually lift the client to a standing position using the hand control on the lift.
7. Use the lift to walk the client or to transfer to a chair.
8. When you are done and client is in the chair, remove transfer belt. Make the client comfortable.
9. Return lift and belt to storage area.
10. Chart completion of the procedure and any abnormal reactions.

NOTE: There are many different types of stand lifts, each one somewhat different from the next one. For safety reasons, do the procedure first with your nurse or a family member before doing it alone.

CAST CARE

Casts are used to immobilize extremities or joints following trauma or fractures, or to correct a body bone/joint defect. Casts may be applied to an extremity or to the entire body. Casts may be made of plaster of Paris, fiberglass, or polyester. Casts promote healing of the injured area, while providing comfort to the client. Procedure 62 demonstrates the proper method to care for casts.

62

Procedure

Caring for Casts

Procedure

1. Observe the new cast every two to three hours for the first two days and then four times daily. Check the skin for signs of irritation such as redness or swelling. Skin areas below the cast must be observed for signs of cyanosis (blue color), unusual coldness, or any unusual odor, which may indicate a serious problem. These signs and any complaints of numbness should be reported to the nurse.
   - Note the color of the skin at the farthest end of cast—normal pink, warm to touch, and movable toes or fingers.
   - Look for edema at both ends of the cast; report and record this information.
   - Observe for response to touch (that is, the response of the nerves to stimulation); report and record this information. Report *any* numbness or tingling that persists.
2. Observe the cast daily for roughness around the edges. This may cause skin irritation and may be filed or covered with soft padding. These rough edges can be covered with plain white tape. This is called petaling and can be done by the nurse.
3. Observe the cast itself, noting any redness that may indicate bleeding or drainage from under the cast. Circle the area with a magic marker, noting the date and time that you first noticed the redness. Also note any unusual odor.

Record and report any abnormal sign or symptom to the nurse.
4. Observe the cast constantly for any cracks. Cracks are unsafe and you should notify your nurse of the crack. You must state the exact location and length of the crack as well as the depth of it.
5. When the cast is near the perineal area, protect it from moisture. Ask your nurse for special instructions on which waterproof or protective device to use. Protect the cast and skin by preventing any dirt, sand, or small articles from getting inside the cast, which could cause an infection under the cast. Note that plaster of Paris tends to crumble and become soft when moist; therefore, this type of cast must always be kept dry.
6. Ask the client if he or she has pain in any particular area under the cast. This may indicate a pressure point and skin breakdown under the cast. Note this area. *Report and record.* Be sure to position your client correctly.

Safety for Client with a Cast

1. Check the house for throw rugs or objects on the floor. Remove any hazard that may cause the client to fall. Remind client to leave a night-light on to prevent a fall in the middle of the night.
2. Remember that at first the client may not have a good sense of balance and may be unsteady in walking. Arrange the furniture so that the client may hold on to furniture or handrails while walking.

3. Assist the client in making changes in eating, dressing, writing, toileting, and walking.

4. Ask the nurse for specific orders for passive range of motion exercises. A physical therapist or occupational therapist may come to assist the client with specific exercises.

5. Determine the composition of the cast by reading the care plan. Plaster of Paris casts take at least 24 hours to dry; polyester or fiberglass casting tape takes 5 to 15 minutes to dry. Be sure you do not touch the wet cast with the fingers because this may leave dents in the cast. Use the palm of the hand to move the cast. Do not allow the cast to dry on a hard surface because this will flatten the cast. Place the entire new cast on pillows and expose to air. Do not allow client to put anything between the cast and the skin if the skin under the cast starts to itch. If itching becomes unbearable, air can be blown in by use of a hair dryer, if the nurse gives you permission to do this. When positioning a client with an extremity cast, elevate the cast on pillows. Generally it is not allowed to have the client lie on the injured side. Instruct the client to wiggle toes or fingers frequently on cast extremity. Do not cover casted extremity because air needs to be allowed to circulate inside the cast.

APPLICATION OF COLD

Heat and cold applications are ordered by a health care provider to promote comfort and healing. Cold applications can ease pain or decrease swelling of localized areas. Heat applications can increase circulation to a body part, relax tension, and relieve pain. Because the application of heat and cold can cause injury and changes in bodily functions, some states and home care agencies do not allow home health aides to carry out these procedures. It is important to follow your employer's policies and procedures. Procedure 63 addresses the proper method for applying a cold application to the client's skin.

63   Procedure

Applying a Cold Application to the Client's Skin

Purpose

• To ease pain
• To decrease swelling of localized area

NOTE: The nurse will tell the aide when to apply ice and how to do it.

All ice applications must be covered with a cloth. Never apply ice directly to the skin. A towel, face cloth, or fitted cover should be used against the skin. If using commercial ice packs have a minimum of two, so you can rotate their use. Ice packs can be bought in many different sizes. Some are very firm on the outside, whereas others are soft and flexible. They should be placed in the freezer until needed.

Procedure

1. Assemble equipment:
   commercial ice pack
   thin cloth to cover ice pack
2. Wash your hands.
3. Tell client what you plan to do.
4. Cover ice pack with thin covering of cloth.
5. Give ice pack to client to apply to affected area.
6. Leave ice pack on for 20 minutes and remove. Check often for signs of redness, whiteness, or cyanosis (blue color).
7. Remove ice pack, wipe with alcohol wipes, and place in freezer.
8. Document completion of procedure and if the application of ice benefited the client. Occasionally, instead of lessening the client's discomfort, cold may increase the pain.
9. Wash your hands.

PERSONAL CARE

Some clients with functional or cognitive impairments may need assistance with personal care, such as dressing and undressing. Procedure 64 demonstrates the proper technique to dress and undress the client.

64 Procedure

Dressing and Undressing the Client

Purpose

- To keep the client clean and comfortable
- To increase client's self-image and well-being
- To reduce client's discomfort and reduce client's risk of strain or injury

NOTE: Do not allow client to remain in nightclothes during the day (unless case manager states it is all right). The client needs to know that it is daytime and needs to dress accordingly.

Procedure

1. Wash your hands and tell client what you plan to do.
2. Assemble clean items:
   undergarments
   clothing—let client select if possible
   stockings and shoes
3. If client is able, help the client to sit at the edge of the bed and dangle his or her legs. If the client is too weak to sit up, have client lie flat on the bed. Place a sheet or robe over client to avoid embarrassing or chilling the client.
4. Assist the client to put on undergarments. (A front closing bra is very convenient for women with limited movement in their arms.) If client has a weak leg, place the weak leg in first, then the other leg. Then put on clothing in the same manner. If the client can stand, pull the pants or slacks up to the waist. If the client must remain on the bed, ask the client to

press the heels into the bed and raise the buttocks. While the client is in this position, quickly slide the pants or slacks up to the waist. Assist the client as necessary. If the client is unable to lift buttocks up, roll the client from side-to-side as you raise the slacks over the hips. Slacks with elastic waist are preferred, as they are put on more easily than pants with zippers and buttons. Cotton jogging suits are becoming a popular option for elderly clients or those with dis-

abilities. They are warm, easy to get off and on, and attractive. They also launder easily.

5. Assist the client to put on a shirt by placing the weaker arm in the sleeve first. Pull the shirt around for the client to place the other arm in the sleeve.

6. When removing a shirt, remove the sleeve of the strongest arm first, followed by the weaker arm. Encourage the client to do as much as he or she is able.

MOBILITY AND EXERCISES

Individuals who become immobile due to illness are very vulnerable to complications. Common effects of immobility are blood clots, pneumonia, kidney stones, atrophy (wasting away) of the muscles, contractures (shortening of the muscles), and loss of motion in the joints of the body. Range-of-motion exercises are performed on clients to prevent the above complications from happening. If the client can do the exercises without the assistance of the aide or another person, they are called active range-of-motion exercises. Refer to Procedure 65 on performing active range-of-motion exercises. If they are done with the support of another person, they are called passive range-of-motion exercises. Refer to Procedure 66 on performing passive range-of-motion exercises. There are special terms used to describe the movements that you will be doing when exercising the client. The following is a list of some of the common terms used in regards to movement of the body:

Abduction—to move a part away from the midline of the body

Adduction—to move a part toward the midline of the body

Dorsiflexion—bending foot toward ankle

Extension—straighten out a joint

Flexion—bend a joint

Opposition—touch each fingertip with the thumb

Internal rotation—turning a joint inward

External rotation—turning a joint outward

Plantar flexion—bending the foot downward

Pronation—turning palms downward

Rotation—turning a joint in a circle

Supination—turning palms upward

Guidelines for doing range-of-motion exercises include:

1. Do only the joints that are ordered to be exercised. Be sure to check the care plan. Today, it is not unusual for the physical therapist to

videotape how the exercises should be done for the client and leave this at the client's home. This is a great tool for aides to see how the professional therapist does the exercises. They can view the videotape frequently if they forget how to do a certain movement.

2. Do the exercises only to the point of pain.
3. Do not exercise the head, unless you are specifically told to do so.
4. Start with the larger joints and work down to the smaller joints (e.g., start with the shoulder joint and end with the fingers).

5. Do one side of the body first and then repeat on the opposite side.
6. Provide privacy for the client and expose only the part of the body being exercised.
7. Do each movement at least three to five times.
8. The exercises can be incorporated when doing other client care procedures such as bathing or walking.
9. Exercise the client's body part in a smooth, gentle, but firm style.
10. Support the extremity above and below the joints being exercised.
11. Exercised can be done either in the bed or chair.

65 Procedure

Performing Active Range-of-Motion Exercises

Purpose

- Increase muscle tone and strength in the client's body
- To restore function to injured parts of the body
- To prevent joint stiffness, contractures, and other complications of immobility

The following are stretch exercises the client can do without the assistance of an aide. The client may need to be reminded to do them. They should be done a minimum of three to five times on each extremity.

1. Chest stretch
   Place both hands on forehead with arms bent at the elbow, bring elbows forward, touching each other, then repeat
2. Shoulder stretch

   Take one arm and stretch it over the opposite shoulder and hold for 10 seconds, then bring arm to the side in extension. Do the same with the other arm.
3. Rotation
   Start with arm in extension on side of body, bring arm up and make circle with arm. Do the same with the other arm.
4. Adduction/abduction
   With arm in extension, bring arm toward midline of body, then bring arm straight out to the side of the body, keeping arm straight. Be sure to do both arms.
5. Extension/flexion
   Extend arm straight out on side of body, bend elbow and touch your shoulder with your hand. Then switch arms and do the opposite arm.

6. Hip adduction
   Lying on your back, with the feet together, try to raise your buttocks by bending the knees, then try to hold buttocks up for 10 seconds.
7. Upper thigh stretch
   Lying down, hold on to one knee using both hands, bend your knee and try to bring your nose to your knee, hold for 10 seconds. Then do the opposite leg.
8. Hamstring stretch
   Sit down on bench, with leg stretched out, bend knee toward upper body as far as you can, hold 10 seconds. Then do the other leg.
9. Quadriceps stretch
   Face the wall, place one hand on wall, bring back opposite leg as far as you can, hold 10 seconds. Then do the other leg.
10. Calf stretch
    Place both arms on wall, bring one leg back about 3 feet from wall with arms stretched out, hold this position for 10 seconds. Repeat with the opposite leg.
11. Lower back stretch
    Lying on the back, bring up one knee as far as you can, hold for 10 seconds. Repeat with the opposite leg.

66 Procedure

Performing Passive Range-of-Motion Exercises

Purpose

- To increase muscle tone and strength in the client's body
- To restore function to injured parts of body
- To prevent joint stiffness and contractures

NOTE: Do not perform the exercises until you have received instructions specific for your client's joints. When possible, support the extremity above and below the joints being exercised. If the client shows pain or discomfort, stop the exercise and document it. The head can be exercised if specifically ordered by the physical therapist.

Procedure

1. Wash your hands
2. Read any special instructions for these exercises for your client.
3. Tell client what you plan to do. Ask client to assist as much as possible.
4. Exercise the shoulder. Turn shoulder; arm bent, move hand toward head—outward rotation (Figure 15-6A). Turn shoulder; arm bent, move hand toward waist—inward rotation (Figure 15-6B).
5. Move arm in circle—rotation (Figure 15-7).

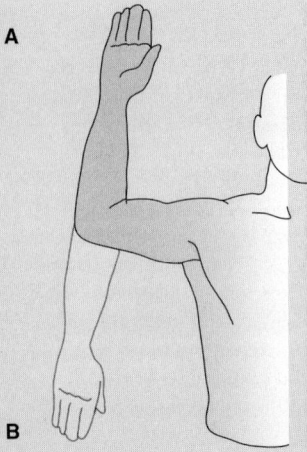

Figure 15-6   Exercise the shoulder. (A) Turn shoulder; arm bent, move hand toward head—outward rotation. (B) Turn shoulder; arm bent, move hand toward waist—inward rotation.

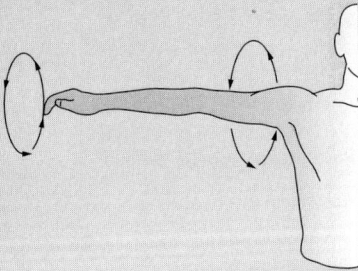

Figure 15-7   Move arm in circle—rotation

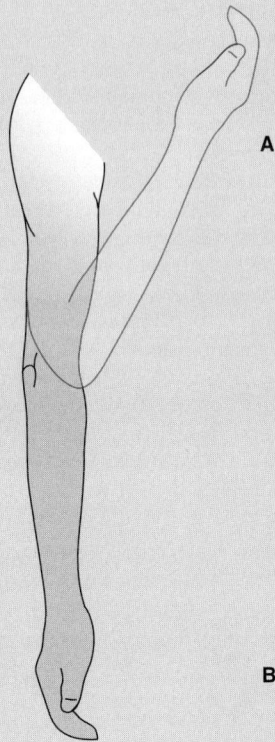

Figure 15-8   (A) Bend elbow—flexion. (B) Straighten elbow—extension

6. Bend elbow—flexion (Figure 15-8A).
7. Straighten elbow—extension (Figure 15-8B).
8. Turn lower arm, palm up—supination (Figure 15-9A).
9. Turn lower arm, palm down—pronation (Figure 15-9B).
10. Straighten wrist—extension (Figure 15-10A).
11. Bend wrist—flexion (Figure 15-10B).
12. Bend fingers—flexion (Figure 15-11A).
13. Straighten fingers—extension (Figure 15-11B).
14. Move fingers apart—abduction (Figure 15-12A).
15. Move fingers together—adduction (Figure 15-12B).
16. Bend thumb—flexion (Figure 15-13A).
17. Straighten thumb—extension (Figure 15-13B).
18. Touch thumb to fingers—opposition (Figure 15-14).

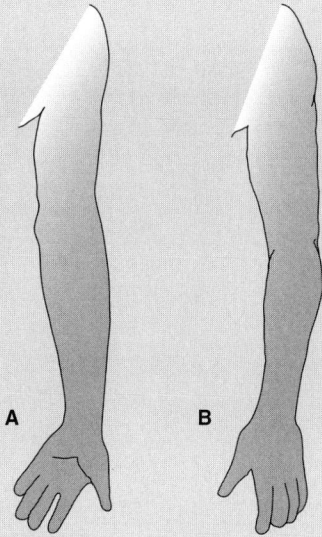

Figure 15-9 (A) Turn lower arm, palm up—supination. (B) Turn lower arm, palm down—pronation.

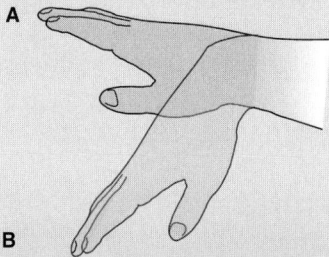

Figure 15-10 (A) Straighten wrist—extension. (B) Bend wrist—flexion.

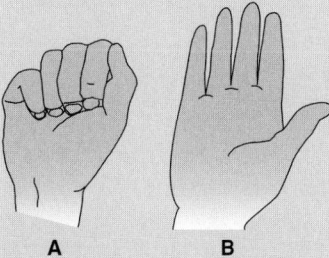

Figure 15-11 (A) Bend fingers—flexion. (B) Straighten fingers—extension.

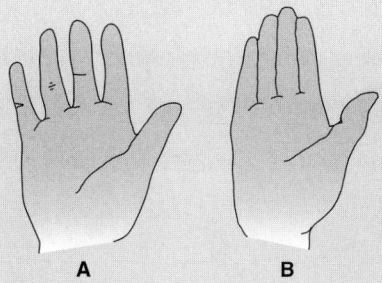

Figure 15-12 (A) Move fingers apart—abduction. (B) Move fingers together—adduction.

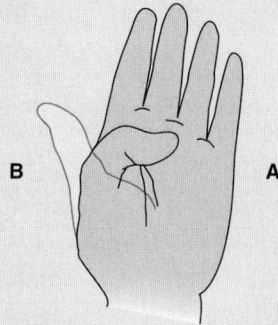

Figure 15-13 (A) Bend thumb—flexion. (B) Straighten thumb—extension.

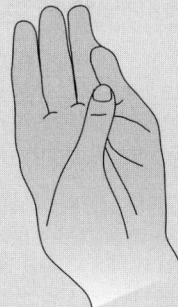

Figure 15-14 Touch thumb to fingers—opposition.

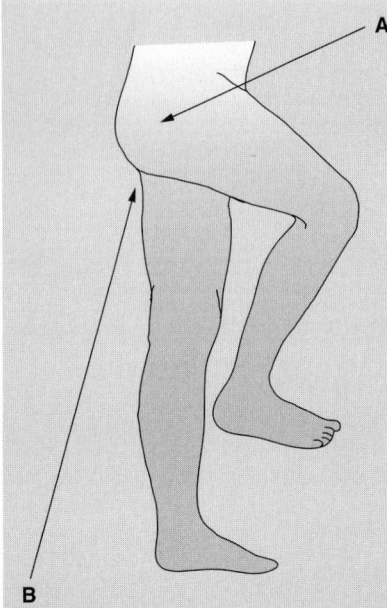

Figure 15-15 (A) Bend hip—flexion. (B) Straighten hip—extension.

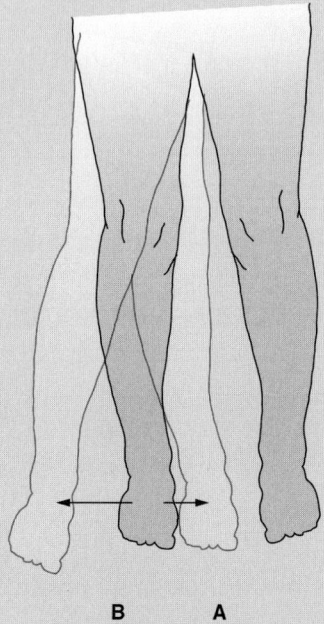

Figure 15-16 (A) Roll leg inward—inward rotation. (B) Roll leg outward—outward rotation.

19. Bend hip—flexion (Figure 15-15A).
20. Straighten hip—extension (Figure 15-15B).
21. Roll leg inward—inward rotation (Figure 15-16A).
22. Roll leg outward—outward rotation (Figure 15-16B).
23. Bend ankle, foot upward—dorsiflexion (Figure 15-17A).
24. Bend ankle, foot downward—plantar flexion (Figure 15-17B).
25. Bend toes—flexion (Figure 15-18A).
26. Straighten toes (Figure 15-18B).
27. Go to other side and repeat movements for each joint.
28. Wash hands.
29. Document completion of exercises and client's reactions.

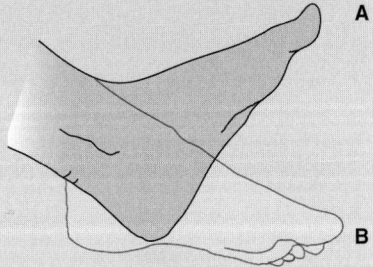

Figure 15-17 (A) Bend ankle, foot upward—dorsiflexion. (B) Bend ankle, foot downward—plantar flexion.

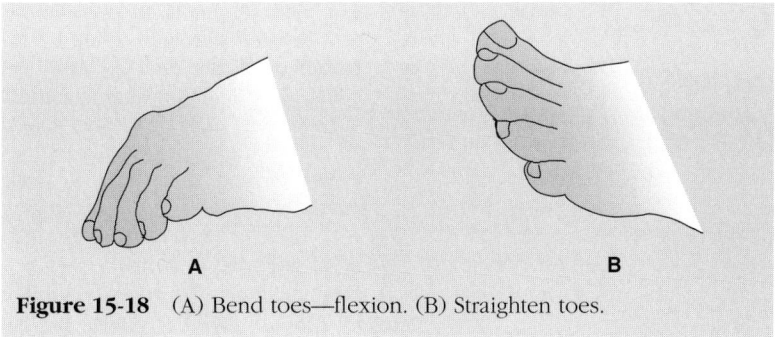

Figure 15-18   (A) Bend toes—flexion. (B) Straighten toes.

NEED FOR REHABILITATION

Part of the care plan for a client may include rehabilitation, which is the restoring of physical abilities to the highest level possible. Most rehabilitation is planned and carried out by a specialist such as the physical or occupational therapist. When physical ability or skill has been lost, the client must relearn it or adjust to coping without it. In some cases the home health aide will be able to assist in the rehabilitation program.

The home health aide may be expected to assist a client with walking. A physical therapist will determine when the client is ready to begin walking again and what types of assistive devices may be necessary to maintain the client's safety. Procedure 67 demonstrates how to assist the client to walk with crutches, a walker, or a cane.

67 ═══ Procedure

Assisting the Client to Walk with Crutches, Walker, or Cane

Purpose
• To provide support and maintain balance as client walks

NOTE: There are three basic walking patterns: nonweight-bearing, partial weight-bearing, and weight-bearing. With a nonweight-bearing pattern, all the weight is placed on the arms and uninvolved leg. A partial weight-bearing pattern means that minimal weight is placed on the toes. However, most weight is still on the arms and the uninvolved leg.

To walk in a nonweight-bearing pattern the client uses crutches. The physical therapist measures the client to select the correct length of crutches. The therapist also teaches the client how to walk with the crutches.

To walk in a partial weight-bearing pattern, the client can use crutches but often uses a walker. The walker is a curved metal frame with four legs. It is a walking aid that gives maximum stability as the client moves. The client steps forward while holding onto the walker with both hands. Some walkers have wheels so that the client does not have to lift up the walker between steps.

A cane is used when the client is strong enough to bear full weight on both legs. A standard cane should not be used as a weight-bearing aid. A special cane with four short legs, called a quad cane, is designed to bear a small amount of weight only. A cane is primarily used for balance. Check rubber tips on the canes, walkers, and crutches because they wear out quickly if used on sidewalks.

Always have client wear good supportive shoes with nonskid soles. Instruct clients to pick up their feet and not to look at their feet, but to look straight ahead.

Procedure

1. Apply transfer belt unless instructed not to.

2. Always walk on the client's weak side.

3. Walk slightly behind the client holding onto the transfer belt from behind.

4. For the client using crutches, hold onto the transfer belt if the client feels uncomfortable using the crutches.

5. For the client using a walker, instruct the client to place the walker firmly before walking. If the client is strong enough, the walker and the weaker leg can be moved forward at the same time.

6. For the client using a cane, instruct the client to hold the cane in the hand opposite the weaker leg. If the right ankle has been injured, the client should hold the cane in the left hand.

7. Balance is a judgmental situation. If the client has poor balance, the aide should support the weak side and use a transfer belt for safety reasons.

8. Document how far the client walked and client's reaction.

While recovering from an illness, clients sometimes become discouraged and depressed and fear they will never feel better. A home health aide must encourage the client, but not raise the client's expectations beyond a reasonable level. It is better to emphasize the client's "abilities" rather than "disabilities." It is important to set realistic daily goals while at the same time working toward a long-term level of physical rehabilitation that can be reasonably expected.

EMOTIONAL ASPECTS OF REHABILITATION

A client with a disability may have lost an ability many of us take for granted. However, he or she can be quite capable in other areas. The home health aide should treat every client, no matter his or her ability, with dignity and respect, enabling the client's right to make decisions, to maximize and support the physical, cognitive, and emotional abilities that do exist.

The aide should report to the case manager, nurse, or physical therapist the client's lack of motivation or interest. The case manager may have some tips on ways to motivate this individual or may want to involve family members in supporting and motivating the client.

REHABILITATION AND ACTIVITIES

The care plan is developed to make the client comfortable and to work toward recovery or to regain as much ability as possible. Several factors influence the care that is planned. The case manager and the home health aide must consider the client's age, condition, abilities, areas where assistance is needed, and personal interests before the accident or illness occurred. The personal habits and the client's personality also enter into the total care plan.

The value of activity must not be overlooked. Activities are useful in helping a client relearn skills that may have been lost because of the illness or accident. They also provide meaningful activity to a client who may be depressed due to the illness. An appropriate activity reminds a client of what he or she is still able to do. Activities are not just structured arts and crafts, or music, but are also sorting socks, washing dishes, planning a meal, dictating a letter, reading a newspaper together, or sorting photos for a photo album. An activity can be used to stimulate reminiscence, to aid in regaining verbal skills after a stroke, or to enhance a relationship.

UNIT 16

Nervous System

NERVOUS SYSTEM

The brain, spinal cord, and nerves make up the nervous system. This system is the communication center that sends messages to all parts of the body. It is the system that enables the body to see, hear, smell, taste, and touch. Sight, sound, taste, smell, and touch are known as the five body senses. The brain (Figure 16-1) is the master control or main switch of the nervous system. Messages are relayed to the brain from all parts of the body. The brain decides how to respond to each message (or stimulus) sent by the nerves. Each area of the brain performs a specialized duty. The brain alerts other control centers in the body so that the body correctly responds to a message.

The spinal cord can be compared to the electrical wiring system in a house. All the major nerves of the body are bound together in the spinal cord and lead into the brain. The spinal cord is protected by the spinal column. If the spinal column is damaged or diseased, the spinal nerves may be affected.

Paraplegia refers to paralysis of the lower part of the body and both legs. Quadriplegia refers to paralysis of both arms and both legs. Both paraplegia and quadriplegia can result from disease or injury to the brain or spinal cord. Hemiplegia is a paralysis of one side of the body. It is frequently the result of a cerebrovascular accident (CVA) or "stroke."

The nerves radiate from the spinal cord to all parts of the body, forming a network. The nerve endings might be compared to the electrical outlets in the house. In the body, the nerves are usually ready to receive stimuli. For instance, the hand touches a hot surface, the nerve sends the message to the spinal cord, and it goes to the brain. The brain sends back the message to move the hand off the hot surface. This entire process takes place in an instant so that one is only aware of the result. The time it takes to respond to a stimulus is known as reaction time. As the human body ages, reaction time often slows down a great deal. It also is affected when part of the brain has been damaged as with a stroke.

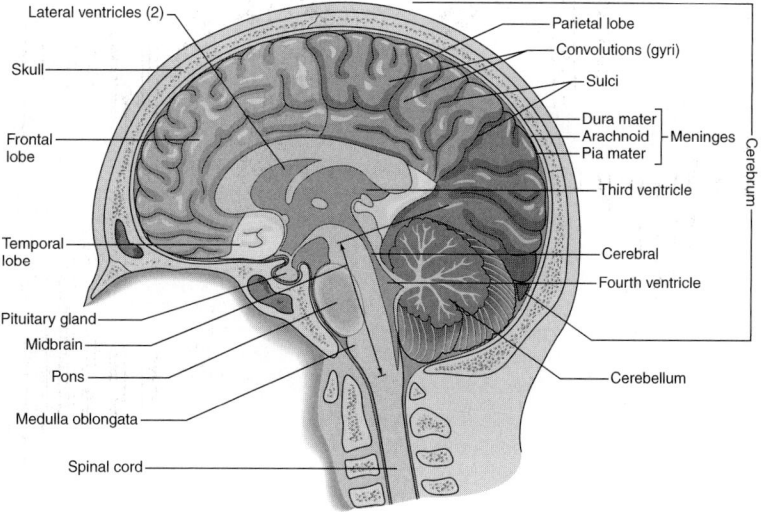

Figure 16-1   The central nervous system—brain and spinal cord

DISORDERS OF THE NERVOUS SYSTEM

Disorders of the nervous system can be the result of disease or injury to the brain or spinal cord. Many of these disorders cause mobility and cognitive problems. For example, shakiness in the extremities (tremors), difficulty walking, and mental changes are common symptoms of nervous system disorders. The home health aide can assist the client who has a nervous system disorder by being aware of the client's limitations, encouraging the client to complete the assigned exercises, and by observing and reporting changes in the client's health status and functioning levels to the health care team.

Parkinson's Disease

Parkinson's disease, first documented by James Parkinson in 1817, is a progressive degeneration of nerve cells in the area of the brain that controls muscle movements. The disease re-

sults from the inability of these nerve cells to produce dopamine, which is necessary for the transmission of signals within the brain. The cause of Parkinson's disease is not yet known.

Parkinson's disease often starts in middle or late life and is progressive in nature, with symptoms worsening over time. Characteristic symptoms of Parkinson's disease include shakiness of the body at rest (tremors), fixated or reduced facial expressions, slowness of movement, shuffling walking pattern (gait), stiffness or rigidity of limbs, and stooped posture (Figure 16-2). In its most severe form, the individual becomes incapacitated by rigidity and tremors. Depression is common among individuals diagnosed with this disease.

Treatment for Parkinson's disease involves drug therapy to restore the brain's supply of dopamine to reverse problems of the disease involving walking, movement, and tremors. Close medical supervision of the drug

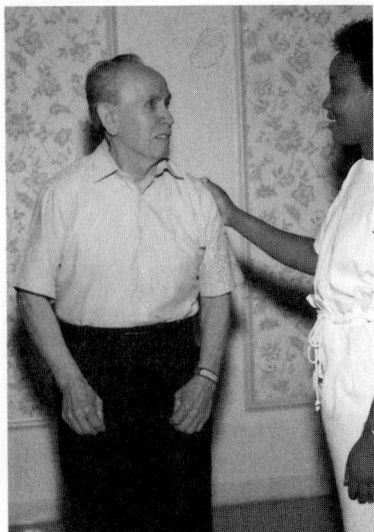

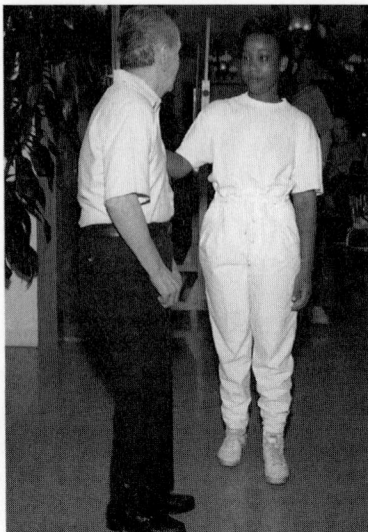

Figure 16-2 Characteristic symptom of Parkinson's disease is a flat, mask-like facial expression.

treatment is necessary. Clients should be monitored for serious side effects such as involuntary movements, nausea, dizziness, and mental changes so that medications can be adjusted to suit the client. Eating a well-balanced, nutritious diet is very beneficial. This can create increased energy, help the body work more efficiently, and help medications work effectively. Regular exercise is another critical part of treatment. However, clients with Parkinson's disease will require many rest periods because their energy levels may go up and down throughout the day.

Multiple Sclerosis

Multiple sclerosis (MS) is a disease affecting the central nervous system, and is generally seen in young adults. In most cases, the disease begins with episodes that last only weeks or months that are separated by periods of remission (absence of symptoms). The cause of MS is not clearly under-

stood. Multiple sclerosis produces a wide variety of symptoms, including poor coordination of muscle movement, numbness or tingling sensations, vision problems, such as blurred or double vision, paralysis of lower extremities, problems with bowel and bladder control, and problems with mental functions. Individuals with MS also suffer from a lack of energy and fatigue easily.

There is no current cure for MS. Three prescription drugs that can be used to treat this disease are Avonex®, Betaseron®, and Copaxone®. Steroid drugs are also used to treat this disorder. Physical and occupational therapy are also an important part of a MS treatment plan. Most people with MS live productive lives and are able to work. Although people with MS are capable of walking, occasionally they may need an assistive device such as a walker or cane. The average life expectancy is 35 years after the onset of the disease.

Amyotrophic Lateral Sclerosis

Amyotrophic lateral sclerosis (ALS) is more commonly known as Lou Gehrig's disease, after the famous baseball player who died from ALS. ALS is a progressive degeneration of the nerve cells in the brain and spinal cord that control the voluntary muscles. Its cause is unknown.

The signs and symptoms of ALS include slow loss of strength and coordination in one or more limbs, muscle twitches, and cramps; increasingly stiff, clumsy gait; and difficulty with swallowing, speaking, or breathing. The onset of ALS begins gradually, first affecting one upper limb and then the next one. Additional muscle areas then become affected and complete paralysis may result. The person's mind stays alert while his or her body wastes away, which is very hard for the family to witness. Following diagnosis, a person generally lives only two to six years.

Epilepsy

Epilepsy is a chronic brain disorder characterized by a sudden episode of intense electrical activity in the brain, which results in seizure activities. Epilepsy takes different forms, with various types of seizures. Seizures are classified as partial or generalized. Partial seizures do not involve the entire brain, only part of the brain. A client having this type of seizure may just stare into space or smack the lips, or pick on clothing. There is no loss of consciousness when having an attack, but the client does not remember doing the particular behavior. An example of the second type of seizure is a grand mal seizure. In this type of seizure, the attack begins with a loud cry, followed by the client falling to the ground and becoming unconscious. The entire body becomes stiff, followed by shaking of the entire body with foaming from the mouth due to overproduction of saliva. Fecal and urinary incontinence may also occur. The attacks last only one to two minutes. After an attack the client may be confused, drowsy, weak, and complain of having a headache. It is important if your client does have a seizure to note what particular behavior the client exhibited. It is also important that the client take the seizure medication as prescribed. If a client refuses to take the seizure medication, be sure to notify the nurse. A client with this diagnosis should also wear a Medic Alert bracelet or necklace. Procedure 68 identifies the proper method for caring for a client having a seizure.

68 Procedure

Caring for a Client Having a Seizure

Purpose
- To protect the client from injury
- To prevent the client from aspirating fluid into the lungs
- To maintain an open airway

During the Seizure
1. Do not try to limit the movements of the client.
2. Protect the client from injuring himself or herself. Loosen the

clothing, if possible, and place a pillow under the head to cushion head.

3. Clear the areas around the client of furniture or other objects.

4. Turn head of client to the side, which will prevent aspiration of fluids into the lungs.

5. Stay with the client until the shaking stops.

After the Seizure

1. If the client has never had a seizure before, has hurt himself or herself, if the seizure lasts more than a few minutes, or if the seizure recurs, call for an ambulance.

2. Always respect the dignity of the client. The client is often embarrassed when he or she regains consciousness.

3. Once the seizure is over, position the client on his or her side. This will allow for normal breathing and for any vomitus, saliva, or blood to drain from the mouth.

4. Confusion may be present for a period of time. Watch the client until there is a complete return of mental function. A client may feel very tired after a seizure.

5. Treat any bumps, bruises, or cuts that may have resulted from the seizure. The client may have become incontinent during the seizure and will want to clean up.

6. Record details of the seizure for the health care provider. It is important to note the duration of the seizure, extremities involved, precipitating factors, and any other characteristics noted.

Muscular Dystrophy

Muscular dystrophy is a progressive disease caused from insufficient nourishment of the muscles. The lack of a key protein essential to muscle function causes the muscles to decrease in size and grow weaker. Muscular dystrophy is a rare disease that is inherited. The disease usually strikes at an early age, usually before 3, and affects only boys. Muscular dystrophy ultimately cripples the person entirely.

Symptoms of the disease are muscle weakness, lack of coordination, clumsy gait, inability to lift the arms over the head, and progressive crippling resulting in a loss of mobility. By the teenage years, most clients require a wheelchair. Many persons with muscular dystrophy die before adulthood. There is no cure. The best treatment regimen involves physical therapy to help minimize deformities.

Spinal Cord Injuries

When a person has an injury to the spinal cord, loss of sensation and function in body parts below the level of that injury often results. Most spinal cord injuries are the result of traffic or industrial accidents, falls, gunshot wounds, and sports injuries. The extent of impairment will depend on where the spinal cord was severed. Many of these clients will spend the remainder of their life in a wheelchair, with little hope of ever walking again.

Cerebrovascular Accident (CVA) or Stroke

Stroke is the common term for cerebrovascular accident (CVA). The blood flow to a specific area of the brain is interrupted, resulting in sudden acute symptoms such as paralysis, vision disturbances, language problems, mental confusion, or a combination of these.

Stroke is caused by a lack of oxygen and nutrients to the brain cells. This interruption of blood to the brain may be due to one of the following three reasons: an aneurysm (a ballooning out of the wall of an artery) that breaks open and causes a hemorrhage; an embolus (a moving blood clot) that causes complete blockage of an artery; or a thrombus (a blood clot that forms inside an artery) that can cause a blockage of blood flow to the brain cells. Brain cells deprived of circulation for even a few seconds stop functioning. If the circulation stops for a few minutes, brain cells die. This causes loss of voluntary motion and results in paralysis, often on one side of the body.

Brain cells die when they are without oxygen for four minutes. Once brain cells are destroyed, they cannot be brought back to life. Unlike other cells in the body, new brain cells do not form to replace damaged ones. The most common cause of a CVA is high blood pressure. A CVA does not necessarily destroy all the brain cells. Remaining cells can compensate by taking over the duties of those destroyed by a CVA.

Risk Factors in Stroke. Often, long before a stroke occurs, there are conditions or symptoms that are now recognized as associated with an increased risk of stroke. These are:

- Hypertension—sustained, elevated blood pressure. This can increase vessel lining damage, accelerating the formation of plaque (fatty deposits) in arteries.
- Atherosclerosis—a disease in which fatty materials containing cholesterol, platelets (blood cells that promote clotting), and calcium accumulate on the interior walls of the arteries. These accumulations can build up to the point where the vessel becomes obstructed.
- Heart disease—coronary artery disease, damaged heart valves
- Diabetes
- Family history of heart disease or stroke

In addition, several conditions also may be controllable risk factors. Among these are high blood fat and cholesterol levels, obesity, physical inactivity, cigarette smoking, use of certain medications such as birth control pills, blood thinners, and steroids, and excessive alcohol intake.

Statistics indicate that although stroke can happen at any age, strokes are more common in older adults. Approximately 66% of strokes that occur yearly are in individuals over 65.

Causes of Strokes. A stroke can be caused by transient ischemic attacks, multi-infarct dementia, cerebral infarction, or cerebral hemorrhage.

Transient ischemic attack (TIA) consists of a brief period of weakness, loss of speech, or loss of feeling that lasts from minutes to hours and then goes away completely. These attacks are caused by a sudden but temporary decrease or stoppage of blood flow to a part of the brain. These attacks are important because they are a reliable warning of possible severe stroke. Another name for TIAs is "small strokes."

Usually a person with TIA reports one or more of the following: the sudden onset of numbness, tingling, or weakness on one side of the body, or in the hand and face on one side; temporary blindness in one or both eyes; severe headache; difficulty understanding words and using them correctly; dizziness; nausea; vomiting; staggering; fuzzy speech; or a combination of these symptoms. During a TIA people do not lose consciousness, and recover with no aftereffect.

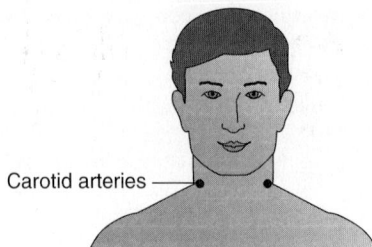

Figure 16-3 The carotid arteries are located on both sides of the neck.

Whenever the symptoms described above occur, it is important that a health care provider be notified, even if the episode seems to pass as quickly as it came. Knowing and heeding these warning signs can help to avoid a future stroke because treatment of the underlying conditions that caused the attack often is possible, either with medications or with surgery.

Most commonly, the site of blockage is in the carotid artery located in the neck (Figure 16-3), where it divides into two large vessels—one going to the brain, the other to the face, jaw, and eye. This site is important because it is accessible to surgery and often the obstruction or plaque can be removed.

Clinical evaluation of TIA usually includes an examination by a neurologist, ultrasound examination of the arteries in the neck, and often an arteriogram. The arteriogram is a series of x-ray pictures that show the flow of blood in the arteries, neck, and head taken after the injection of dye into the artery. The dye causes the arteries to stand out clearly in the x-ray picture, allowing the health care provider to identify sites of obstructions. This allows the health care provider to determine whether surgical correction of an obstruction is

possible. One of the tests done on new stroke clients is called magnetic resonance imaging (MRI). This test can pinpoint where the problem lies in the brain. Another test often done is called computed tomography (CT). These two tests give the health care provider adequate information as to what might have caused the stroke and what treatment is indicated. If there is a clot in a particular area in the brain, a health care provider who is trained in this type of emergency can administer a drug to dissolve the clot and, hopefully, the client will recover with few aftereffects.

Multi-infarct dementia is a common form of dementia that is the result of multiple strokes that damage brain tissue. This condition may occur suddenly or develop gradually over time. Signs seen in a person consist of a deterioration of mental function, confusion, memory loss, poor judgment, and changes in personality. These symptoms are progressive.

Cerebral infarction is the term used to describe a stroke in which a portion of the brain dies when an artery becomes blocked and blood is prevented from reaching that part of the brain. The blockage can be the result of hardening and eventual blockage of the artery (atherosclerosis), or be caused by a blood clot in the vessel, or other substances plugging a vessel (emboli). The portions of the brain thus starved of blood, die and cannot function. The effects of the stroke, weakness, paralysis, and loss of feeling, become evident in those parts of the body controlled by the affected part of the brain.

Risk factors that singly or in combination increase the chances of stroke caused by the interruption of blood flow to the brain, resulting in cerebral infarction, are the same as for TIA.

Cerebral infarction is the most common form of stroke and is responsible for most of the partially or completely disabling strokes.

Cerebral hemorrhage means bleeding into the brain, which destroys or disrupts brain tissue. Normally, blood flows to the brain through arteries under high pressure. In vessels with weakened walls, the pressure may cause a rupture and blood will escape into the brain. Under high pressure, blood can spread rapidly in all directions from the point of rupture and may disrupt or damage a large area of the brain, causing weakness, paralysis, loss of sensation, and, frequently, loss of consciousness.

High blood pressure is the main risk factor for hemorrhage into the brain because almost all cerebral hemorrhages occur in clients with high blood pressure.

Possible Aftereffects of Stroke. Stroke can affect an individual in many different ways, depending on which part of the brain has been damaged. Among the possible deficits and problems are:
- Physical Deficits
  —Paralysis or complete loss of strength or mobility in a part of the body, usually the arm, leg, and face on one side.
  —Weakness in a part of the body. Usually weakness is more marked in the hand than in the arm, and the arm is more affected than the leg.
  —Loss of sensation (feeling) in parts of the body, usually on one side
  —Loss of bladder and bowel control
  —Difficulty in swallowing
  —Loss of coordination, such as unsteady gait
- Perceptual Cognitive (thinking) Deficits
  —Loss of awareness
  —Speech and language disability. Difficulty thinking of and saying words or difficulty using or understanding words
  —Denial or neglect of the right or left part of the body and environment
  —Inability to understand time
  —Difficulty performing tasks in proper sequence
  —Disrupted sleep-wake cycles
  —Uncontrolled laughter or crying
  —Confusion, forgetfulness, memory loss, impaired judgment
- Personal Family Problems
  —Loss of job
  —Inadequate financial resources
  —Loss of independence. Dependence on others who may or may not be willing or capable of accepting the new responsibility for continuing care.
  —Loss of sexual capacity
  —Loss of self-esteem
- Psychological Problems (mood)
  —Depression, apathy
  —Anger, hostility
  —Euphoria
- Environmental Problems
  —Architectural barriers in the home
  —Lack of accessible transportation
Not all of these problems happen to each individual. When any of them do happen, there are degrees of difficulty. Most of these problems can be improved. However, after a stroke, the person will always have limitations.

Signs and Symptoms Immediately After a Stroke. The person who suffers a stroke usually loses consciousness and becomes incontinent of urine and feces. In addition, breathing becomes labored or difficult. If consciousness is not lost, the client may complain of a severe headache, slurred speech, and blurred vision. After a stroke there is usually a weakness or paralysis on one side of the body. This one-sided weakness or paralysis is known as hemiplegia. The use of muscles is temporarily or permanently lost when paralysis occurs. Thus, the client may have difficulty in speaking, eating, swallowing, and even hearing. Vigorous therapies need to be started as soon as the client is stable. The majority of the improvement will occur in the first six months after a stroke.

Rehabilitation After a Stroke. A care plan will be developed by the home health team for each individual client. The plan will be implemented once the client has returned home. The goal of the plan is to have the client return to the highest level of function as possible. The client will need to be encouraged continuously to do as much as possible with as little assistance as possible from others. At times it may be easier for an aide to dress or feed the client, but it must be remembered that the goal of care is to have the client do it, not the aide.

After a stroke the client will most likely have one-sided weakness. The client will need to do exercises to regain strength and function to the side of the body that is weak. If the client is unable to do the special exercises, called range-of-motion exercises, the aide will need to do the exercises. The nurse or physical therapist will train the aide to do the exercises. Exercises will be helpful in the prevention of contractures and will improve the client's self-image.

Ambulation is important in the rehabilitation of a person after a stroke. The client may need to have a brace applied to the weak leg for support before ambulating. Check to see if the brace fits properly and does not cause skin irritation. Occasionally a client's sight may be affected after a

stroke. Be sure when you walk a client there is a clear pathway without obstacles in the way. You, the home health aide may see these obstacles, but your client may not.

Dressing is another area in which the client may need assistance. If you need to assist the client to put on a shirt, remember to put the shirt on the weak arm first and then the strong arm. If the client is unable to button the shirt, Velcro closures can be substituted in place of buttons. Elasticized waist slacks will be easier to slip on and off than pants with buttons and zippers.

Oral care is of special importance for the client with a stroke. Before mealtime, it is important to do routine oral care, and if the client has dentures, encourage the client to wear them. The client may need assistance in eating or the client may need to use one of the many assistive feeding devices now available. An occupational therapist may work with the client in restoring the ability to eat without the assistance of others. It will be the home health aide's job to follow through with the plan designed by the occupational therapist. Be sure to check the inside of the weak side of the mouth for food particles after the client has finished eating. The client does not have feeling on the paralyzed side and often food becomes lodged in the cheek and the client may not know it.

Bowel and bladder retraining may also be part of the rehabilitation of a stroke client. The aide should follow the schedule in the care plan.

Communication Problems. The client with a stroke often has a great deal of trouble communicating. The home health aide must be patient and understanding regarding the client's speech problems. Aphasia is a condition in which the ability to speak is impaired. Aphasia is common after a client has had a stroke. Aphasia can affect the ability to talk, listen, read, or write. The client's speech may be slurred, distorted, and slowed. A client who has receptive aphasia does not understand words someone else says. In this case, it may be better to have a communication board to point to (Figure 16-4). In a few cases the client might understand all words coming into the brain, but he is unable to respond appropriately. An example of this might be when an aide asks him if he is hungry and he responds with "no" and in reality he wanted to say "yes" but the answer came out just the opposite of what he wanted. This is extremely frustrating to both you and the client. This type of aphasia is called expressive aphasia because the client is unable to express himself correctly. In the majority of cases in which the client just recently suffered a stroke, a speech therapist will be assisting with communication problems. The speech therapist will inform the aide of the client's type of aphasia and how to communicate more effectively. Sometimes the only words a stroke client uses are curse words or nonsense syllables. This is called automatic speech (involuntary speech). The client's use of curse words can be somewhat embarrassing, since the client never used these words before he or she had a stroke. If your client does use curse words, do not take it seriously because the majority of the time the client has no knowledge of what he or she is saying. In speaking to a stroke client, the aide should use simple sentences that require only short and simple answers from the client. Speaking clearly and simply aids the client's understanding.

Clients who normally wear glasses should continue to wear them even if their sight has been affected by the stroke. This makes the client feel less changed in outward appearance. The same is true if the client wears dentures or a hearing aid.

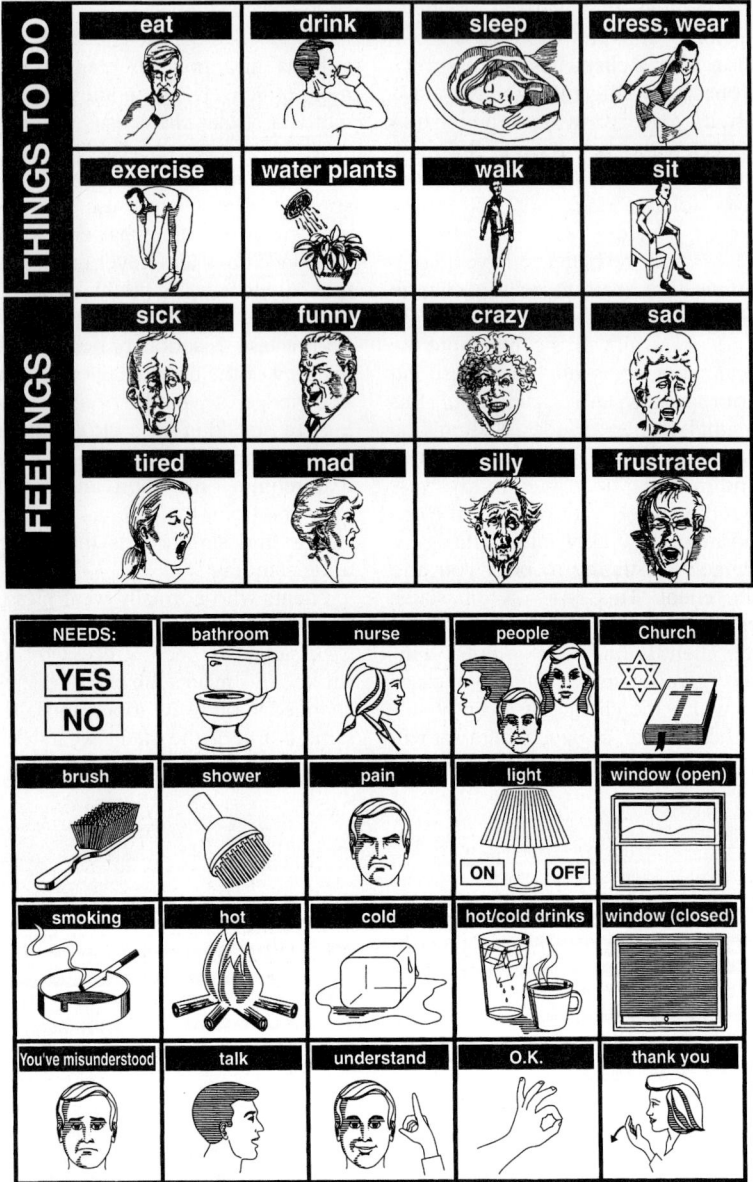

Figure 16-4 A communication board is often used to increase communication with a client who has aphasia.

UNIT 17

Circulatory System

The organ that provides power to the body system is the heart. The heart is a hollow muscular organ about the size of a closed fist (Figure 17-1). Although it is one of the most important organs in the body, it has only one job—to pump blood throughout the body.

CIRCULATORY SYSTEM

The heart has four chambers, the right and left atria and the right and left ventricles. The right atrium receives oxygen-poor blood from the tissues. This blood is pumped to the lungs by the right ventricle, where carbon dioxide is exchanged for oxygen from the lungs. The oxygenated blood is received by the left atrium, which then pumps it to the left ventricle; it is then pumped out to all parts of the body.

Connected to these chambers are the largest blood vessels in the circulatory system. There are three kinds of blood vessels. The arteries carry blood away from the heart to the body cells. The arteries join the tiny blood vessels, called capillaries. The capillaries meet the veins. The veins carry the blood back to the heart. It takes 1 minute for blood to leave the heart, travel through the arteries, capillaries, and veins and return to the heart. This is a cycle that continues each minute of the day.

As the heart contracts (squeezes together) and expands (relaxes), it pushes the blood into the arteries. The arteries contract and expand in the same rhythm as the heart. The pulse measured at the wrist is the expansion of the radial artery. The blood carried in the arteries is a rich, bright red color. Venous blood is a darker red because it is low in oxygen.

RISK FACTORS

Because of the many deaths due to heart problems, many research studies have been conducted on individuals with heart problems. Research has documented the following as major risk factors in heart disease.

- Heredity—Children of parents with heart problems have a greater risk of developing heart conditions.
- Male sex—Men have greater risk than premenopausal women and have heart attacks earlier in life.

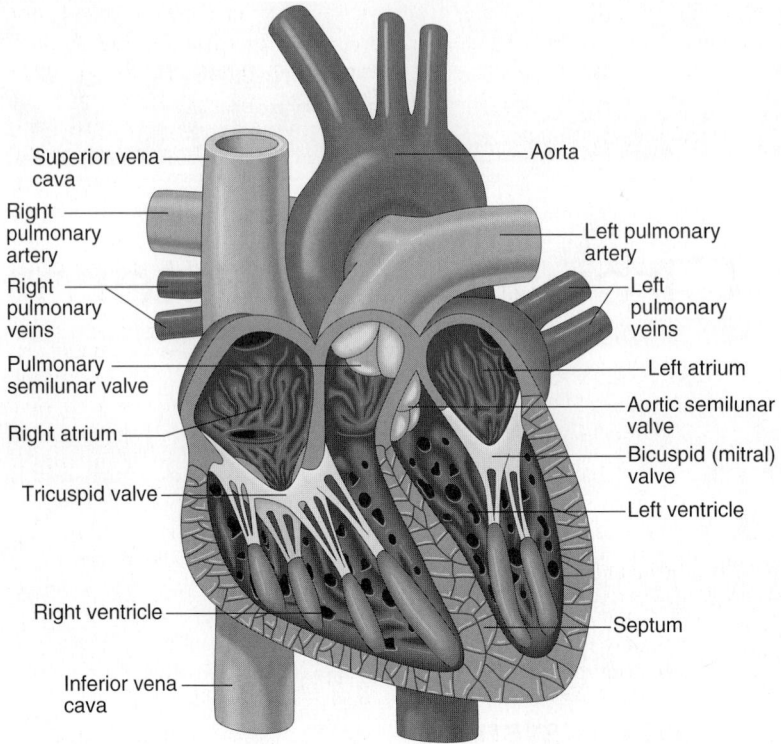

Figure 17-1 The heart is a hollow muscular organ about the size of a closed fist.

- Increasing age—Majority of all heart attacks occur in individuals who are 64 or older.
- Cigarette smoking—Smokers have twice as many heart attacks as nonsmokers.
- High blood pressure—High blood pressure increases the heart's workload and weakens the heart and also the blood vessels in the brain, which eventually can cause either a heart attack or stroke.
- High cholesterol levels—As cholesterol levels increase, the risk of having a heart disease increases.
- Diabetes—People with diabetes have a greater incidence of heart attacks.
- Obesity—Individuals who are 30% overweight have a greater incidence of heart disease.
- Physical inactivity—Lack of exercise combined with obesity and high cholesterol levels will definitely increase the person's chances of having heart disease.
- Stress—There is an increased risk of heart disease in people who are under continuous stress in their lives.

DISORDERS OF THE HEART AND CIRCULATORY SYSTEM

The number one killer of individuals in the United States is heart disease. Circulatory problems affect people of all ages. If an infant is born with a heart defect, it is called a congenital heart problem. The majority of individuals who survive after a heart attack will need some type of medical care and also assistance with activities of daily living (ADL). A home health aide has an important role to play in the recovery of these clients. Some of these clients will need assistance with ADL for the rest of their lives.

The aide may be assigned to help clients with heart problems. Certain conditions require clients to reduce their activity. Clients may need assistance with household duties or child care. The health care provider's orders explain a safe range of activity.

Angina Pectoris

Angina pectoris is a symptom of a condition called myocardial ischemia, which occurs when the heart muscle (myocardium) does not get an adequate supply of blood and oxygen to do its work. Lack of blood supply is called ischemia. Angina pectoris is a mild pain in the chest radiating to the left arm and up through the neck area; or a feeling of fullness, pressure, aching, burning, squeezing, or painful feeling in the chest, back, or jaw. This condition results from lack of oxygen in the heart muscle due to constricted blood vessels. An attack can last from a few seconds to several minutes. It may occur after physical exertion or it may occur after eating, excitement, and exposure to cold. The client becomes pale and ashen and the body stiffens. Blood pressure increases dramatically (hypertension). The client becomes flushed and perspires heavily.

Immediate treatment for angina is physical rest. If this is not the first angina attack, the client is likely to have medication on hand. A common

emergency medication used for angina is nitroglycerin. Nitroglycerin may be taken sublingually, in which case the tablet is placed under the tongue. A spray is also available today that can be sprayed under the tongue. It can also be applied topically in the form of a nitro-patch placed on the skin. The nitroglycerin is absorbed through the skin; a patch provides 24 hours of medication. Old nitroglycerin patches should be removed and the area of skin under the patch cleansed before a new patch is applied. This is to prevent a buildup effect from residual nitroglycerin. Application sites should be alternated daily to prevent skin irritation.

Nitroglycerin opens the blood vessels to increase the blood flow. The effects of the drug occur within 2 to 3 minutes. The pain from angina is usually relieved in 5 to 10 minutes. If three tablets taken over a time span of 15 minutes do not provide relief, emergency care is required. Nitroglycerin is one of the medications that can only be used for a specified period of time because it loses its potency and effectiveness. The aide should check the expiration date. This drug must be kept in the original bottle and out of the light to maintain its potency.

Tests used to diagnose this condition are echocardiogram (determines how the heart is pumping and what areas are not pumping), exercise stress test (heart rate is monitored while client is exercising), and electrocardiogram (heart electrical activity is recorded).

Myocardial Infarction

Myocardial infarction is more commonly known as a coronary, or a major heart attack. A myocardial infarction is a condition in which a blood vessel of the heart muscle closes or is blocked by a blood clot.

The client may go into shock and collapse. Prompt emergency treatment is needed and is begun in the ambulance and continued in the hospital. In the hospital the client will be treated for a heart attack. The need for specialized treatment or surgery will be determined. A coronary angiogram can be done, whereby the health care provider can see inside of the coronary arteries to detect any blockage. Another procedure done today to clear a blockage in the heart is called an angioplasty. In this procedure a catheter with a balloon at the end of it is threaded through the client's coronary artery. When the blockage is located, the balloon is inflated and the plaque or obstruction is flattened and the artery is reopened. One common operation is called coronary artery bypass grafting, or CABG. After release from the hospital, treatment at home may include increased activity with periods of rest and a special diet.

Anticoagulants and other drugs may be part of the treatment when a client has had a coronary attack. Anticoagulants are drugs that reduce the ability of the blood to clot. A home health aide should observe and report any signs of side effects from the use of anticoagulants. These may include bleeding from the gums or bruising of the skin.

Congestive Heart Failure

Congestive heart failure is a condition in which the heart does not pump effectively. This condition can affect the right or left side of the heart, or even both sides at the same time. This is most often caused by heart muscle damage. Thus, the heart's pumping action is weakened. A client with congestive heart failure may have one acute attack and then develop a chronic condition. The signs include a cough, shortness of breath (dyspnea), bluish tinged skin and nails (cyanosis), dizziness, weakness, rapid and irregular heartbeat, and retention of fluid (edema). Fluid (frothy pink sputum) may accumulate in the lungs, causing pneumonia.

Diet control is an important part of the treatment for congestive heart failure. Diets usually are low in sodium and fat.

Arteriosclerosis

Arteriosclerosis is a condition in which the arteries become hard and lose their soft, rubber-like stretchiness. It is caused by a buildup of fatty deposits on the inside walls of the blood vessels. This disease takes many years to develop and once symptoms appear, the disease is fairly well advanced. Individuals who smoke and have high cholesterol and high blood pressure are at the greatest risk.

Phlebitis

Phlebitis occurs when the lining of a vein becomes inflamed, causing a clot to form in the vein. This usually occurs in one leg, which may become swollen and painful to touch. The area may feel warm. The health care provider may order antiembolism stockings or elastic bandages to be applied to the affected leg or to both legs. Refer to Procedure 69.

69 — Procedure

Applying Elasticized Stockings

Purpose

- To prevent swelling of feet and ankles
- To prevent formation of blood clots in legs
- To increase blood circulation in the legs

NOTE: It is better to apply the elastic hose in bed rather than in the chair. Elastic hose should be removed and reapplied every 8 hours. Elastic hose come in a variety of sizes and lengths. They need to be supportive but not too tight. If they are too loose, they lose their effectiveness. The nurse usually measures the client's legs and orders the stockings. The stockings are usually washed by hand and placed in the bathroom to dry overnight. Do not wash in hot water, as that will damage the elasticity of the stockings. Other names for this type of stocking are TEDS® hose and Ace stocking.

Procedure

1. Wash your hands.
2. Tell client what you plan to do.
3. With client lying down, expose one leg at a time.
4. Turn stocking inside out to heel by placing your hand inside stocking and grasping heel (Figure 17-2A).
5. Position stocking over the foot and heel of client, making sure the heel of stocking is in the proper place. If the client just had a bath, apply a thin coat of powder on the legs to make application easier (Figure 17-2B).

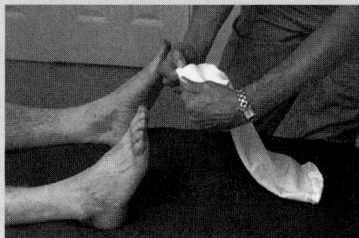

Figure 17-2A   Turn stocking inside out to the heel.

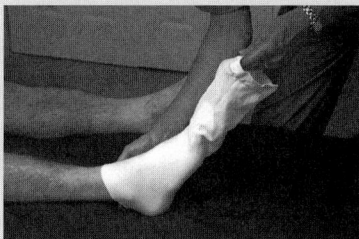

Figure 17-2B   Position stocking over the foot and heel of client, making sure the heel of stocking is properly placed.

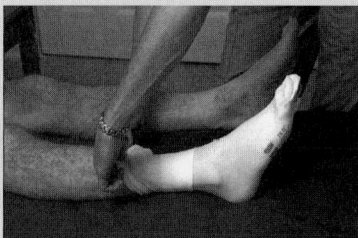

Figure 17-2C   Slide stocking over foot and heel.

6. Slide the remaining stocking over foot and heel (Figure 17-2C).

7. Continue to pull stocking over calf or thigh. The stocking can be either full length to the thigh or knee length, which ends just above the knee (Figure 17-2D).
8. Check to be sure stocking is applied evenly and smoothly and there are no wrinkles.
9. Repeat procedure on opposite leg.
10. Wash your hands.
11. Document completion of the procedure and any unusual observations such as swelling of the ankle.

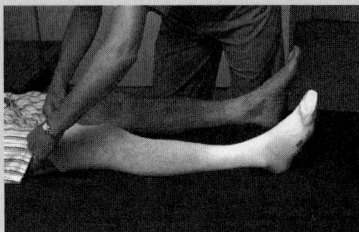

Figure 17-2D Pull and stretch stocking over calf or thigh. Stocking can be either full length to the thigh or knee length, which ends just above the knee. Check to see that there are no wrinkles in the stocking.

Venous Insufficiency

Venous insufficiency is due to damage of the veins that return blood to the heart. The symptoms are chronic aching, edema, and discoloration of the lower extremities. The client may develop leg ulcers due to lack of oxygen available to these tissues. Clients with venous insufficiency are at-risk of developing thrombophlebitis, which occurs when the vein becomes inflamed and a clot forms. The symptoms of this condition are tenderness, redness, warmth over the vein, and pain in the calf of the leg when the client flexes his or her foot. As part of the treatment for this condition the aide may have to assist clients with the application of elastic stockings, which promote venous blood return. Refer to Procedure 69. The client should be discouraged from standing or sitting for any prolonged period of time. The symptoms of pulmonary embolus are shortness of breath, chest pain, and increased heart rate. This is a life-threatening condition that requires immediate medical attention.

Arterial Insufficiency

Arterial insufficiency results from a narrowing of the arteries that deliver blood to the lower extremities. When a client walks any distance, exercise increases the demand for oxygen to the tissues and muscles of the legs. Because of the narrow arteries, the blood flow is not sufficient to meet the demand. The client experiences cramping pain in the calf of the leg or thigh. This is called intermittent claudication. This pain should subside after the client rests for a few minutes. If an artery should become completely obstructed and blood not restored in four to six hours, the client is in danger of losing a limb. Signs of complete obstruction are severe pain, pallor, absence of pulse in foot and lower leg, numbness, paralysis, and coldness of limb.

Gangrene

Gangrene is death of body tissue brought on by lack of adequate blood supply to the area. Signs of gangrene are fever, pain, darkening of the skin, and unpleasant odor. Those at risk for developing this infection include diabetics and other people with poor circulation. The lower extremities are most often affected. The home health aide must look carefully for any signs of skin breakdown, especially in diabetics, and report any sign of skin breakdown to the nurse.

DISORDERS OF THE BLOOD

Blood is the life stream of the human body. Blood performs many tasks, and no part of the body can live without it. Blood supplies the cells of the body with the food and oxygen they need for work and growth. It carries waste products to specific organs that remove them from the body, or breaks them down into harmless substances. Blood also fights germs that enter the body. Blood has four main parts:

1. Plasma (the liquid part of the blood)
2. Red blood cells (carry oxygen and carbon dioxide to and from the lungs and body tissues)
3. White blood cells (fight infections)
4. Platelets (help to clot the blood)

Disorders of the blood can occur as a result of a malformation or malfunction of a part of the blood.

Anemia

Anemia occurs when there are not enough red blood cells. It may result from an excessive loss of blood, from malformation of blood cells, or from a lack of essential nutrients. If blood loss is excessive, hypotension (low blood pressure) may occur.

Iron Deficiency Anemia. Iron deficiency anemia causes shrinkage of the red blood cells, leading to weakness, headaches, loss of color, and loss of concentration. Iron deficiency is the most common nutrient deficiency in the world. Treatment includes taking an iron supplement or

eating iron-rich foods such as red meats, beans, dark leafy vegetables, and fortified breads and cereals.

Pernicious Anemia. Pernicious anemia is a vitamin B_{12} deficiency caused by the body's inability to produce the intrinsic factor, which helps with vitamin B_{12} absorption. Red blood cells and the nervous system can be damaged with this anemia. Treatment involves a monthly injection of vitamin B_{12}.

Sickle Cell Anemia

With sickle cell anemia the client's red blood cells are crescent shaped, like a sickle. The cells do not carry enough oxygen in them, causing anemia. This is an inherited disease for which there is no cure. In the United States, this disease is usually found only in African Americans.

Leukemia

Leukemia is a condition in which there are too many immature white blood cells. These excess white blood cells block the normal transport of oxygen to the body's tissues. They may also affect production of new red blood cells. Leukemia may also be called cancer of the blood. Leukemia clients are very prone to infections and must be protected from outside sources of infection such as crowds of people and especially those with colds.

Hemophilia

Hemophilia is an hereditary disease characterized by spontaneous hemorrhages due to a deficiency of a clotting factor in the blood. The classic form of the disease affects males only. If an individual starts to bleed, a special preparation can be given to stop the bleeding. These individuals must be protected from injury by use of helmets, elbow pads, and kneepads.

UNIT 18

Respiratory System

The respiratory system consists of the nose, pharynx, larynx, trachea, bronchi, and lungs (Figure 18-1). Through effective air distribution and gas exchange, the respiratory system helps maintain a constant balance in the body, enabling the cells to function properly.

RESPIRATORY SYSTEM

The respiratory system is closely linked to the circulatory system. Blood is supplied with fresh oxygen by means of this system. Fresh air is inhaled into the body and carried to the lungs. The oxygen from the air is carried to all parts of the body by the circulatory system. As oxygen is delivered to the cells of the body, waste gases are picked up and carried back to the lungs, where they are exhaled from the body. The most plentiful waste gas is carbon dioxide.

MAJOR RESPIRATORY ILLNESSES

Diseases of the respiratory system have now been classified together as chronic obstructive pulmonary disease (COPD). COPD refers to the decreased ability of the lungs to perform their ventilation function, which may result from an acute infection, such as pneumonia, or a chronic condition, such as bronchitis or asthma. An example of a COPD is emphysema. Clients with breathing difficulties will need more frequent rest periods because they tire easily. In addition, they will need more time to accomplish their activities. Often, clients who experience difficulty breathing will be anxious. It is important that the aide remain calm and help the client to stay calm as well.

Clients with breathing difficulties may use inhalers, bronchodilators, nebulizers, compressors, or portable oxygen containers. These treatments are prescribed by a health care provider. A respiratory therapist or nurse will train the client on the proper use of equipment and medication. The home health aide may be instructed to coach the client through a breathing treatment or to simply be supportive of the client who is self-administering a breathing treatment.

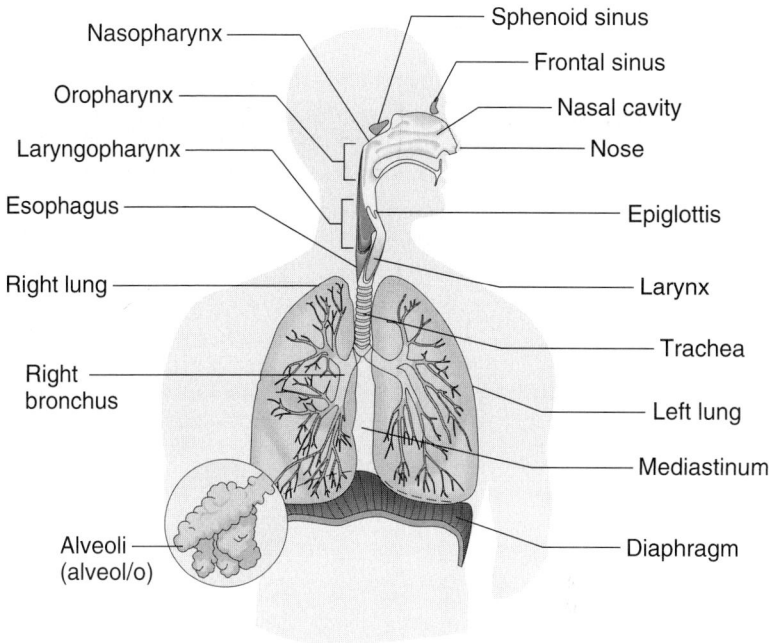

Respiratory System

Figure 18-1   The respiratory system. Primary organs of the respiratory tract are the nose, pharynx, trachea, bronchi, and lungs. The upper respiratory tract refers to anything outside the chest cavity. The lower respiratory tract refers to within the chest cavity.

A nebulizer is a device that is usually power-driven by a compressed air machine. It changes a liquid medication into a fine mist. The lungs can then absorb the medicine more effectively. A nebulizer can be used for treating respiratory problems in infants, children, and adults.

A sputum specimen may be required to diagnose a respiratory infection and to provide a method to monitor the client's ongoing respiratory condition. Procedure 71 describes the proper technique for collecting a sputum specimen.

71

Procedure

Collecting a Sputum Specimen

Purpose
- To provide a sputum specimen for a diagnostic test
- To monitor the client's ongoing condition

NOTE: Do not have client use mouthwash before collecting a sputum specimen. Specimen should be from the lungs and not saliva from the client's mouth.

Procedure

1. Assemble supplies:
   - disposable gloves
   - specimen container, cover with label completed
   - tissues
   - disposable plastic bag
   - mask (optional)
2. Wash hands and apply gloves. Wear a mask if client has an infectious disease.

3. Ask client to cough deeply and bring up sputum from the lungs. Have client expectorate (spit) into the container. Collect 1 to 2 tablespoons of sputum unless otherwise directed. Be sure to have client cover mouth with tissue to prevent the spread of droplets in the air. If excess sputum contaminates the outside of the container, wipe off right away. Cover specimen container and place in plastic bag.
4. Remove gloves and wash hands.
5. Document collection of sputum and when transported to laboratory.

Pneumonia

Pneumonia is an inflammation of the lungs due to an infection by bacteria or viruses. The incidence of pneumonia increases in infants and adults. The disease is diagnosed by a chest x-ray and sputum analysis. Pneumonia is also named after the part of the lung that is affected such as right lower bronchial pneumonia or right lower lobar pneumonia. If caused by bacteria, pneumonia can generally be treated using antibiotics. The type of pneumonia seen in frail older adults and postsurgical clients is called hypostatic pneumonia. This type of pneumonia is due to inactivity of the lungs. If a person has surgery, doing deep-breathing exercises (refer to Procedure 72) can prevent this type of pneumonia.

72   Procedure

Assisting with Cough and Deep-Breathing Exercises

Purpose
- To prevent congestion or infections in the client's lungs
- To expand the lung capacity

Procedure

1. Wash your hands.
2. Explain the procedure to the client.

3. Assemble equipment:
   - disposable gloves—optional
   - pillow case—covered pillow
   - tissues
   - optional: incentive spirometer
4. Have client in a sitting position.
5. If the client has recently had surgery, a pillow placed over the incision site may reduce muscle

movement in the area and reduce discomfort.

6. Ask client to take as deep a breath through the nose as possible and hold it for 5 to 7 seconds and then exhale slowly through pursed lips.

7. If using an incentive spirometer have the client inhale air through the mouthpiece of the incentive spirometer and try to get the ball up as far as he or she can and hold it for 6 to 7 seconds and then exhale slowly after removing the mouthpiece.

8. Repeat exercise about five times.

9. Give client tissues and instruct client to take a deep breath and cough forcefully twice with mouth open. Collect any secretions that are brought up in tissues. Protect yourself from secretions and droplets.

10. Slip on gloves if you will be touching or handling the tissues.

11. Dispose of tissues in plastic bag and assist client to comfortable position.

12. Remove gloves and wash hands.

13. Document procedure completed, your observations, and client's reaction.

NOTE: Frequency of these exercises can vary according to the health care provider's orders and the client's medical condition.

Pneumonia is a leading cause of death in the United States. Because many older adults already have preexisting conditions and chronic illnesses, they are more vulnerable. It is critical to understand that many older adults do not always have severe early symptoms, but then can become acutely ill very quickly. It is recommended that older adults get a flu shot, because the flu can lead to pneumonia. Another preventive measure is to get the pneumonia vaccine, which will protect the elderly from a common type of pneumonia called pneumococcal pneumonia.

Chronic Bronchitis

Chronic bronchitis often occurs in middle-aged or elderly persons. It can result from a number of acute conditions such as asthma, bronchitis, cigarette smoking, and air pollution.

Bronchitis is an inflammation of the bronchi. This condition is seen most often in the elderly, people who are obese, and smokers. This includes, in particular, elderly individuals with a history of chronic lung disease. The treatment plan is devised to relieve symptoms.

Symptoms include fever (usually low grade) with coughing spells that produce thick, white, greenish or yellowish phlegm, and lethargy, malaise, and breathlessness. Treatment includes rest, fluids, and cough medication to loosen secretions. Medications to dilate the bronchi and facilitate more effective breathing are also ordered. Encourage clients to elevate both their head and chest to facilitate better breathing. Refer to Procedure 72 on the proper method to assist with cough and deep-breathing exercises.

Asthma

Asthma is a condition that affects the bronchial tubes or airways of the lungs. It is usually caused by an allergic reaction, although there are other causes. Often the specific substance causing the asthma cannot be determined. Symptoms may include coughing, difficulty breathing, whee-zing, and a feeling of tightness in the chest.

Asthma strikes more adults than once thought. Primarily asthma is as-sociated with constriction of large and small airways causing spasms. Swelling in the airway and increased mucous productivity result in these symptoms: severe difficulty breath-ing, wheezing, sweating, feelings of suffocation, and anxiety. The care plan includes resolving immediate respiratory distress, elevation of client torso, and encouraging the client to inhale through the nose and exhale through pursed lips. Remain calm and help client stay as calm as pos-sible. Provide adequate humidity. Have client avoid the potential aller-gens (the substances causing allergic reactions) if they are known.

Emphysema

Emphysema is a lung condition in which the air sacs within the lung lose their elasticity. Breathing is diffi-cult for the person affected by this disease. Medications can relieve the symptoms of emphysema, but there is no cure.

Care plan includes oxygen as or-dered to facilitate breathing. A posi-tion used often by emphysema clients is to sit up in a lounge chair with a small table placed across the chair with pillows on top of the table. Em-physema clients often sleep in this position because they have problems breathing in a supine position in bed. Refer to Procedure 73 on the method to assist the client with oxygen ther-apy. The care plan also includes edu-cation regarding healthier lifestyle and abstinence from smoking.

73 Procedure

Assisting the Client with Oxygen Therapy

Purpose

- To assist the client to receive cor-rect amount of oxygen
- To avoid misuse of oxygen equip-ment and careless practices that risk causing fires, explosions, or injury
- To aid in breathing

Procedure

1. Check the meter of the oxygen tank or reservoir. If low, check to see if there is a spare tank. If there is not a spare tank, call for a re-placement. **NOTE:** An oxygen

concentrator removes the oxygen from the air. This device is usually ordered for clients who will be on oxygen for a long period of time. A long tube is connected to the device, giving the client greater freedom of movement. Another method of delivering oxygen is through a nebulizer. The nebu-lizer delivers fine mists with a high degree of humidity. When nebulizers are used, large tubing should be used to connect the nebulizer to the oxygen device.

2. Wash your hands.

3. Check to see if the client's oxygen mask or cannula is placed properly. The straps on the cannula should be secure but not too tight. Check top of ears for signs of irritation. Check for signs of irritation where the prongs touch the client's nose. Be sure both prongs are in the client's nose.

   If a mask is being used, check to see whether the mask is over both nose and mouth. If inside of mask is wet, remove and dry inside.

4. Check the gauge to see if the oxygen is being given at correct amount of liter flow (Figure 18-2). (Oxygen therapy is delivered in liters.) The client's care plan should state the liter flow to be administered to the client. Follow any special instructions listed in the care plan. A typical order would look like this: O$_2$ @ 4L prn. O$_2$ is the abbreviation for oxygen, L is the abbreviation for liter, and prn means as needed.

5. Check the client's position. If in bed, elevate the head with three pillows to assist the client in breathing.

6. Do frequent mouth care for clients receiving oxygen therapy. The client's mouth can become dry and have an unpleasant taste. Apply water-soluble lubricant to lips if they become dry.

7. Check that all safety precautions are being observed.
   • Do not smoke in room where client is receiving oxygen. Post "No Smoking" sign, if

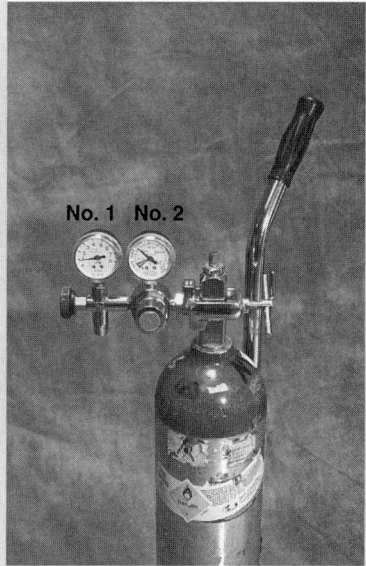

Figure 18-2   No. 1 gauge notes the liter flow. No. 2 gauge notes the amount of oxygen left in the tank.

necessary, to warn visitors not to smoke.
   • Do not use matches, candles, or open flames where oxygen is used or stored.
   • Do not use electrical appliances during oxygen therapy. Avoid sparks. If you need to shave the client, turn off the oxygen while using the electric razor, or use a disposable razor.

8. Wash your hands.

9. Document the liter flow and the device being used, your observations, and client's breathing pattern.

Reproductive System

REPRODUCTIVE SYSTEM

The reproductive system consists of the external and internal sex organs of the male and female. The male organs include the scrotum, a saclike organ that contains the testes and other tubules; the testes, which produce sperm, the hormone testosterone and fluid; and the penis, which contains the urethra for transporting urine and sperm (Figure 19-1).

The female external organs are the genitalia (vulva) and breasts. The internal organs include the vagina, which functions as the birth canal and leads to the cervix and uterus; the cervix, which is the mouth of the womb; the uterus, located behind the urinary bladder (which functions as the womb that receives the fertilized egg and developing fetus); the ovaries, located on either side of the lower abdomen, which produce estrogen and progesterone hormones as well as egg cells; and the fallopian tubes, which carry the egg cells from the ovaries to the uterus (Figures 19-2 and 19-3).

The female has a menstrual cycle approximately every 28 days, by which the uterus is prepared to nurture the fertilized egg into a viable fetus. However, if the egg cell that is produced midcycle is not fertilized by the sperm cell, the uterine lining is sloughed off, and bleeding occurs for approximately 3 to 5 days. This is called menstruation.

The reproductive system is important in maintaining sexual characteristics. The hormones that produce male characteristics (such as broad shoulders, facial, chest, and pubic hair) and female characteristics (such as rounded hips, enlarged breasts, and pubic hair) are also thought to help maintain function in other systems of the body. Illness or malfunction of the reproductive system can cause emotional and physical problems.

COMMON DISORDERS OF THE REPRODUCTIVE SYSTEM

Some common disorders of the reproductive system include dysmenorrhea, vaginitis, and sexually transmitted diseases. Many of these disorders may be caused by infections or sexual activity with an infected person, and may require medication for treatment.

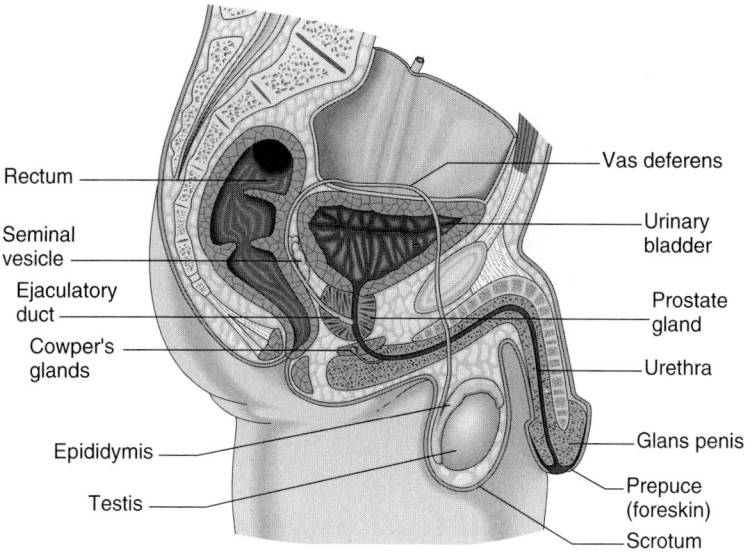

Rectum

Seminal
vesicle

Ejaculatory
duct

Cowper's
glands

Epididymis

Testis

Vas deferens

Urinary
bladder

Prostate
gland

Urethra

Glans penis

Prepuce
(foreskin)

Scrotum

Figure 19-1   The male reproductive system

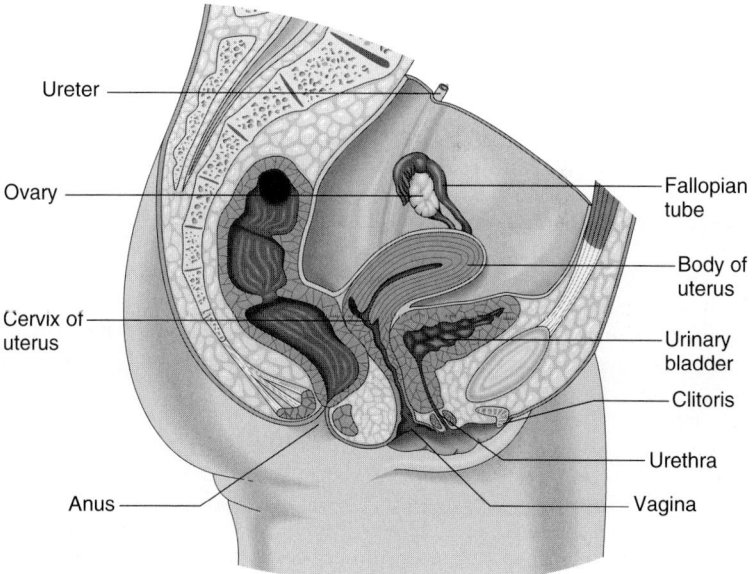

Ureter

Ovary

Cervix of
uterus

Anus

Fallopian
tube

Body of
uterus

Urinary
bladder

Clitoris

Urethra

Vagina

Figure 19-2   The female reproductive system

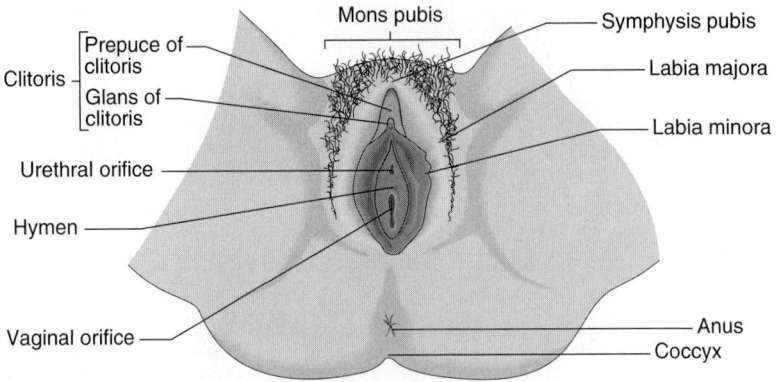

Figure 19-3   The female external genitalia

Dysmenorrhea

Dysmenorrhea refers to pain that sometimes accompanies the menstrual flow. Although a large percentage of women experience some minor discomfort during menstruation, it should be emphasized that menstruation is a normal process. However, any severe cramping or persistent pain should be reported to a gynecologist, a health care provider specializing in women's reproductive health.

Vaginitis

Vaginitis is an infection of the vagina (birth canal), which may be caused by bacteria, viruses, or yeast; or may result from changes in vaginal secretions after menopause (the permanent end of menstruation). There is usually a whitish, odorous discharge with itching and burning. Treatment consists of wearing cotton underwear, avoiding garments that hold heat and moisture, eating yogurt, and treating the infectious organisms with drugs. In older women, vaginal creams containing estrogen may be used.

SEXUALLY TRANSMITTED DISEASES

Infections spread by sexual intercourse are called sexually transmitted diseases (STDs). These are common worldwide, especially among young adults. In developed countries, syphilis and gonorrhea declined after World War II, increased in the 1960s and 1970s, and declined in the 1980s, and are rising again.

Common symptoms of sexually transmitted diseases occur in or near the vagina or penis and include: unusual discharge; lumps, bumps, or rashes; sores that are painful, itchy, or painless; itchy skin; and burning on urination. In most cases both partners need to be tested and treated. If only one person is treated, that person can be reinfected again, if his or her partner is not treated.

Chlamydia

Chlamydia is a disease caused by bacteria that is spread when infected fluid from the sex organ or rectum contacts the penis, vagina, mouth, or anus. Women may have an inflammation of the cervix with a foul-smelling discharge, burning on urination, and itching around the sex gland. Men have similar symptoms. Chlamydia may also have a silent beginning, whereby there will be no symptoms exhibited until the infection has spread to the pelvic area and caused pelvic inflammatory disease (PID). It is the most common cause of STDs and is a common cause of infertility. Chlamydia can be treated with antibiotics. If left untreated in a pregnant woman, the disease can be passed from mother to infant during birth. The infant may have eye, lung, or other health problems.

Pelvic Inflammatory Disease

Pelvic inflammatory disease (PID) is an infection of the upper female reproductive tract. Bacterial organisms such as *Chlamydia* or gonorrhea cause the disorder. Diagnosis is based on analysis of the cervical or vaginal secretions. It can be treated with antibiotics. If not treated, PID can cause severe damage and scarring of the reproductive tract. Complications include chronic pelvic pain, infertility, and abnormal menstruation. Scarring in the fallopian tubes can block passage of the fertilized egg, increasing the risk of an ectopic (tubal) pregnancy, a condition in which the egg implants outside the uterine cavity.

Nongonococcal Urethritis

Nongonococcal urethritis, also known as nonspecific urethritis, is urethral inflammation caused by an infection other than gonorrhea. This infection is among the most prevalent of all STDs. Symptoms usually start 1 to 3 weeks after exposure. In women, the main symptom is vaginal discharge. Men, as a result of inflammation of the urethra, commonly experience discharge from the penis and pain when urinating. Infection

may cause scrotal pain and swelling. Treatment consists of antibiotics.

Gonorrhea

Gonorrhea, a bacterial infection, causes a discharge of pus from the penis or sometimes the vagina, and pain on urination. The main sites of infection are the urethra and, in women, the cervix, from where organisms can spread to the uterus, fallopian tubes, and ovaries. The rectum can also be affected. A pregnant woman risks passing the infection to her baby during childbirth. In men, it infects the urethra, and then spreads to the testes and prostate. This can cause pain, swelling, and scarring. Gonorrhea is treated by antibiotics, but in some parts of the world resistance has developed to most drugs.

Syphilis

Syphilis is a bacterial disease. Syphilis progresses in three stages and becomes more severe in each stage. It is treated with antibiotics. The earliest symptom of syphilis is usually an ulcer (chancre) on the genitals. However, an ulcer can also develop in the mouth or anus. A rash, mouth ulcers, and enlargement of the lymph nodes follow. Later effects include brain, heart, and bone disorders. A pregnant woman can pass the infection to her baby.

Genital Herpes

One of the most common STDs is genital herpes, and its reported incidence has increased over recent years in some countries. Caused by an organism known as herpes simplex virus, genital herpes tends to recur. The first episode is the most severe, with subsequent occurrences decreasing in severity and frequency.

During an episode, crops of small blisters form on the penis or around the vagina, then develop into shallow, painful ulcers. The first attack of herpes may be accompanied by headache, fever, and pain in the groin, buttocks, and legs.

There is no cure for genital herpes. Painkillers and keeping lesions clean and dry, as well as not scratching them, can relieve symptoms. Certain drugs can provide pain relief and speed healing during an attack. Prolonged use of the antiviral drug, acyclovir, may reduce the number and frequency of occurrences.

Genital Warts

Viruses cause genital warts. These warts may appear as bumps or small pink or red growths, or be flat and difficult to see. They can be painful and irritating. The warts can grow in, on, or near the penis, vagina, cervix, rectum, or throat. Using chemicals, freezing, or laser therapy can remove them. More than one treatment is usually needed. These warts can continue to reappear, and just removing them does not mean the disease is cured. Even when condoms are used during sex, the virus can be spread through contact with the skin of the infected partner, which the condom does not cover.

Prevention of STDs

To prevent STDs, sexually active people should, ideally, have a single sexual partner, always use a latex condom when engaged in penetrative sex, and avoid practices that could damage the delicate lining of the vagina or anus. People with symptoms of an STD or who are being treated for an STD should abstain from sex, and their partners should be checked for infection and also treated.

UNIT 20

Endocrine System and Diabetes

ENDOCRINE SYSTEM

The endocrine system is composed of many glands scattered throughout the body. The **endocrine glands** are ductless glands that secrete substances within the body called hormones (Figure 20-1). The glands do not have ducts (little tubes) and are, therefore, unlike tear and sweat glands. Hormones are chemicals that are secreted directly into the bloodstream. They are carried throughout the body to regulate and control specific body functions. They are powerful substances and direct the functions of other systems. Each hormone has a special job to do (Figure 20-2). It only takes a small amount of hormone to trigger a body reaction. Most scientists agree that the brain sends messages to the endocrine glands. These messages cause the gland to secrete the hormone needed by the body.

HYPERTHYROIDISM AND HYPOTHYROIDISM

The thyroid weighs less than an ounce but all aspects of metabolism, from the rate at which your heart beats to the speed at which you burn calories, are regulated by the thyroid hormones. Some people have an overactive thyroid and their food metabolizes quickly (hyperthyroidism). They usually have a rapid heartbeat and tend to be restless and irritable.

About 7 million Americans, mostly women over the age of 40, are affected by an underactive thyroid (hypothyroidism). Early symptoms of an underactive thyroid, such as sluggishness and fatigue, are often vague.

DIABETES MELLITUS

Diabetes mellitus is a chronic disease with no cure. The disease is primarily managed through diet, exercise, and drug therapy. The pancreas either does not produce any or produces an inadequate amount of a hormone called insulin.

The functions of insulin are to enable the body to use glucose (sugar), to aid in the storage of nutrients, and to make possible the metabolism of carbohydrates and protein. When insulin is not manufactured or cannot be used correctly, a condition called **diabetes** develops. In diabetes, the person's blood sugar level is elevated (hyperglycemia) because the sugar remains in the blood instead of being

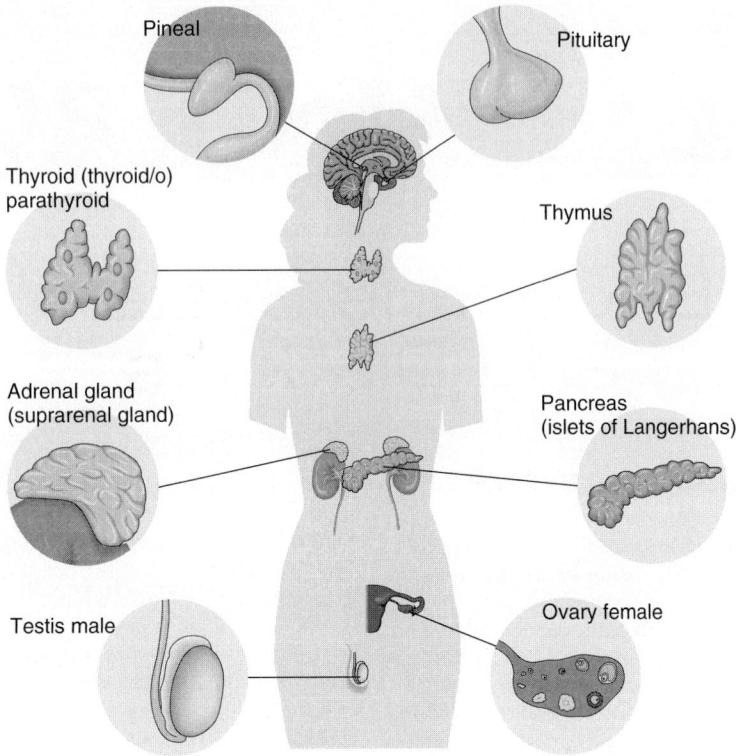

Figure 20-1   Location of the endocrine glands

absorbed into the cells and used for food. The buildup of sugar in the blood is unhealthy for a number of reasons. It disturbs the fluid balance in the body because it causes kidney problems. Diabetes suppresses the immune system and this allows infections to flourish. Sugar buildup in the blood vessels results in restricted circulation because of damage to the blood vessels. The lack of adequate blood supply to certain body areas causes many problems in the brain, extremities, eyes, kidney, and heart.

Diabetes is a double risk for clients with heart disease. Cardiovascular disease is the most lethal of possible complications of diabetes. It claims about 65% of people with this metabolic disorder. According to the National Diabetes Education Program, adults with diabetes are two to four times more likely to have heart disease or suffer a stroke than those without the condition. High blood pressure is also associated with diabetes. Diabetes promotes plaque formation in the arteries. Few people are aware of these risks. Early identification and management of cardiovascular complications in clients with diabetes is important.

Classifications

Diabetes can be classified into several types.

- Insulin-dependent diabetes mellitus (IDDM) Type I: usually occurs before age 25. The pancreas no

Pituitary gland	Once called "master gland" of the body; secretes a number of hormones that regulate many bodily processes. The pituitary is completely controlled by the hypothalamus, a part of the brain.
Thyroid gland	Helps to regulate the metabolic rate and growth process.
Parathyroid glands	Regulate metabolism of calcium and phosphorous.
Thymus gland	Regulates immunity to infectious diseases during infancy and early childhood; becomes smaller as body ages.
Adrenal glands	Adjust body to crisis and stress; increase blood pressure; speed reactions; metabolize carbohydrates and proteins.
Pineal gland	Regulates the secretion of the hormone melatonin. Light inhibits melatonin secretions, while darkness stimulates melatonin production. This hormone regulates sleep and waking cycles.
Pancreas	Produces insulin needed to burn sugar in body. (Too little insulin causes diabetes; too much insulin causes hyperglycemia). Also produces glucagon to raise blood sugar.
Ovaries	Produce ovum (egg) for reproduction; secrete estrogen and progesterone that develop and maintain secondary sexual characteristics (breasts, pubic and underarm hair, etc.).
Testes	Produce sperm to fertilize ovum; secrete male hormone called testosterone.

Figure 20-2   Functions of the glands of the endocrine system

longer produces any insulin and this person needs daily insulin injections.

- Non–insulin-dependent diabetes mellitus Type II diabetes: usually develops after the age of 40 and is commonly seen in older adults. Insulin is produced, but may be insufficient or ineffective in preventing hyperglycemia. This person is unable to use this insulin effectively to change glucose (sugar) into energy. People with Type II diabetes may need to use insulin, but usually take oral medication.

- Gestational—Type III: Occurs during a woman's pregnancy and usually returns to normal after delivery. However, these women often will develop diabetes later in life unless changes are made in diet and exercise.

Signs and Symptoms

Signs and symptoms of diabetes can come on slowly and will only be detected by a physical evaluation and blood tests. Occasionally it is caused by infection or stress and will come on suddenly. Some of the signs and symptoms to watch for are:

• Weakness
• Sudden weight loss
• Unusual thirst
• Frequent need to urinate
• Crankiness
• Itching
• Sores that do not heal
• Repeated infections

Testing

Routine testing for glucose (sugar level) during a physical examination is important for early diagnosis and detection. Common tests used in the diagnoses and care of diabetes are:

• Fasting blood sugar (FBS): Blood sample tested for sugar in the blood content; normal range is between 70 and 120 mg.

• Urinalysis: Urine sample is tested for presence of sugar or ketones.
• Glucose tolerance tests: Series of tests done on blood within designated time periods. Blood is tested while fasting and then after drinking a high-glucose solution at different time periods.
• Glycosylated hemoglobin (HbA_{1c}): Blood test that will give the average blood sugar over a period of 6 to 12 weeks.

Once diagnosed with diabetes, clients are taught how to test their blood. Testing the blood gives a reading of what the blood sugar value is at the moment. Blood testing kits are readily available at any pharmacy. Blood testing equipment (glucometer) has been greatly improved in the last few years and, although the cost may be high, it is the best method to monitor blood sugar levels. Medicare will now pay for testing supplies for diabetics, if the client is enrolled in the program. Procedure 73 outlines the method for testing blood.

73   Procedure

Testing Blood

Purpose

• To determine the blood sugar level

Testing procedures for blood sugar vary according to the type of glucometer the client has purchased. The instructions must be followed carefully to avoid an inaccurate reading. It is also important if you assist with the procedure that you follow standard precautions. *Always check with your agency to see if you are allowed to do this task.*

Procedure

1. Gather necessary equipment:
   • disposable gloves
   • glucometer (Figure 20-3A)
   • blood lancet (needle)
   • alcohol swab

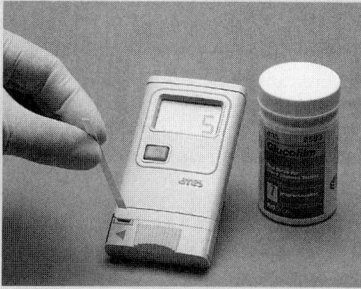

Figure 20-3A   Diabetic blood testing equipment: glucometer and blood testing strips

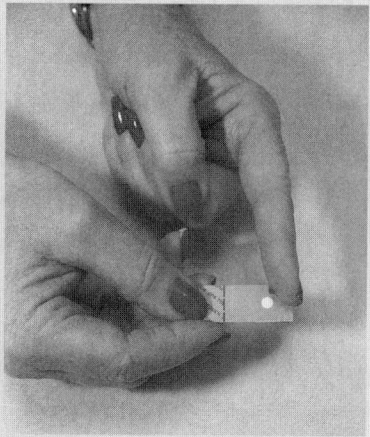

Figure 20-3C   Drop of blood from client's finger on blood testing strip

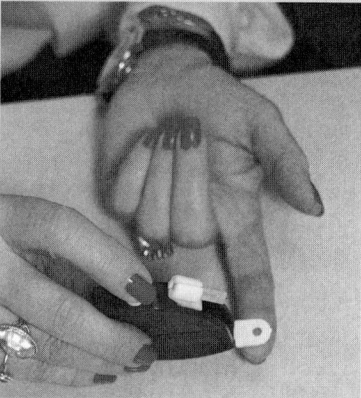

Figure 20-3B   Client pricking finger

- blood strips—be sure you have blood strips that correspond with your glucometer.
2. Wash hands and apply gloves.
3. Have client wipe finger with alcohol wipe; then have the client squeeze

and prick the finger with the lancet (Figure 20-3B). The client may use a special apparatus to prick the finger. Rotate fingers. Use the side of finger that has less use.
4. With palm facing down, firmly apply pressure to the pricked finger until a large drop of hanging blood forms. Bring the blood strip to the finger and touch the blood strip to the drop of blood (Figure 20-3C). Completely cover the test zone of the strip with the blood.
5. Insert blood strip into machine and observe read-out.
6. Discard blood strip and lancet in proper container.
7. Remove gloves and wash hands.
8. Record reading.

Some machines have the ability to talk the client or the caregiver through the procedure. It is important to know when the blood sugar reading is high or low. When taking a reading, you must be aware of when the client last ate or drank anything to accurately know if the blood sugar reading is high. Your nurse will advise you when to call to report abnormal readings. A reading of 200 might be normal for one client, but it might be abnormal for another. It is the responsibility of your nurse to interpret the reading.

Emergency Treatment

Insulin shock and diabetic coma can be life-threatening situations for the client. The home health aide needs to be familiar with the signs of each condition. Be alert to the signs of each and report them immediately to the case manager. If your client is a diabetic, know where the juice or other easily absorbed carbohydrates are stored. If either condition is not corrected immediately, coma or death can occur.

Hypoglycemia or Insulin Shock.

If the blood sugar goes too low, a condition called hypoglycemia occurs. This is also called insulin shock. Normal blood sugar is between 70 mg to 110 mg. This condition occurs when there is an imbalance between food intake and the appropriate dosage of hypoglycemic drug therapy—oral drugs, insulin, or both. Exercise, intake of alcohol, or decreased kidney or liver function can aggravate this condition. The signs of hypoglycemia are:

- Change in mental functioning
- Fast heart rate
- Cold, clammy skin
- Hunger
- Shaking
- Seizures

If it is confirmed that the blood sugar is below 50 mg, this is an emergency. If the client is alert, give some form of concentrated sugar such as hard candy, honey, or glucose tablets. If the client becomes unresponsive, call 911 and begin your emergency protocol—A, airway; B, breathing; C, circulation.

Hyperglycemia or Diabetic Acidosis/Coma.

If a client's blood sugar is high, this is called hyperglycemia. The blood sugar is usually over 250 mg. This should be confirmed by a blood sugar check. This condition can also be called **diabetic coma** or **acidosis.** This condition occurs because of overeating, too little insulin medication, emotional stress, or lack of activity. The signs of hyperglycemia are:

- Increased thirst, hunger, and urination
- Weakness
- Abdominal cramps
- Generalized aches and pains
- Nausea and vomiting
- Fruity odor to breath

This is a serious condition. Your case manager should be contacted immediately. If the person is unresponsive, you should call 911 or begin emergency protocol. Insulin is needed as well as a fluid replacement and blood tests to evaluate the client's metabolism. If either insulin reaction or acidosis is not corrected immediately, coma or death can occur.

Diet

Diet is the cornerstone to the management of diabetes. The diet should contain necessary elements of good nutrition, maintain blood sugar levels, and be acceptable to the client's preferences. The diet needs to contain a defined number of calories and consist of 50% to 60% carbohydrates, 12% to 20% protein, and 30% to 36% fat. The food intake should be distributed throughout the day and accommodate the client's lifestyle, activity, and diabetic medication. Because 90–95% of diabetics are classified as type II diabetics, they will also need to have their carbohydrate intake limited. Of all the different components of a client's diet (carbohydrate, fat, and protein), carbohydrates have the most effect on blood sugar levels. The American Diabetes Association has developed exchange lists of foods that can assist the aide and the client in meal planning.

An important duty of the aide is to prepare meals using the diet prescribed by the dietician and exchange list. The aide needs to encourage and reinforce the importance of abiding by this diet. A diabetic client also needs to remember to eat meals and snacks at the same time every day.

Obesity and poor nutrition are two common problems in diabetes.

Exercise

Regular exercises are often recommended in the daily routine of clients with diabetes. The benefits of exercise are many. Exercise can improve the client's circulation, assist in maintaining ideal weight, increase the client's well-being, and improve control of glucose in the body. A home health aide should encourage and assist the client in doing the prescribed exercises.

Drug Therapy

Treatment of diabetes depends on the type of disease. For example, a type I diabetic is always treated with insulin injections. However, a person with type II diabetes may need to take oral hypoglycemic drugs (which stimulate the pancreas to make more insulin), insulin injections, or both.

Type I Diabetes.   Type I diabetes is always treated with a drug called insulin, which needs to be injected subcutaneously (under the skin). It cannot be taken orally because the stomach juices will dissolve the drug. The client with diabetes is taught where, when, and how to inject the medication (Figure 20-4). If a diabetic client is unable to self-inject, another member of the family might be taught to give the injections.

CAUTION: A home health aide is *not* permitted to inject insulin. The aide's responsibility is limited to bring-

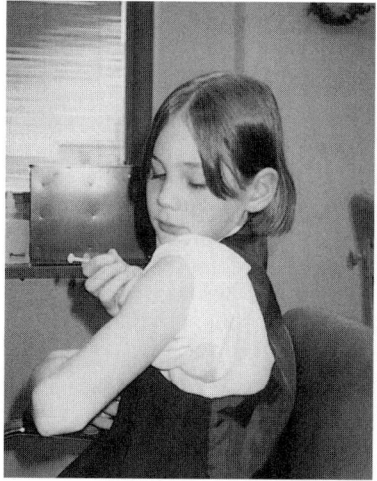

Figure 20-4   This young diabetic is self-injecting insulin into the upper arm. (Courtesy of The Diabetes Center of Albany Memorial Hospital, Albany, NY)

ing the medication and necessary supplies to the client.

The three most important factors to remember about insulin are:

1. Measurement must be *accurate.*
2. The drug must be taken at the same time every day.
3. Sterile technique must be maintained when injecting the drug.

The health care provider may prescribe different kinds of insulin. Some insulins are fast acting and some are slow acting. The health care provider will prescribe the type of insulin needed, the frequency, time, and amount of insulin.

Sites recommended for injections include the abdomen, upper arms, buttocks, and thighs. Most clients are encouraged to rotate injection sites on a daily or weekly basis to avoid changes in the skin tissues, which can alter the rate of absorption of the drug. It is a good idea to keep a record of where the injection was given to assist the client in rotating sites.

The use of the insulin pump is limited because of the cost of the equipment and the vigorous participation that is required by the client for safe maintenance and monitoring. Insulin pumps are popular among young adults and older adolescents. The pump is the size of a cell phone and continually delivers insulin through a tube inserted into the abdomen. This pump can lower the risk of the client's glucose from going too high or too low. Another benefit is that the client does not have to inject insulin through the skin numerous times a day. A control button or a switch allows the client to adjust the release of insulin. This device may be implanted in diabetic clients just as pacemakers are now implanted into clients with heart disease.

Experiments are now being conducted with pancreatic transplants. The purpose of the transplant is to replace non–insulin-producing cells with insulin-producing cells. Newer advances in insulin therapy are coming in the future, such as the insulin pill, oral sprays, inhaled insulin, and a combination of these therapies.

Type II Diabetes.   Type II diabetes can be treated in three ways. One way is by diet alone. Once individuals have reached their ideal weight and eat the proper foods, they may be able to maintain their blood sugar level without drugs. The second way is by taking oral hypoglycemic drugs daily.

As a home health aide you need to remember to encourage your client to take the prescribed drug as ordered. Generally, the drug is taken once a day, but it is not uncommon for a health care provider to order the drug two (bid) or three (tid) times a day.

The third way of treating type II diabetes is with insulin injections. There is another class of drugs whose purpose is to assist with the utilization of glucose. These drugs can be used alone or in conjunction with hypoglycemics or insulin.

Long-term Complications

Untreated or improperly treated diabetes can lead to many physical problems. Abnormal conditions that occur after a person develops diabetes are called diabetic complications. In some cases, even a well-cared-for diabetic may develop serious complications. The most common complications are vascular (blood vessel) disease and a high risk of infections.

Special Considerations for the Home Health Aide

Because diabetes can have serious consequences, it is important that the home health aide be particularly observant for signs and symptoms of health problems in the client.

Neuropathy in the Diabetic.   Neuropathy is defined as a destructive disorder of the nerves. Diabetic neuropathy is the loss of sensation in nerves. These individuals may be unable to feel pain or differentiate between hot and cold temperatures. This can be extremely dangerous. For example, a diabetic injures a foot or leg and, because no pain is felt, continues to use the limb. An infection can occur and the diabetic does not even realize there is a problem. Cuts or wounds not felt and thus not cared for can become infected. A home health aide carefully and routinely must check the client's feet and legs for any sign of redness, any "warm" area, any swelling, or any open cuts. Many diabetics have poor eyesight, or have difficulty bending their legs, and are unable to see to check their feet. They rely on the aide to do the checking.

Foot Care.   The home health aide should give special attention to the diabetic's feet every day. A client's feet and legs need to be examined daily for signs of dry, scaly, itching, or cracked skin; blisters; corns; infections; blueness and swelling of the ankles; and discolored nails.

Any abnormality must be reported to the nurse. Feet are bathed and soaked in warm water with mild soap and then dried with a soft towel. A good lanolin-based lotion is then applied starting at the client's toes and working toward the ankles. This helps stimulate the blood circulation to the feet. If the areas between the toes are moist due to perspiration, a very small piece of lamb's wool or cotton can be placed between the toes. Bunions and corns must be treated by a podiatrist (health care provider who specializes in foot problems).

In the older adult, the nails become thick and difficult to cut. Nail care (both fingernails and toenails) must be carefully done by a nurse or someone who has been taught to do it correctly. **CAUTION:** The aide may NOT cut the diabetic client's nails. There is danger of infection from skin cuts around the nails. In addition, improper cutting may cause ingrown toenails, which easily can lead to infection. If the client's feet are well cared for and examined daily, infection is unlikely to develop. The following foot care guide will help reduce injury to the feet:

- Bathe the feet daily in warm, not hot, water.
- Pat the feet dry with a soft towel, especially between the toes.
- Massage the feet to increase circulation.
- Wear clean white cotton socks and change daily.
- Do not apply iodine or carbolic acid to cuts on feet.
- Avoid walking barefoot.
- Always wear comfortable, well-fitting, leather shoes.
- Do not use commercial corn pads.

Vision Loss.   Loss of vision is a common problem of clients with diabetes. A few older adults may have vision problems and be unable to read directions to do blood sugar testing or to read the numbers on the insulin syringe. Because of these vision problems, the home health aide may need to read the directions to the client and also double-check the readings. The majority of clients will be able to do their own insulin injections and their own blood testing.

Prevention of Infections.   Clients with diabetes are very susceptible to any type of infection. If they do get the flu or a cold, their blood sugar levels usually decrease and increase erratically. Diabetic clients need to have their blood sugar monitored closely if they have even a mild cold or fever.

Diabetic persons also have problems with small cuts or abrasions healing. Special attention by the aide to keep the cut or abrasion as clean as possible will assist in the healing process. Slow healing is due in part to poor circulation.

When blood vessels are injured or diseased, the surrounding cells die from lack of nutrition and oxygen. A large area of dead tissue is called gangrene. Gangrene is a serious condition because it is easily infected with certain bacteria. Gangrene is a form of an infection.

The aide should check the client's feet and broken skin areas for signs of gangrene. The first sign is a hot and reddened skin area. This area becomes cold and bluish (cyanotic). After the tissues are dead, they turn black and flake off. Drainage from the area may be bubbly and emit a strong, foul odor.

Identification Tag

All diabetics should wear a Medic Alert identification tag. The ID is a labeled tag worn as a bracelet or necklace. The ID tag should be worn by the diabetic individual at all times. The label indicates the person's:
- Name
- Address
- Telephone number
- Medical condition
- Health care provider's name

In emergencies, the Medic Alert ID informs emergency personnel, police, health care providers, and others of the diabetic's medical condition. A diabetic who develops acidosis or insulin shock needs immediate help. The ID tag notifies health personnel that the person's emergency is possibly a diabetic condition. If the person is unconscious, the tag may provide information necessary to save the person's life. Medic Alert tags are also worn by clients with epilepsy and with allergies to certain drugs.

Clients Requiring Special Care

Unit 21
Caring for the Client Who Is Terminally Ill

Unit 22
Caring for the Client With Alzheimer's Disease

Unit 23
Caring for the Client With Cancer

SECTION 6

Caring for the Client Who Is Terminally Ill

Most people in our society feel uncomfortable talking or thinking about death. This is more true today than in earlier times in history. Gathering in the room of a dying relative was a custom practiced no more than 40 years ago. Death was accepted as the natural end to life. Children openly shared the final moments of life with a dying grandparent, parent, or sibling.

This is the first time in society that three or four generations of one family are living at the same time. Death experiences in some families have been rare. For many individuals, death is extremely difficult to deal with.

HOSPICE PROGRAM

Hospice care is a choice for clients who have been given a diagnosis that death will most likely come within the next six months. Hospice care involves a team of professionals such as nurses, home health aides, clergy, health care providers, and volunteers. Their goal is to assist the client and the family to make the dying process as pain-free and comfortable as possible. The client no longer seeks a cure for his or her illness. The hospice team also helps the client with social, financial, and spiritual concerns.

The primary concern of hospice is quality of life and not prolonging the client's life.

ADVANCE DIRECTIVES

Medical science has made treatments more available and more effective. Because of these and other changes, people can expect to live for many years. Diseases once incurable have been conquered. New medicines and surgical techniques have been developed that save thousands of lives daily. Most of these medical advances improve the quality of life. Because of problems with the making of decisions regarding use of life support machines and other life-prolonging measures, in 1991 the Patient Self-Determination Act was passed. This law requires home health agencies receiving Medicare and Medicaid to implement procedures to increase public awareness regarding the rights of clients to make choices. The law is concerned primarily with advance directives, papers that specify the type of treatment clients want or do not want under serious medical conditions in which they may be unable to communicate their wishes to the health care provider or family.

Advance directives can be done by a living will or by durable power of attorney. Before you start caring for a client, the decision may already have been made by the client what he or she wants done when seriously ill. One of these forms has probably been completed already by the client. Your case manager will inform you of your client's wishes.

Changing attitudes toward death have appeared partly as a result of increased life expectancy. People seem to fear death as never before. They want to hold on to life and try not to think about death. Children are sometimes protected from the facts of death. When a beloved grandparent dies, children may be told that the grandparent has gone away. Because families are often separated by great distances, some children believe that their grandparents have just moved. How a family deals with death is a personal matter. A home health aide must respect the wishes of the family in dealing with the death of a family member.

STAGES OF GRIEF

Dr. Elisabeth Kübler-Ross has made careful studies of dying persons and their families. She has described a general pattern common to persons facing death. The pattern may apply to both the dying person and the person's family. Dr. Kübler-Ross has noted five stages of grief. Clients may go through the five stages at different times. Sometimes the client may repeat the stage or bounce back and forth through the stages. The aide must listen and closely observe the client and try to recognize what the client is communicating.

1. Denial—This can't be happening to me; perhaps someone else, but not me.

2. Anger—An extension of denial; feeling that this death is unfair; bitterness and loss of faith; fighting against death or loss of a loved one.
3. Bargaining—Starts bargaining for more time to live: "I promise to live a better life if I can just get better now."
4. Depression—Clients come to full understanding that they might die. Display brooding, withdrawal, lack of communication; thoughts of suicide—"I'd rather kill myself than die from this disease."
5. Acceptance—Calmly facing what is to be or feeling a sense of peace; looking forward to release from pain and sorrow; hoping for the release of a loved one to a better world.

Home health aides who are in an environment of expected death may see these patterns develop or may find themselves experiencing these stages. The aide should be understanding, kind, and empathetic. By knowing what to expect in the way of reactions, the home health aide is better prepared to adjust to the situation.

Sometimes a client may die suddenly and unexpectedly. Other times death is preceded by a long illness. Some people are relieved that life is ending. Some clients become comatose (unconscious) just before death. Of the five senses (hearing, taste, touch, sight, smell), the last to be lost is hearing. For this reason when working with an unconscious client, the home health aide should be careful what is said in the client's presence. It would be cruel if the last words a client heard were, "Well, she's almost gone; she'll be dead by morning." The home health aide's first duty is to keep the client clean and as comfortable as possible. The client should be treated with kindness and dignity at all times. In addition, the aide should provide emotional support to the client and the family. Good communication skills are needed when dealing with the dying client and the family.

Home Health Aide Responsibilities in Caring for the Dying Client

As a home health aide, you will be working with the client more than the other members of the health team. You will see the client often, and it is important to create and maintain a trusting relationship with the client. When the client knows there is no cure for his or her illness, the care given to this client is called palliative care. This type of care emphasizes quality of life, not prolonging life. The physical pain arising from a terminal illness such as cancer can be unbearable, terrifying, and dehumanizing. There are many medications available to keep the client as pain-free as possible. The majority of clients do experience anxiety and depression over their diagnosis. A little distress is normal, but if it is prolonged the aide should report this, as the client may need some counseling or may need medication for depression. As the disease progresses in the body other physical problems need to be addressed such as nausea, constipation, and breathing. The client may need antinausea medication for the nausea, enemas or suppositories for constipation, and oxygen to help with breathing. It is of utmost importance to keep the nurse informed on the status of the client and any changes occurring with the client. This will assist the nurse in deciding when and what to do for the client to keep the client as comfortable as possible. As death gets closer, nursing responsibilities become greater. The duties of the home health aide will need to be carried out in a quiet and

efficient manner. The home health aide will need to pay particular attention to the comfort measures. The client will need:

- Position changed every two hours
- Mouth care performed every two hours
- Lip moisturizer applied often
- Artificial eyedrops instilled in eyes because eyes may cease to blink
- Vital signs monitored
- Skin kept clean and dry
- Small sips of water given often

If the home health aide has time, the aide can just sit and hold the client's hand, or read from the Bible or other books that might be available. Another suggestion is to play soft music. Clients generally will like a quiet, softly lit room, but soft music is often welcomed.

Signs of Approaching Death

Certain signs indicate that death is approaching. These signs are:
- Moist respirations (rales)
- Breathing will stop (apnea) and then breathing will be labored (dyspnea), known as Cheyne-Stokes respirations
- Pulse is irregular, rapid, and weak
- Incontinence of bowel and bladder
- Cool, moist, and clammy skin
- Eyes do not respond to light
- Body relaxes and jaw drops
- Diminished sense of pain
- Skin becomes pale and mottling (discoloration) can occur

The dying client will normally try to hold on, even though it may bring prolonged discomfort, in order to be sure that those who survive will be all right. When a client is ready to die, allowing family members or friends to say good-bye is a final gift of love and achieves closure to life.

When death occurs, family members may be highly emotional. The

1. Call the case manager. Write down the time the client stopped breathing and you felt no pulse. The case manager will call the health care provider, family, and funeral director. A death certificate will be completed by the health care provider.
2. Do not touch the client until the case manager states it is all right to do so.
3. Clean the client's body and remove all tubings. The funeral director will come to the home to pick up the body.

Figure 21-1   What to do when a client dies

home health aide must remain calm because many details must be taken care of. Death is a legal event that calls for certain formalities. A health care provider must complete a death certificate that states the cause of death, and formally register the death. Figure 21-1 lists the duties of a home health aide when the client dies.

RELIGIOUS AND CULTURAL INFLUENCES

Cultural and family differences will influence the death and dying process, including the public behavior of grieving.

Among some Jewish families, burial occurs within 24 hours after death. Jewish religious practice forbids embalming (treating the body with preservatives to prevent decay) the body and requires that the casket remain closed. After the funeral the family may have a period of formal mourning.

In other Jewish families and in Catholic or Protestant families, the body is usually taken to a funeral home. Friends and family meet at the funeral home during the one or two days before the body is buried.

Religious practices differ from one group to another and even from family to family. Most people do recognize the need for sharing grief. This is part of the final acceptance of death.

Some people weep, others are angry. Some are very quiet. As people work through their emotions, they come to accept the loss. Many believe that the death of an older person is less tragic than the death of a younger person. A death that is sudden is more difficult to accept than one following a long, painful illness. Mixed emotions may be felt by families when a client dies after a long illness. On the one hand, families are glad that their loved one is no longer suffering, yet on the other hand, their loved one will be missed.

The grieving process is the physical and emotional response to a loss, and the process of accepting it. The grief process can take a long time, and it is hard work. It can take from several months to a year to readjust to the loss of a loved one. Often, the first several months are the most difficult. Although all people cope with grief in different ways, grief needs to be expressed, or processed, so it can be healed. If grief is not expressed, symptoms of erratic behavior or failing health may appear. Today there are special support groups for individuals to assist them in the grieving process. Your agency's social worker can help the family find support groups in your area.

UNIT 22

Caring for the Client With Alzheimer's Disease

ALZHEIMER'S DISEASE

Alzheimer's disease is the most common form of dementia (loss of mind). When a client has dementia of any type, the results are similar. The client will experience impaired thinking, inability to comprehend, loss of memory, loss of reasoning ability, and loss of judgment. Alzheimer's disease affects an estimated 4 million American adults. Risk factors for the disease are being female, old age, Black ethnicity, having high blood pressure, and family history. The disease strikes 10% of people over the age of 65, and 50% of those are over the age of 85. Only 10% of all individuals with dementia have "early onset" dementia, which is seen in individuals under the age of 65. Signs and symptoms come on gradually and include memory loss, decline in the ability to perform routine tasks, disorientation, personality changes (Figure 22-1), difficulty in learning, and loss of language skills. Figure 22-2 identifies the 10 warning signs of Alzheimer's disease. The time from onset of symptoms until death can range from 3 to 20 years.

In the advanced stage of the disease, clients are totally dependent on others for activities of daily living.

Diagnostic tests used to confirm the diagnosis are magnetic resonance imaging (MRI) and computed tomography (CT). Documenting and recording of the client's behavior by a friend or family member over time will assist the health care provider in the final diagnosis. Recently, new drugs are being used in the beginning stages of the disease, and they do help delay the progression of the disease.

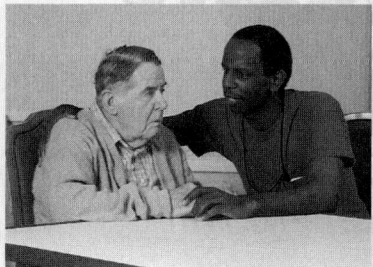

Figure 22-1 The first sign of dementia is the loss of spontaneity and change in personality.

261

Ten Warning Signs of Alzheimer's Disease
To help you know what warning signs to look for, the Alzheimer's Association has developed a checklist of common symptoms (some of them also may apply to other dementing illnesses). Review the list and check the symptoms that concern you. If you notice several symptoms, the individual with the symptoms should see a health care provider for a complete examination.

1. **Memory Loss That Affects Job Skills**
   It's normal to occasionally forget assignments, colleagues' names, or a business associate's telephone number and remember them later. Those with a dementia, such as Alzheimer's disease, may forget things more often, and not remember them later.
2. **Difficulty Performing Familiar Tasks**
   Busy people can be so distracted from time to time that they may leave the carrots on the stove and only remember to serve them at the end of the meal. People with Alzheimer's disease could prepare a meal and not only forget to serve it, but also forget they made it.
3. **Problems With Language**
   Everyone has trouble finding the right word sometimes, but a person with Alzheimer's disease may forget simple words or substitute inappropriate words, making his or her sentence incomprehensible.
4. **Disorientation Of Time And Place**
   It's normal to forget the day of the week or your destination for a moment. But people with Alzheimer's disease can become lost on their own street, not knowing where they are, how they got there or how to get back home.

(continues)

Figure 22-2 The 10 warning signs of Alzheimer's disease (Courtesy of The Alzheimer's Association)

Stages of Dementia

No two clients are alike with this disease. One client will progress quite quickly through the various stages, while another client will go slowly through each stage. The five basic stages of the progression of dementia are as follows:

1. Mild cognitive impairment—The client may experience some memory problems but is able to live independently.
2. Mild dementia—The client starts experiencing short-term memory loss and has problems with everyday thinking skills. The client will need assistance in financial matters, grooming, dressing, meal planning, and cooking. The client becomes somewhat

5. **Poor Or Decreased Judgment**

   People can become so immersed in an activity that they temporarily forget the child they're watching. People with Alzheimer's disease could forget entirely the child under their care. They may also dress inappropriately, wearing several shirts or blouses.

6. **Problems With Abstract Thinking**

   Balancing a checkbook may be disconcerting when the task is more complicated than usual. Someone with Alzheimer's disease could forget completely what the numbers are and what needs to be done with them.

7. **Misplacing Things**

   Anyone can temporarily misplace a wallet or keys. A person with Alzheimer's disease may put things in inappropriate places: an iron in the freezer, or a wristwatch in the sugar bowl.

8. **Changes In Mood Or Behavior**

   Everyone becomes sad or moody from time to time. Someone with Alzheimer's disease can exhibit rapid mood swings—from calm to tears to anger—for no apparent reason.

9. **Changes In Personality**

   People's personalities ordinarily change somewhat with age. But a person with Alzheimer's disease can change drastically, becoming extremely confused, suspicious, or fearful.

10. **Loss Of Initiative**

    It's normal to tire of housework, business activities, or social obligations, but most people regain their initiative. The person with Alzheimer's disease may become very passive and require cues and prompting to become involved.

(Courtesy of The Alzheimer's Association)

Figure 22-2   The 10 warning signs of Alzheimer's disease (Courtesy of The Alzheimer's Association)—*continued*

confused when in public or around large crowds. The client will experience problems remembering everyday events and handling money. The client will start to have problems with dressing and may need someone to pick out his or her clothing. If left alone, the client would not know how to cook a meal.

3. Moderate dementia—The client has severe memory loss and has problems talking with others and understanding what other people are saying. The client can no longer live alone and needs

assistance with all activities of daily living. Behaviors such as wandering, sleeplessness, and shadowing become more evident.

4. Severe dementia—The client experiences severe problems communicating with others. The client becomes incontinent of urine and then feces, and requires care 24 hours a day. The caregiver is required to bathe, dress, and assist the client with feeding and toileting. Often in this stage, the family seeks out long-term care arrangements for the client.

5. Profound dementia—Body functions slowly shut down. The client is able to say about six words, loses ability to walk, then loses the ability to sit up, then loses the ability to smile, and finally is unable to hold the head up.

CARING FOR THE CLIENT

Taking care of a client with Alzheimer's disease is difficult and requires a great deal of patience, empathy, and understanding of the disease process.

The majority of clients with dementia you will be caring for in the home will be moderately impaired. There are support groups in many communities. Family members can meet to share common problems and learn more about how to cope with their parent or relative as well as face up to their own feelings and fears. The Alzheimer's Association can link families with resources in their community to help them cope with this disease. The national toll-free number to the Alzheimer's Association is 1-800-272-3900, and the Web address is www.alz.org.

In some areas there are special day-care centers where Alzheimer's disease clients can be taken for a few hours a day. These centers provide activities, and clients will often enjoy talking, playing cards, playing the piano, or singing with others. Because the progression of the disease varies, clients may have "good" days or weeks when they function reasonably well at such centers. On the other hand, if the group activities have a negative effect on the client and make the person more agitated or fearful, the activity should be stopped immediately.

The home health aide helps the family members by providing respite care. That is, while the home health aide provides care, the family may take advantage of these few hours to take care of errands or just experience freedom from caregiving responsibilities.

Keeping the home environment safe is an important role for the home health aide, especially when working with a client who suffers from memory problems or who may wander away.

BEHAVIORAL CONSIDERATIONS

An Alzheimer's patient who is confused, frightened, or in pain might demonstrate behavior that would be troublesome. If possible, the aide should identify and remove the cause of problem behavior. Sometimes when behavior management does not work, a health care provider may order medication or physical restraints to control the problem behavior. If a client is put on medication, the time, dose, and side effects of the drugs should be closely monitored.

Wandering

Wandering is the most common agitated behavior among people with Alzheimer's disease. Frustration, fear, confusion, fatigue, and discomfort of the client can increase wandering. Often, the client is looking for something, for example, the bathroom, food or drink, a remedy for pain and suffering, a place to lie down, or a familiar face. Other times the client may wander because he or she is playing out an old routine, such as leaving work for home or going to get a loved one.

Safe Return Home Program is a national program that a person with dementia registers for. In this program, if the client wanders away and gets lost, the program will assist the client with a safe return home.

INTERVENTIONS

At the present time there is no cure for Alzheimer's disease. However, good planning, medical care, and a well-structured, calm environment can ease the burden to the client and family. For example, it is a good idea to consider health directives for the Alzheimer's client in the early stages of the disease, while the client still has the mental capacity to make choices. Physical exercise and good nutrition will help maintain the client's health.

Validation Therapy

Validation therapy is a communication technique that is used for moderately to severely disoriented clients with diagnosed dementia. The goal of this therapy is to increase self-esteem and validate the client's feelings. The basic premise is that if the client wishes to remain in the past, that should be allowed and no attempt should be made to reorient the client. Figure 22-3 identifies some useful techniques for communicating with a client with dementia.

Reminiscence

From the time of diagnosis until the end of life, the clients with Alzheimer's disease and their families are victims, suffering from pressures and strains of this disease. These clients have poor short-term memory, but long-term and deep-seated memories may remain. These memories, whether pleasurable or sad, can be recalled by reviewing past life history. Reminiscence helps the client with Alzheimer's disease experience being cared for with compassion.

Family involvement can be an important part of this therapy. This time for reclaiming the past creates connectedness. The present moment of a relationship increases family and client satisfaction. Sharing of information might be done by reviewing old movies, videotapes, pictures, songs, popular radio programs, or even using scrapbooks in which to write and draw.

Habilitation

Habilitation is the term used to describe care for the client, which focuses on what the client can do, not what the client used to do. This is recommended for the middle stages of the disease. The aide or caregiver is directed to move into the client's "current world" rather than the "real world."

Reality Orientation

For those clients with mild to moderate memory loss, and particularly for those who continue to understand words, it may be helpful to provide simple memory aids to assist the client in day-to-day living. For example, a prominent calendar, lists of daily tasks, written reminders, signs, labels, and clocks can help to orient the client to the present. It is also recommended to have photos of close family members placed where the client can see them daily. This process of orienting the person to the present moment is known as **reality orientation.** This technique would not be

1. Make sure you have your client's attention *before* you begin to speak: make sure that she can see and hear you, and that she knows that you are talking to her.
2. Face your client when you speak to her, and speak slowly and clearly.
3. Do not talk too much! Give one instruction at a time.
4. Speak in positives instead of in negatives. Your client will respond better to, "Come with me," than she will to "Come away from there!"
5. If necessary, repeat the statement or question—do not change the wording.
6. Lead the client in answering if the client cannot find the right words—point to objects to provide clues.
7. Listen carefully to what your client is saying. She may be telling you something important.
8. Respond to your client's feelings, not just to her words.
9. For clients with severe memory loss, focus on validation, not on reality orientation.
10. Be aware of body language—yours and your client's.
11. If your client is frustrated by not being able to make you understand her, then reassure her that you still care about what she feels: "I'm sorry I can't understand what you are saying. Why don't you wait a while and try to tell me later?" Then, move on to another activity.
12. *Never* ask, "Do you remember . . . ?" It may embarrass your client if she can't remember. Instead, tell your client what you want her to remember: "We went to your health care provider's office on Tuesday, and he said that you need to drink more water."

Figure 22-3 Tips for communicating with a client with dementia

appropriate, however, for someone with a more severe memory loss and may cause frustration, agitation, and loss of self-esteem. The home health aide must use imagination, patience, kindness, and understanding to give the Alzheimer's client the service and care that best meets the individual's needs.

Caring for the Client With Cancer

CANCER

Cancer is the uncontrolled growth of abnormal cells. In healthy tissue, body cells grow, die, and are replaced by new cells. This is a normal process that goes on day after day. Sometimes cells do not follow the rules of the body; they begin to divide quickly, stealing nourishment from surrounding cells, and pushing normal cells out of the way. They prevent normal cells from doing their regular jobs. Finally, these cells cause changes in the body, which produce signs and indicate something is wrong. Any individual experiencing one of the warning signs listed in Figure 23-1 should see his or her health care provider as soon as possible.

A substance or agent that produces cancer is called a carcinogen. The general group of carcinogens are chemicals, environmental factors, hormones, and viruses. A chemical could be ingested with food such as red dye #2. The chemical could be inhaled as tar or asbestos. Environmental factors include such physical agents as x-rays, sunlight, or trauma. Hormones may be cancer causing because of their excess, deficiency, or imbalance. Viruses seem to upset the functions within a cell. Certain forms of cancer are inherited or have a familial tendency such as cancer of the breast and colon.

Benign tumors develop and tend to be encapsulated (confined within a capsule) (Figure 23-2A). The tumors generally stay in one area, and if removed, they rarely reoccur. Malignant or cancerous tumor cells spread rapidly and infiltrate other areas of the body (Figure 23-2B). Cancer cells appearing under a microscope vary in size, are disorderly, and do not form tissues as normal cells do. These cancer cells do spread to other body tissues through a process called metastasis. The cancer cells are carried to other sites by either the blood or lymph system. If the spread of cells is not controlled, the effects on the body can be cachexia (marked wasting away of the body) and death. A **biopsy** (sample) of the body tissue is done if the health care provider suspects the individual has cancer. This biopsy is done to confirm the diagnosis and to find out what stage of cancer the tumor is. Other tests are also done such as body scans, x-rays,

Warning Signals

C	Change in bowel or bladder habits
A	A sore that will not heal
U	Unusual bleeding or discharge
T	Thickening or lump in the breast or elsewhere
I	Indigestion or difficulty swallowing
O	Obvious change in wart or mole
N	Nagging cough or hoarseness

Figure 23-1   Warning signs of cancer

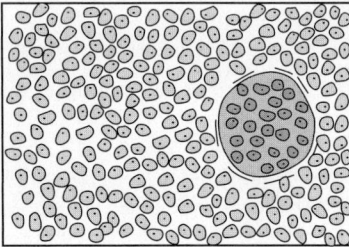
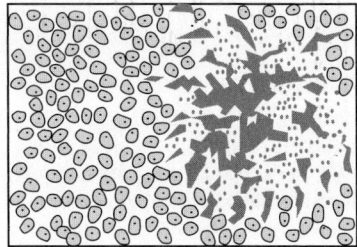

A   **B**

Figure 23-2   Growth of cancer cells. A. Benign tumor growth (with capsule around it). B. Malignant cancer growth (no capsule with random growth).

and blood tests to determine what stage the cancer is in. If the cancer is Stage I, it is in the very beginning of development, whereas Stage IV cancer is well developed in the body. Treatment is more successful in the earlier stages than in the advanced stages of the disease. When cancer is treated early and does not reappear for five years, the cancer is considered to be cured or in remission. Remission means no longer growing or spreading.

It has been estimated that in the United States alone more than 1,400 people a day die from some form of cancer. Since 1949, there has been a sharp rise in the number of men who develop cancer. Cancer of the pros-tate, lung, colon, and rectum occur most often among men. Cancer of the breast, lung, colon, and rectum occur most often among women. There are more than 100 types of cancer. Cancer is second only to heart disease as the leading cause of death each year. However, statistics also show that deaths due to cancer are increasing, whereas those due to heart conditions are decreasing. Research continues into the causes and possible cures for cancer.

CANCER TREATMENTS

Several kinds of treatments may slow or stop the growth of cancer cells. Surgery, chemotherapy, or radiation can be used. These can be used in combination or alone. A client may have a tumor surgically removed from her breast and then need to go through a series of radiation treatments. Home health aides are often employed to care for a client temporarily when the client is recovering postoperatively, undergoing chemotherapy, or having radiation treatments.

If your client is undergoing radiation therapy, the area receiving treatment is usually outlined in black ink or may even be outlined in tiny tattoos. After a few treatments the skin in the enclosed area may become dry, red, itchy, or scaly. It is important that the client follow certain guidelines while receiving treatment and for three weeks after completion of the treatment. Remember these are just general guidelines, and a client must follow the guidelines given by his or her primary health care provider. Suggested guidelines are as follows:

• Wash the area receiving radiation gently. Use your hand to cleanse the area rather than a washcloth. Do not wash off markings.
• Rinse well, making sure all soap residue is removed.
• Pat areas dry, do not rub the area dry.
• Limit baths and showers to one-half hour per day and use warm water rather than hot water.
• If skin cream is ordered, apply to area after washing off previous layer of cream.
• Increase fluid intake unless the health care provider has ordered differently.
• Avoid clothing that will increase friction and rubbing in the outlined area. It is better to wear loose cotton clothing.
• Do not use tape on the affected area.

If your client is receiving drugs or medications to treat the cancer, this process is called chemotherapy. These drugs can be given orally, intravenously, or intramuscularly. It is important that the client and home health aide follow the precautions listed below after the client has received chemotherapy. The precautions are:

• Wash hands often.
• Do not use a hard toothbrush or floss teeth.
• If skin becomes dry, soften it with cream.

The following are done for 48 hours after treatment:

• The home health aide should wear gloves when handling body fluids, soiled linens, or clothing.
• If the client needs to vomit, have the client attempt to do it directly into the toilet. If an emesis basin is used, dispose of the contents directly into the toilet. Close the lid and flush at least three times. Rinse the emesis basin thoroughly.
• If the client uses the commode, dispose of the contents directly into the toilet, close to the water to restrict splashing. Close the lid and flush three times.
• If the client is wearing adult briefs, the briefs need to be double-bagged and disposed of in the regular trash.

Whether the client is receiving chemotherapy or radiation therapy, the client will experience some unpleasant side effects. However, one needs to remember that the side effects need to be weighed against the benefits of the treatment—the destruction of the cancer cells. The most common side effects are:

• Nausea and vomiting
• Loss of hair
• Fatigue
• Sore mouth and throat
• Loss of appetite
• Increased susceptibility to infections

Some general guidelines to follow with the client relating to some of the above side effects are:

- Avoid food or juices high in acid content such as tomato, orange, or grapefruit juice.
- Avoid salty or spicy foods.
- Rinse the mouth with 1 teaspoon of baking soda mixed with warm water. Have the client hold the rinse in the mouth for about a minute.
- Avoid commercial mouthwashes.
- Use an electric razor for shaving to avoid cuts that may cause bleeding.
- Use lip balm.
- Minimize contact with birds and their cages and cats and their litter boxes.
- After each bowel movement, clean the rectum gently and thoroughly.
- Avoid large groups of people to limit the client's exposure to other infectious diseases.
- Space activities with rest periods to avoid extreme fatigue in the client.

So-called miracle cures for cancer are sold in many forms. Most people who market these products are only interested in making a profit from the misfortune of others. Some people with cancer choose to take experimental drugs. However, a person is wiser and safer to follow the advice of a trustworthy health care provider. The best treatment plans are based on sound research.

CARING FOR A CLIENT WITH CANCER

When a cancer client becomes too weak to care for himself or herself, a home health aide is often employed to assist the client with activities of daily living. Generally, the client who has cancer in the later stages or is just receiving treatment needs to focus on increasing protein and calories to prevent malnutrition and fluids to prevent dehydration. The food texture may need to be modified due to sores in the mouth and the inability to chew. High-fiber foods are usually eliminated from the diet. The client is advised to eat in small amounts, and have high-calorie snacks available. The client should avoid an empty stomach, as this will prevent nausea from occurring. Sipping fluids throughout the day rather than drinking large amounts of fluids at one time is helpful. Another useful tip is to have the client suck on ice chips, Popsicles, or hard candy, if the client's mouth is sore. Occasionally, a client may have "upbeat" times during the day when he or she may feel like eating. The home health aide should take advantage of these times and offer the client high-calorie foods to eat.

If the client with cancer is terminal, the client will slowly become weaker and weaker. As the cancer spreads throughout the body, the client may have a distinguishing odor due to the death of body cells. In these cases, room deodorizers can be used to mask the odor.

Pain management at every stage is an important concern, and the generous use of various painkillers and noninvasive techniques that promote relaxation and distractions is encouraged. The goal of care in the final stages is to keep the client as comfortable as possible. As cancer spreads throughout the body, the pain may become more severe and less tolerated by the client. It is important that the home health aide assist the nurse in monitoring the pain level in the client. If the pain medication is not working, the aide needs to inform the nurse. Sometimes, the client may choose to enter into hospice care. Hospice is designed to relieve the physical and emotional suffering of terminally ill clients. This is usually done in a long-term care facility or at home. The main goal is to provide comfort, peace, and dignity to the dying client and emotional support to the family and loved ones.

CANCER OF THE FEMALE REPRODUCTIVE SYSTEM

All women should have an annual physical examination, including a Pap smear. A Pap smear detects early cellular change in the cervix.

Cancer of the Breast

Another area in which women develop cancer is the breast. An excellent method of detecting breast cancer is self-examination. Each woman should self-examine her breasts monthly about 7 to 10 days after each period. She checks for changes in the shape of each breast, swelling, dimpling of the skin, or changes in the nipple.

CANCER OF THE MALE REPRODUCTIVE SYSTEM

Prostate cancer is the most common cancer in older men. The signs of this cancer are silent at first. It is important that the male have a routine physical examination done to detect this cancer in the early stage of the disease. The tests for prostate cancer include the prostate-specific antigen (PSA) and a digital rectal examination by the health care provider.

Testicular cancer is a primary cancer of young men. As in most cases, signs of this cancer are silent at first. Health care providers promote a monthly testicular self-examination for men to detect any abnormality of the testes early. The American Cancer Society recommends the following method to perform the examination. The best time to perform this exami-

nation is during or after a shower or bath when the scrotum is relaxed. The man should hold the penis out of the way and examine each testicle separately. He then holds the testicle between the thumbs and fingers with both hands and rolls it gently between the fingers. He should look and feel for any hard lumps or nodules or any change in the size, shape, or consistency of the testes. If any abnormality is felt, he should see his health care provider as soon as possible.

CANCER OF THE RESPIRATORY SYSTEM

Many infections and disorders can affect the respiratory system. Everyone has had a common cold. Flu, pneumonia, bronchitis, and upper respiratory infections are some of the illnesses affecting this system. Cancer, too, can start to grow in the lungs. Signs of lung cancer are:

- A persistent, hacking cough
- Tiredness
- Sudden weight loss
- Coughing up blood
- Recurrent bronchitis or pneumonia
- Difficulty swallowing
- Clubbing of fingers and toes
- Hoarseness
- Shortness of breath
- Loss of appetite
- Swelling in neck and face

The most common cause of cancer of the lung is smoking.

If a biopsy shows cancer cells, surgery can sometimes be done to remove all or part of a lung. Removal of part of the lung is called a **lobectomy.** Removal of the entire lung is called a pneumonectomy. Radiation and chemotherapy are also used to treat the cancer, but rarely is it cured. Lung cancer grows slowly at first. However, by the time it is diagnosed, 7 of 10 clients are not helped by surgery. A person with lung cancer must be kept as comfortable as possible. Most clients with lung cancer are cared for in the home setting. The client will require oxygen therapy 24 hours a day.

Cancer of the Larynx

The larynx (voice box) is located at the top of the trachea (windpipe or airway between the nasal passages and the lungs). Cancer of the larynx occurs in men more often than in women. In addition, 75% of the people who develop cancer of the larynx have been heavy smokers. A common treatment for cancer of the larynx is surgical removal of the larynx, called a laryngectomy. To remove the larynx, a tracheostomy must be performed. A tracheostomy is a surgical opening made into the trachea below the larynx. The tracheostomy is an artificial airway that can be used to supply oxygen to the lungs. A tracheostomy tube is placed into the artificial airway to keep it open (Figure 23-3). The client, if capable, will be taught how to clean the tube and dressing and, if need be, how to suction out the opening. If the client is not capable of cleaning the tube and dressing, a nurse will come to the home to change the dressing and clean the tube.

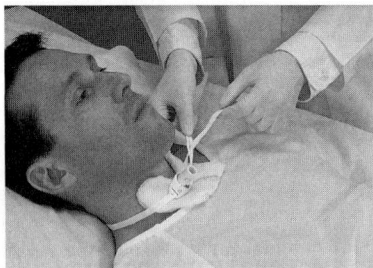

Figure 23-3 A tracheostomy tube provides an airway for the client.

After the tracheostomy has been done, the second part of the surgery is completed and the cancerous larynx is removed. The tracheostomy tube remains in place permanently in a laryngectomy client. After the client has recovered from surgery, rehabilitation starts.

Speech therapy is needed to teach the client how to talk. One of the methods is to gulp air in through the tracheostomy tube, swallow it, and then burp out words. It takes a great deal of practice to relearn speaking. Another method the laryngectomy client may use to aid speech is an artificial larynx. A battery-powered vibrator is one type of artificial larynx. When wishing to speak, the client places the vibrator against the side of the neck. The vibrator vibrates the air inside the client's mouth as the client tries to make sounds.

GASTROINTESTINAL CANCER

More new cases of gastrointestinal (stomach and colon) cancer occur in the United States every year. At least 93% of these individuals are over 50 years of age. Women are slightly more likely than men to develop the disease. Only lung cancer exceeds colon cancer in the number of new cases and number of deaths each year. Early detection of such cancer is an important factor in survival. Signs of colon cancer are:
- Change in bowel habits
- Blood in or on the stool
- Unexplained anemia
- Unusual stomach or gas pain
- Fatigue
- Vomiting

SKIN CANCER

Skin cancer is becoming a common type of cancer, especially among older adults. Skin cancer is caused by heredity and overexposure to sunlight, sunburn, tanning, and environmental factors in the younger years. The lesions can be either benign or malignant. Definite signs to watch for on the client's skin include changes in color, shape, size, and texture. If the home health aide notices any of these signs while bathing or dressing a client, the aide should report the lesion to the nurse. If detected and treated early enough, the prognosis is good.

Common types of skin cancers are basal cell and squamous cell. The first sign of skin cancer is a sore on the skin that does not heal. The sore may look like a lump. The lump can be smooth, shiny, waxy, red, or reddish brown. The lump can feel rough or scaly. If removed in the first stage of the disease, it rarely reoccurs because it is usually benign. The type of skin cancer that is malignant is a melanoma, which can quickly metastasize to other areas of the body. This type of lesion may have an irregular border and be multicolored such as red, blue, black, or brown. On men, the lesion is more often found in the area between the shoulders and hips. On women, the lesion may be found on the arms or legs.

Maternal/
Infant Care

UNIT 24

Maternal Care

The goal of every expectant mother and the professionals who care for her is the delivery of a normal, healthy baby. A key element in normal fetal development is an expectant mother in good physical and emotional health.

DISCOMFORTS OF PREGNANCY

Pregnancy today is regarded as a normal and natural stage of a woman's life cycle. A normal fetus will grow in a woman's uterus for approximately 280 days from the last menstrual period. An ultrasound test is done usually in the fourth month of pregnancy to check the growth of the fetus. At the same time, the woman must realize that extra demands are being placed on her body by the growing fetus. Prenatal (before birth) care should be sought as soon as a woman realizes she is pregnant and should continue throughout the pregnancy. Even with regular prenatal care, often discomforts are involved with pregnancy. Most women experience at least one of the discomforts listed below at some point during their pregnancy.

Frequent Urination

Frequent urination is caused by pressure of the enlarged uterus on the bladder. This usually subsides by the second or third month of pregnancy, when the uterus rises in the abdominal cavity. However, in the last week of pregnancy, when the uterus drops into the pelvic cavity—a condition known as engagement—both urgency and frequency of urination can be noted.

Morning Sickness

Morning sickness is one of the most common symptoms of pregnancy. It is characterized by nausea and, sometimes, by vomiting. Although it usually occurs in the morning, it can happen at any time of day, most often lasting for a 4- to 12-week period during the first trimester. Hormonal changes can contribute to morning sickness.

Some techniques for alleviating nausea include remaining in bed and resting for half an hour after awakening. During this period the expectant mother should try to eat dry toast or a cracker, or sip on soda or juice.

Heartburn/Flatulence

Diminished gastric motion during pregnancy may cause stomach contents to back up into the lower esophagus. This is commonly called **heartburn.** Nervousness and emotional upsets can contribute to this symptom. Fried and fatty foods should also be avoided. Sitting up for 30 minutes after eating will also help to alleviate this condition. Antacids should be used only with a health care provider's permission.

Feelings of gassiness, referred to as **flatulence,** may also be present because of gas-forming bacterial action in the intestines. One way to alleviate gassiness is to eat slowly, chew food thoroughly, and avoid gas-forming foods, such as beans, corn, and fried foods. Yogurt will help to inhibit gas formation. If gas or flatus becomes very uncomfortable, lying with the knees toward the chest may bring relief from the cramping.

Constipation/Hemorrhoids

Constipation can result from the pressure of the uterus on the intestines. Pressure exerted by the pregnant uterus can interfere with circulation in the veins. In the anal area, coupled with constipation, this can result in **hemorrhoids** (enlarged varicose veins around the anus). Suppositories or other medications, including those available over the counter, should be used only when ordered by the health care provider.

Varicose Veins

Varicose veins (swollen veins) can develop during pregnancy. This can be caused by pressure on the great veins of the pelvis, a hereditary predisposition, constrictive clothing, and prolonged standing, and can affect the lower extremities. The woman should be encouraged to elevate her legs often and wear elastic support hose.

Breathlessness

The pressure of the enlarged uterus on the diaphragm can cause respiratory discomfort. The expectant mother should be reassured that, with the birth of the infant, or even before, the symptom will resolve itself. About 2 to 3 weeks before the onset of contractions, the fetus descends into the pelvis. This process is called lightening and usually alleviates respiratory discomfort of the mother.

Backache

Backache is a common complaint of pregnant women and results from adjustments in posture caused by carrying the baby's weight, the changes in the mother's center of gravity, and the relaxation of the joints at the base of the spine. Wearing flat, firmly balanced shoes and a properly fitting maternity support garment may help, as well as practicing good posture, proper body mechanics, and getting adequate rest.

Leg Cramps

Leg cramps or spasms of the lower leg and foot muscles are a common and painful experience during pregnancy. The cramp may occur without warning, sometimes in the middle of the night. The calf muscles in one leg may feel like a "knotted ball." Sometimes leg cramps are related to an insufficient intake of calcium or an excess of phosphorus in the diet. Phosphorus is found in milk and dairy products but also in soft drinks and many processed snacks. The best treatment for the cramps is stretching the muscles. It is helpful to massage or knead the leg to try to relax the muscles. The lower leg may remain tender for several hours after the cramp.

Edema

Edema, or swelling, of the lower extremities can also occur, particularly in warm climates and when standing for too long. Swelling of the woman's fingers may also occur. The fingers may become stiff and rings may be too tight to wear. Rest, elevation of the legs, abdominal support such as a girdle, elastic support hose, soaking the feet and hands in cool water, and limiting salt intake may help the edema.

Vaginal Discharge

It is normal for women to have a pale yellow, thin vaginal discharge during pregnancy. If the discharge becomes irritating, odorous, excessive, is yellow or green, and is accompanied by vaginal itching, the health care provider should be consulted. One or all of these signs may indicate an infection, which if left untreated could cause premature delivery of the infant. Among the possible causes could be bacteria, fungi, or a sexually transmitted disease.

COMPLICATIONS OF PREGNANCY

Although the vast majority of pregnancies progress quite naturally, occasionally complications may develop. Complications of pregnancy may be the result of the age of the mother, the use of harmful substances during pregnancy, or certain medical factors. Complications of pregnancy can affect the health of the mother and the baby. For this reason it is important that women receive prenatal care throughout the pregnancy.

High-Risk Pregnancies

When physical, emotional, or environmental situations compromise the mother's well-being, a high-risk pregnancy can result. These pregnancies can cause low birth weight, premature or brain-damaged babies, and maternal complications. These complications increase the chances of infant and maternal mortality (death).

The age of the mother can have a significant influence on the outcome of the pregnancy and its identification as a high-risk event. Statistically, women over age 35 are more likely to give birth to babies with Down syndrome, a form of retardation. Prenatal (before birth) tests are offered to pregnant women in high-risk categories. These prenatal tests include ultrasound, amniocentesis, and blood tests that can determine the development of the fetus.

Pregnant women are advised against drinking alcohol during their pregnancy. Drinking alcohol during pregnancy can result in several serious complications known as **fetal alcohol syndrome (FAS)**. This condition produces infants who are born underweight, usually mentally deficient, and with multiple deformities. Cigarette smoking can also lead to a variety of pregnancy complications. Tobacco use is one of the causes of prenatal problems, such as vaginal bleeding, miscarriage, and early delivery. If the expectant mother is a substance abuser, her chances of problems during pregnancy are increased. Drug-addicted women can, and often do, give birth to drug-addicted babies.

Women can be placed in the high-risk group because of medical factors, such as having a history of spontaneous abortions, stillbirths, premature births, or difficult pregnancies in the past.

Hypertensive Disorders of Pregnancy

Prenatal care is very important during pregnancy. Each time a pregnant woman comes in for a checkup by the obstetrician or midwife, the woman's blood pressure is taken and the urine is checked for sugar and protein. The reason for the frequent blood pressure checks and urine checks is to screen the woman for potential hypertensive disorders of pregnancy. This is the new term for toxemia or elevated blood pressure during pregnancy. Signs and symptoms of this disorder are swelling in the hands and feet upon rising in the morning, elevated blood pressure, and protein in the urine. If the woman is diagnosed with this disorder, bed rest may be ordered. If so, the woman may need home health care for herself and assistance in child care if she has small children. If the home health aide is allowed and trained to measure blood pressure, the aide will need to measure the woman's blood pressure each time the aide is in the home. The woman will also need to be weighed frequently, and she may need to check her blood sugar. The pregnant woman will require a diet with adequate calories, protein, and fluid. The health care provider or midwife will watch her and the fetus closely for further complications.

Danger Signals

Many expectant mothers fear miscarriage during their first trimester of pregnancy. Some possible signs of miscarriage include bleeding associated with abdominal cramping, severe abdominal pain that does not go away, heavy vaginal bleeding or light spotting that continues for several days, and passing blood clots or grayish pink material.

CARING FOR THE EXPECTANT MOTHER

In many parts of the country, demand for home health care services for the expectant mother and for new families is growing. Home health care services for a pregnant mother can occur if a pregnancy is high risk, the mother is under unusual stress, or the mother is on limited activity.

When taking care of a pregnant woman in the home setting, some important things for the home health aide to remember are:

- Encourage a balanced diet; this is important for the mother and especially for the growth of the fetus.
- Encourage regular prenatal check-ups.
- Follow the care plan carefully, which will include activity orders. Bed rest is sometimes ordered for high blood pressure or vaginal bleeding.
- Make sure the nurse is aware of *any* medication the mother-to-be might be taking because birth defects can result from taking certain medicines.
- Discourage smoking and drinking of alcohol.
- Observe the mother-to-be carefully for signs of bleeding.
- Encourage good personal and dental hygiene and exercise.
- Try to help the mother-to-be feel as optimistic as possible; provide a calm environment to help promote a general feeling of well-being.
- Help her maintain a good fluid intake.

Exercise is important in moderation. Age, physical condition, previous exercise history, and the stage of pregnancy all influence the type and amount of exercise allowed.

While meeting the expectant mother's medical needs is important, her personal needs relative to good hygiene and lifestyle cannot be neglected. As her body changes, she needs to feel good about herself and the way she looks. Attractive nonrestrictive clothing will help her feel physically and emotionally comfortable. An abdominal support may be necessary in the last stages of pregnancy to prevent fatigue and backaches.

CARING FOR THE POSTPARTUM MOTHER

Labor and delivery are exhausting physical and emotional experiences. In the past, new mothers remained in the hospital for 5 to 7 days after delivery. Today, new mothers are released to their homes within 24 to 48 hours after vaginal deliveries and in 3 to 4 days after cesarean sections. As a result, many new mothers are choosing to employ home health aides to assist them during the first several weeks postpartum. The postpartum period is defined as the period after childbirth, usually lasting 6 weeks.

Postpartum Discomforts

Frequently, first-time mothers are unprepared for the discomforts of the postpartum experience. The home health aide should be supportive and reassure the new mother that her feelings—physical and emotional—are considered normal postpartum experiences. The home health aide should be aware of common postpartum discomforts that new mothers may experience. Many new mothers experience these discomforts (listed below) following the birth of an infant.

Exhaustion. The postpartum mother is usually exhausted as a result of labor and delivery and her role as a new mother. She should be encouraged to get as much rest as possible so that she can regain her strength.

Lochia. Lochia is the bloody vaginal discharge that is secreted by postpartum women. Although bright red at first for several days, it should turn light pink, brown, then yellow by the end of two weeks. Sanitary pads should be used to absorb the flow. Excessive bleeding should be reported as well as lochia with a foul odor. Pads should be changed frequently and the area should be kept clean.

Incisional Pain. Incisions (episiotomy or cesarean section) can be quite painful. Encourage and assist the client with cool sitz baths to ease the pain, and offer ice packs to reduce swelling and numb the pain. A health care provider will determine what, if any, pain medication should be used.

Breast Engorgement. A few days after delivery, breast milk comes in, causing breast engorgement. If bottle-feeding, this can be a painful experience for postpartum women. A sports bra or a tight wrap and ice packs will minimize the pain. Reassure the client that engorgement should last only 12 to 24 hours. A health care provider may prescribe pain medication. If breast-feeding, warm showers and compresses will help the milk flow.

Difficulty Walking and Sitting. Assist with walking and sitting. Remind client to walk as upright as possible and, if desired, to sit on a foam cushion.

Abdominal Cramping. Abdominal cramps are believed to be caused by the uterus as it contracts to its normal size. Cramping will be felt more during nursing as the sucking initiates the uterus to contract.

Difficult Urination. Difficulty with urination is a common postpartum condition. This temporary condition should last only a short time. Kegel exercises can also help the woman control her urination better. If the woman continues to have problems urinating, the nurse should be contacted because the woman may have a urinary infection.

Depression/Mood Swings. Postpartum blues, or postbaby blues, are experienced by many women during the first few weeks after delivery. Some women feel anxious, tired, and weepy or experience mood swings. The home health aide should provide support and reassurance. If the post-partum mother feels that she is likely to hurt herself or her baby, professional assistance should be sought.

The following are factors to be considered when caring for the new mother:

- Encourage the new mother to get as much rest as possible to regain energy.
- Emotional changes may range from depression to elation in both parents; the mother may be irritable and weepy at times; be understanding and patient.
- Involve the family in care of the new baby to help in family adjustment.
- Help with home management activities as needed.
- Encourage the mother to eat a balanced diet, get adequate rest and exercise, interact with the family unit, and take time to get to know her baby.
- Watch for signs of infection (pain, elevated temperature, or foul odor of the vaginal discharge) and report any of these signs or symptoms to the nurse.

- Watch for vaginal bleeding; the discharge should change from bright red to pink to white within several days; report excessive bleeding immediately.

Nutrition and Breast-Feeding

If a mother is planning to breast-feed her baby, she will need to pay close attention to her diet. The mother's diet will influence both the amount and quality of the milk she produces. Some tips to maintain the best nutrition for a breast-feeding mother are:

- Eat three regular meals and a bedtime snack. Avoid going too long between meals.
- Additional protein in the diet is needed; eat generous servings of meat, milk, eggs, or cheese.
- Additional calcium will help meet vitamin D needs.
- Calcium, iron, and vitamin supplements may be continued.
- Avoid trying to lose weight too quickly after the baby's birth.
- Caffeine and alcohol are passed from the mother's blood into the milk and should be avoided.
- Some drugs are passed from the mother's blood into the milk, and should only be taken if prescribed by a health care provider.
- Drink plenty of fluids.

Infant Care

INFANT CARE

The birth of a baby is a time of adjustment for both the baby and the new parents. During the first year of life, the child is totally dependent on the care of others. Physical and emotional well-being are intimately related to each other. The individuals who meet the infant's primary needs significantly influence his or her physical and emotional development. Caring for a newborn baby can create anxiety for the new parents. The home health aide should try to reduce these anxieties by becoming familiar with basic infant care procedures, such as feeding, burping, bathing, caring for the circumcised or uncircumcised penis and the umbilical cord. The majority of new mothers go home with little need for a home health aide, as they have help from either their husband or their family. The new mothers who may need assistance from a home health aide are very young single mothers, mothers with emotional problems, and mothers with multiple births or premature infants.

FEEDING THE INFANT

The newborn infant will approximately triple his or her birth weight during the first year of life. The nutritional needs during this rapid growth period are greater than at any other time in its life. Feeding the infant should be an enjoyable, relaxing time. Hold the infant close, cuddle, and make eye contact while feeding. There are two ways to feed the infant: breastfeeding and bottle-feeding. Either method can be used independently or in combination.

Breast-Feeding

Human milk is the best possible food for any infant. Its major ingredients are lactose (sugar), protein (whey and casein), fat, and numerous vitamins, minerals, and enzymes, all appropriately combined to suit an infant's nutritional needs. Breast milk has infection-fighting properties. When breast-fed infants get an infection, the infection is less severe. The home health aide should assist the new mother with the breast-feeding technique, as outlined in Procedure 74.

74 Procedure

Assisting with Breast-Feeding and Breast Care

Purpose

- To provide for cleanliness
- To protect the nipples from cracking or soreness
- To protect the infant from infection
- To provide for the mother's comfort
- To nourish the infant
- To promote mother-infant interaction

NOTE: Assist the mother to establish a routine, preferably in a calm environment. A rocking chair is a great place to nurse an infant. While nursing it is helpful to have a small nursing pillow to support the infant in the mother's lap, and a small stool to elevate the mother's feet to ease the strain on her back.

Procedure

1. Gather supplies:
   clean, moist washcloth
   nursing pads
   disposable towelettes
   clock or watch to time nursing
   period
2. Wash your hands.

3. Give the mother towelettes or a moist washcloth to wash her hands.
4. Have the mother open the front of her dress or shirt top.
5. Have the mother sit in comfortable position in a rocking chair with armrest and footstool to support the feet.
6. Bring infant to mother. Make sure infant's nose is not pressed against the mother's breast. The nostrils must be free so the infant can breathe as it nurses. The infant should be square on the breast, the mouth facing the nipple. There are three positions for breast-feeding: side-lying, football hold, and cradle hold (Figures 25-1A–C). Rotate positions to reduce tenderness in one particular area.

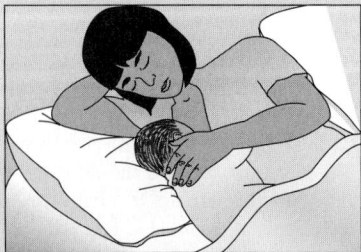

Figure 25-1A Side-lying position for breast-feeding

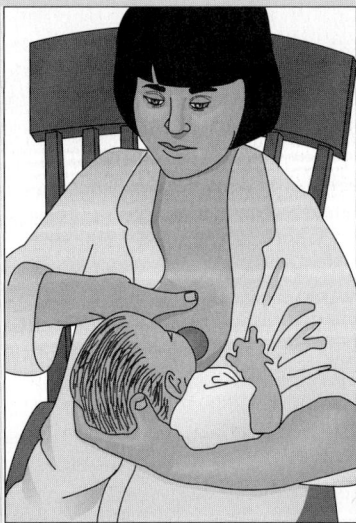

Figure 25-1B Football hold position for breast-feeding

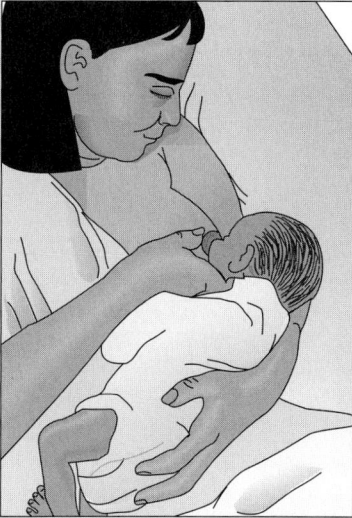

Figure 25-1C Cradle hold position for breast-feeding

7. The nursing period is gradually increased from just a few minutes to about 20 minutes. Some mothers prefer to let the infant nurse at both breasts during one feeding. Others will feed the infant only at one breast for each 20-minute feeding and alternate breasts at different feedings.
8. To remove the infant's mouth from the breast, have mother insert finger in infant's mouth to break suction.

9. Have the mother burp the infant. When the mother is finished nursing, take the infant and place in the crib with the infant lying on the back, or in an infant seat. Check to see if the diaper needs to be changed. If the infant is getting enough breast milk, the infant should be wetting a diaper almost hourly until the infant is 3 months old. The infant should be having at least three bowel movements each day by the time the infant is 2 weeks old. The first stools the infant will have are called meconium stools. The stools will be thick and sticky in consistency and either yellow, green, or brown in color.
10. Wash your hands.
11. Help the mother with her bra, putting fresh nursing pads over the nipples. If nipples are sore or cracked, use breast milk as a cream, and air-dry the nipples. Wash the mother's nipples only with water. An ointment or medication may be prescribed. Report these problems to the nurse. An over-the-counter ointment called Lanisol may also be used for sore or cracked nipples.
12. Return supplies to storage.
13. Wash your hands.

After nursing it is important to keep the nipple as dry as possible. Exposing the nipple to air is recommended and reduces the risk of developing cracked nipples and breast infections. Cracked nipples are common among breast-feeding women. Sometimes the nipple may bleed, making nursing painful. Germs can enter the breast through the cracked nipple and lead to an infection. Signs of a breast infection include red, tender, or painful swelling or lumps in the breast. In addition, swollen glands in the armpit or fever can also signal a breast infection. If a nursing mother has a cracked nipple, contact the health care provider, who can recommend a soothing lanolin cream that can be applied several times daily (not before nursing). This type of cream can help the nipple heal within a few days.

Bottle-Feeding

Infant formula used in bottle-feeding combines all the nutrients found in breast milk; however, it does not provide the antibodies found in the mother's breast milk. When preparing the infant's formula all equipment must be cleaned properly, as the infant's immune system is still immature and may be unable to fight off food-borne illnesses. The correct measurement of formula and water is also essential. Once the formula is mixed, it must be refrigerated and used within 48 hours. Bottle-feeding allows all members of the family to participate in the feeding process. The home health aide can feed the infant or assist the new parents, following the guidelines outlined in Procedure 75.

75 Procedure

Bottle-Feeding an Infant

Purpose

- To provide nutrition
- To give the infant the security of being held, cuddled, and bonded
- To observe infant's responses, color, skin condition, etc.

Procedure

1. Wash your hands.
2. Prepare formula as directed and pour into baby bottle (Figure 25-2). Put lid on bottle (Figure 25-3). Test the temperature of the formula before feeding (Figure 25-4).
3. Change infant's diaper, if soiled, so infant will be comfortable, clean, and dry while eating. Wrap infant loosely in a clean receiving blanket. Leave infant in crib with side rails up.
4. Wash your hands.
5. Bring warm bottle of formula to a comfortable rocker or armchair.
6. Support the infant's head and back when picking the infant up from the crib. Sit comfortably in chair, holding infant securely in a comfortable position for taking

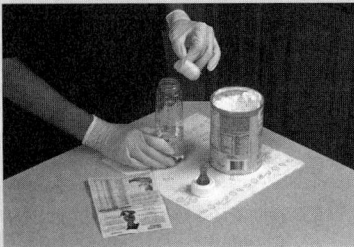

Figure 25-2 Prepare formula as directed. Be sure all equipment is clean before using.

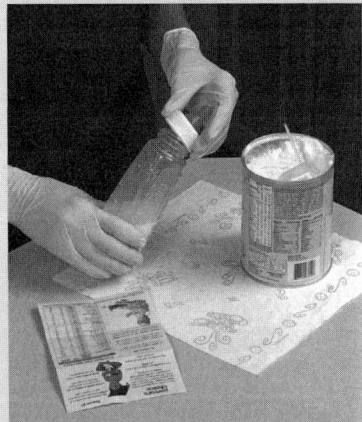

Figure 25-3 Put lid on bottle.

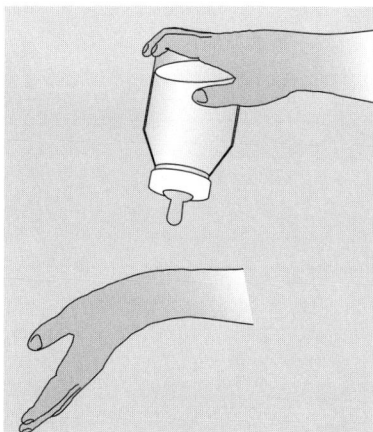

Figure 25-4 Test bottle temperature by shaking a few drops on your wrist.

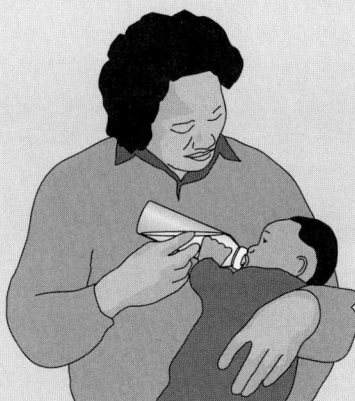

Figure 25-5 Infant should be held while feeding.

nipple; start to feed the infant. Keep the nipple full of formula. Do not prop bottle (Figures 25-5 and 25-6).

7. When infant has had 2 to 3 ounces, burp the infant.

8. Continue feeding and burping until infant is finished or shows no interest in eating. Do not force infant to take more than infant wants. If the infant drinks a partial bottle, throw the rest away.

9. When the infant is finished, burp the infant once more, then place in the crib, the infant lying on the side or back. *Do not place the infant on his or her abdomen!* Exceptions are in the cases of:
—Premature infants

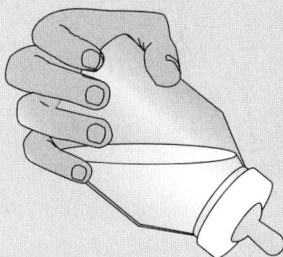

Figure 25-6 Be sure the neck of the bottle is covered with formula.

—Excessive spitting up or vomiting
—Facial deformities that make infant susceptible to airway blockage

10. Wash your hands.

Spend as much time as you can with the infant and interact with the infant (Figures 25-7, 25-8, and 25-9).

Burping the Infant

Both bottle-fed and breast-fed infants swallow air while feeding. Infants may fuss or become cranky if they need to burp. It is a good idea to burp the bottle-fed infant after the infant drinks 2 to 3 ounces and the breast-fed infant between breasts. If the infant does not burp after several minutes, continue feeding and try again when the infant is finished. Refer to Procedure 76 for techniques for burping an infant.

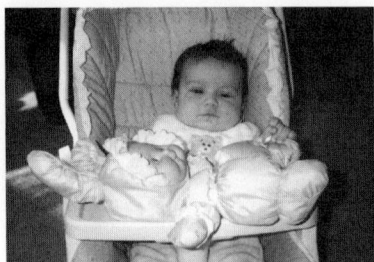

Figure 25-7 It is good to place an infant in an infant seat occasionally, as it will give the infant a chance to sit up.

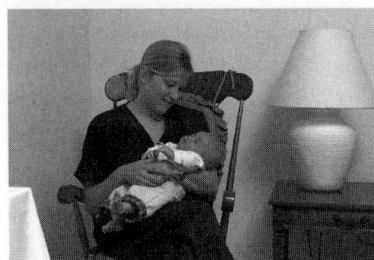

Figure 25-8 Infants need to be held and talked to often.

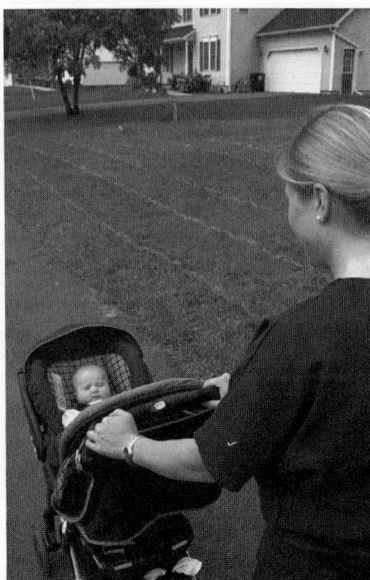

Figure 25-9 A stroller ride is an enjoyable occasion for both caregiver and infant.

76 Procedure

Burping an Infant

Technique A—The Sitting Position

1. Sit the infant in your lap.
2. Support the infant's head and chest with one hand.

3. Pat or rub the infant's back gently with the other hand (Figure 25-10).

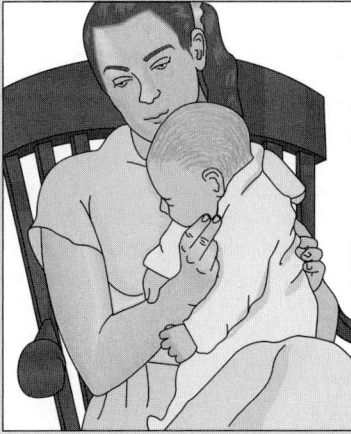

Figure 25-10   Sit the infant on your lap, supporting the chest and head with one hand while patting his or her back with your other hand.

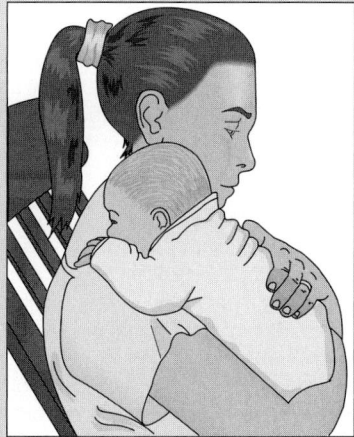

Figure 25-11   Hold the infant upright with the head on your shoulder, supporting the head and back, while you gently pat the back with your other hand.

Technique B—The Shoulder Position

1. Put the burp cloth or pad on your shoulder.
2. Hold the infant upright, with the head on your shoulder (your shoulder will provide support for the infant's head and neck).
3. Gently pat or rub the infant's back (Figure 25-11).

Technique C—The Lap Position

1. Place the burp pad in your lap.
2. Place the infant in your lap, face down, with his or her head turned to one side.
3. Support the infant's head so that it is higher than the chest.
4. Gently pat or rub the infant's back (Figure 25-12).

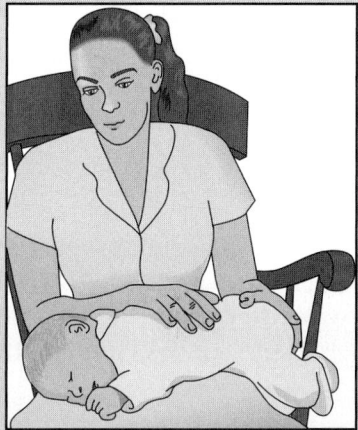

Figure 25-12   Lay the infant on your lap, on the infant's abdomen. Support the head so it is higher than the chest, and gently pat or rotate your hand on the infant's back.

CARING FOR THE NEWBORN INFANT

In addition to feeding and burping the infant, the care of an infant will include bathing, care of the penis, and care of the umbilical cord.

Bathing an Infant

The newborn infant does not require much bathing as long as the diaper area is cleaned thoroughly during diaper changes. If the infant wears disposable diapers, use infant disposable wipes to clean the perineal areas each time you change the diaper. The wipes not only clean the perineal area but also cover

the area with a protective coating, which will prevent the perineal area from breaking down. Generally, there is less chance of diaper rash with disposable diapers than with cloth diapers. Do not use powder on the perineal area or dispose of the diaper in the toilet. Disposable diapers usually work better if they are the correct size. The majority of disposable diapers have color tabs in the middle of them, which change color when the diaper needs to be changed. Sponge baths should be given until the stump of the umbilical cord has fallen off and the circumcision is healed (for males). Refer to Procedure 77 on how to bathe an infant.

77 Procedure

Bathing an Infant

Purpose

- To clean and refresh the infant
- To observe skin tone, activity, and signs of abnormality or unusual changes in behavior

Procedure

NOTE: Use a sponge bath until the infant's umbilical cord falls off. For small infants, place a towel in the bottom of the sink or tub so that the infant does not slip. Have bathing supplies, infant's clothes, and towels ready ahead of time and keep the phone within arm's reach. Never leave the room for any reason while giving the infant a bath. It is recommended not to bathe infants daily, as it dries out their skin.

1. Gather supplies:
   warm water in basin or sink
   soft towel and washcloth

diaper
baby soap and shampoo
baby lotion
change of clothing
disposable gloves

2. Wash your hands and apply gloves (optional).

3. Bring infant to bathing area.

4. Place infant on towel and remove clothing (Figure 25-13). Roll soiled diaper up. **CAUTION:** Never leave the infant unattended. Never leave the infant to answer the phone.

5. Check bathwater and place infant into basin, which is one-third to one-half full of warm water (Figure 25-14). If the infant does not have good head control, be sure to support the neck and head. Keep hold of the infant throughout the complete bath.

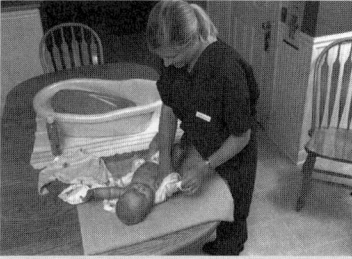

Figure 25-13 Undress the infant before the bath.

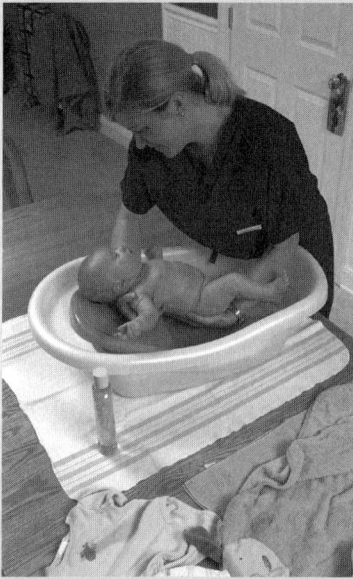

Figure 25-14 Slowly place the infant into basin half filled with warm water. Be sure to test the water before placing infant in basin.

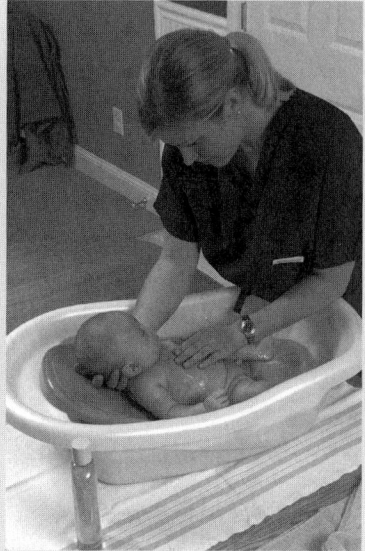

Figure 25-15 Wash the infant's body with your hands.

Use soap very sparingly, as it dries out the infant's skin.

7. Talk or sing to the infant during the bath—make it a fun time for both you and the infant.

8. Continue to move down the body and do the hair last. You may use your hands to wash the rest of the infant's body (Figure 25-15). The reason for doing the hair last is that a great deal of body heat is lost through the head, so it is best saved to last.

9. Before washing the infant's hair, bundle him or her in a towel. To shampoo the infant's hair, hold the infant in your arms like a football. Use a warm, wet washcloth to dampen hair. Gently apply shampoo or soap and rinse carefully to avoid getting soap in the infant's eyes. Massage the scalp gently to prevent the formation of cradle cap.

6. Carefully support the infant with one hand, use your free hand to wash the infant's face with plain water, no soap. Pat face dry. Clean ears with ends of washcloth. Do not use cotton swabs to clean the insides of the ears. Pat dry. Wash and rinse neck.

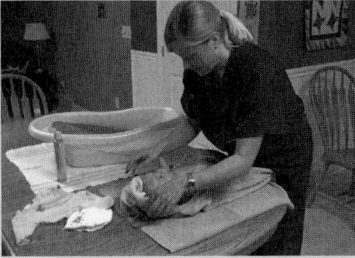

Figure 25-16 Cover the infant's head with a towel as soon as you are finished shampooing the hair.

10. Cover the infant's head with a towel as soon as you are finished shampooing the hair (Figure 25-16).
11. Apply baby lotion sparingly, if needed. Dress infant and apply clean diaper (Figure 25-17).
12. Place the infant in a crib or infant seat.
13. Return supplies to storage area. Place soiled clothing in hamper. Dispose of diaper in proper receptacle.

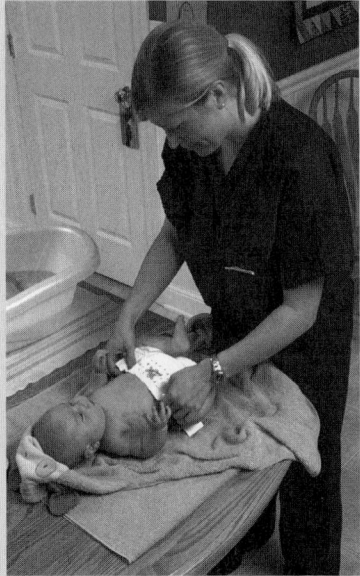

Figure 25-17 Apply the diaper and finish dressing the infant.

14. If wearing gloves, remove the gloves and wash your hands.

Care of the Penis

At birth, the boy's foreskin is attached to the glans (head) of the penis and cannot be pushed back. Urine flows through the small opening at the tip. Circumcision is a procedure in which the connections between the foreskin and the glans are separated, and the foreskin is removed, leaving the glans visible. Parents may choose to have their sons circumcised in the hospital, one to two days after birth. Some Jewish parents may have circumcision done during a religious ceremony seven days after birth.

Caring for the Circumcised Penis.

A light gauze with petroleum jelly or an antibiotic ointment applied will be placed over the glans of the penis after the circumcision procedure. At each diaper change, the dressing should be changed, as recommended by the nurse (usually two to three days, or until healed). The area should be kept clean. The tip of the penis may appear red, and a yellow secretion may be noticed. This indicates the normal healing process. The redness and secretions should disappear within a week. If there is swelling, the redness persists, or crusted yellow sores appear, there may be an infection. The nurse should be notified. The penis requires no special care after the circumcision has healed.

Caring for the Uncircumcised Penis. During the first few months, the uncircumcised penis should be cleaned with soap and water. The foreskin is connected by tissue to the glans so it should not be pulled back.

Care of the Umbilical Cord

When the baby is born, the umbilical cord is cut about 2 inches from the baby's abdomen. The remaining stump of the cord begins to dry up and then falls off within 12 to 15 days after birth, leaving the navel. Care of the umbilical cord is easy. In fact, many health care providers advise not to cover the area at all and to keep the area dry. When diapering the baby, fold the top of the diaper over so that it does not cover the navel. This will promote the healing of the site.

Employment

Unit 26
Job-Seeking Skills

UNIT 26

Job-Seeking Skills

CONTACTING PROSPECTIVE EMPLOYERS

Your first step toward finding a job is to research your community's job market. Local and national agencies in most areas are listed in the telephone directory. Your instructor may also be able to provide you with a list of possibilities. You can look in the employment section of your local newspaper; you can contact your local department of social services; and you can see if area hospitals have a registry service or home health agency where you may apply. Another place to check for possible home care positions is through the Internet.

Make a list of those places you plan to contact; then keep a record of the date you called and any appointments you may set up. Remember, you may register at several agencies and you may work for more than one agency on a part-time basis. When you telephone for an appointment, know what you want to say. "I am a graduate of the ABC home health program, and I am looking for work. May I have an appointment to discuss job opportunities in your agency?"

THE JOB INTERVIEW, APPLICATION FORM, AND JOB OFFER

Demonstrating a professional attitude and appearance throughout the job search process will help you in your job search. The interview provides you an opportunity to discuss your skills, but also helps you to learn more about the company and the people with whom you may be working. Completing the application form and negotiating a job offer are also important steps in the job search process.

The Interview

When you go to your appointment remember that first impressions are vital. Dress neatly and look your best.

It is better to go alone to the interview. Bringing someone with you to the interview may give the impression that you are not able to make decisions alone.

Before you go to the interview, research all you can about the agency. (Check in the yellow pages to see what services they offer, ask employees about what type of clients they serve, etc.). Before the interview collect the following items and bring them with you for the interview: certificates of completion of programs (e.g., CPR, First Aid, Home Health Aide), skills checklist, driver's license, and Social Security card. If an automobile is required for the position, the agency may ask for verification of auto insurance. If possible, have the latest record of your immunizations, including hepatitis B and the result of a tuberculosis test. It is also good to familiarize yourself with typical interview questions and decide how you will answer them. Practice answering typical interview questions. Some sample interview questions are:

- Have you had previous homemaker/home health aide work experience?
- Tell me about yourself.
- Can you tell me about your previous employment?
- Explain any time gaps between jobs.
- Why did you leave your last job?
- Why are you interested in this job?
- What did you like most/least about past jobs?
- What are your strengths/weaknesses?

Determine what you will wear. Dress neatly and conservatively—remember you only have one chance to make a good first impression. Avoid excessive jewelry, cologne, perfume, and makeup.

Arrive at least 15 minutes early. This will tell your prospective employer that you are prepared to arrive on time for your assignments if you are hired. Make sure you know the name of the interviewer and that you know how to get to the appropriate location.

Introduce yourself to the interviewer by name, with a smile and *firm* handshake and eye contact. Always be polite, speak clearly, sit or stand straight, and use correct grammar—no slang. Do not chew gum or smoke during the interview. Answer all questions truthfully and with more than one word. Be ready to talk about the training and experiences you have had. Be positive about former employers and working conditions. Be honest about the kind of cases you prefer. The interview is the employer's opportunity to get to know you. It is also the time for you to learn about the employer. Prepare a list of questions before going to the interview. The interviewer may ask if you have questions. It is good to ask questions; it shows that you prepared for the interview. Some suggested questions are:

- How far will I need to travel to and from each client? Is public transportation available or will I need to have an automobile?
- What shift or shifts will I be expected to work?
- If the position is part-time, is there a possibility of a full-time position soon?
- Is there a mechanism in place for advancement or additional training?
- Is overtime available?
- What are the fringe benefits? Is health insurance available and for what cost? Do I get holiday or vacation pay? Do I get sick days? Is there a pension plan available?
- Is child care available? If so, at what times and what is the cost? Do they take infants?
- If traveling is required between clients, is mileage paid? If so, how much per mile?

Listen carefully to your interviewer. Do not immediately ask about salary or benefits unless the employer brings it up first. This information is usually supplied by the interviewer toward the end of the interview. If you are unclear about information on the position, ask questions.

You should not anticipate receiving a definite indication of a job offer or rejection at the end of the interview. The interviewer will usually let you know when you will be contacted. Remember to thank the interviewer as you leave.

After the interview, send a thank-you letter and again express an interest in the position. Try to evaluate the interview to discover ways to improve for the next one. It is all right to call the agency in a few days to inquire about the status of the position.

The Application Form

Have an information sheet with you listing some facts that usually appear on an application form. This will save you time and you will not make foolish errors when you fill out the application.

If you do not have a telephone, you should leave the number of a neighbor or friend who has agreed to take messages for you. Personal references may not be relatives, but may include your past employers, supervisors, or instructor(s). Be sure that you have permission from those people you list as references to use their names. If possible, obtain letters of recommendation from these people before you go for a job interview. This will save time for the agency, and the person who is giving the recommendation only has to write one letter of reference. The agency can then make a copy of your letters of reference and confirm them by telephone.

Each agency will have its own application form. It is always a good idea to read the application form carefully before completing it. It may include special instructions, such as asking the applicant to type or print all information. Fill out each item neatly and completely. Do not leave any items blank; if the item does not apply to you, write "N.A." (not applicable). Take care to spell words and to punctuate sentences carefully.

Bring a pocket dictionary if you have difficulty spelling. Do not write in spaces marked "office use only." Review your application before submitting it to the employer. Remember to bring your own black or blue pen.

The Job Offer

If you are offered the job, you have the choice of accepting the agency's terms, thinking about it for a few days, or looking elsewhere for a position. Once you have accepted a position with an agency, be realistic in your goals. As in any kind of employment, this is a system of progression where the new employees must prove themselves. It is possible that an agency may test you by calling you for weekend or holiday part-time work. Many employers think it is a sign of dedication if you accept the assignments offered. After you have worked for a while, the agency will have a better idea of your abilities and strengths and will work you into a regular schedule.

When you are employed by an agency, you may be asked to sign a document. This document will indicate the policies and rules of the agency and the consequences to employees for breaking the rules (infractions) or for incidents of misconduct. Read it carefully and be willing to accept and abide by the conditions included in it.

The majority of states now require restrictive codes for agencies providing home health care services. To be qualified to operate, agencies must meet exacting standards set by both the Department of Health and the Centers for Medicare and Medicaid. Included in the standards required by states are:

- A grievance procedure for an agency's employees
- A client's bill of rights that *must* be explained to the client (or client's family) in the presence of a witness

- Documentation of certification of all employees
- Proof of an annual physical examination by employees
- Proof of employee's attendance at a minimum number of *in*-service programs each year
- Proof of citizenship or verified alien registration

- Satisfactory completion of an approved home health aide program
- No legal record of client abuse or misuses of client's property in a caregiver's situation, verified through a state criminal background check.
- Proof of being on the state registry for home health aide in the state in which you are applying for a position

APPENDIX A

Emergency Procedures Guidelines

This appendix identifies emergency situations and the procedures that should be followed by the home health aide in emergencies.

First aid is care given to clients who suffer from accidents or sudden illnesses until more help is available. A client should be treated physically and emotionally, and may need reassurance as well as physical care. The whole environment must be evaluated to prevent further injury. First aid is **immediate care** that must be given after the **emergency medical system (EMS)** in your area has been notified.

In the home, emergency phone numbers should be posted by the telephone. Include the local emergency squad, fire department, police, ambulance, poison control center, and family or friends the client wants contacted in case of an emergency. If someone needs immediate help, the home health aide may need to evaluate the situation and give emergency care according to the priority of needs.

Do not leave someone who requires immediate help. Have someone else call for help. When clients need immediate help and there is no one in the home, home health aides should assess each situation and respond based on their knowledge, abilities, training, and experience. Several emergency situations and the appropriate home health aide responses will be covered in this appendix.

When a client needs help, but not **immediate** care to sustain life, the aide's responsibility is to prevent more injury, seek medical help, and keep the client calm. For example, if a client's skirt caught fire and burned her legs, you would put the fire out before getting help for the burns. **Good judgment** is needed to give good emergency care. The whole situation must be evaluated to see what help is needed first and what further problems could arise.

Because this appendix covers only some life-threatening situations, it is advisable to take a course in cardiopulmonary resuscitation (CPR) and have current first aid books readily available for handling emergencies. Check with your agency regarding its emergency procedure policies.

BLEEDING

1. Wear gloves and follow the principles of standard precautions for a client who is bleeding.
2. Cover wound using a clean cloth, gauze, or hand.
3. Place your hand over bandage. Apply firm pressure for approximately 5 minutes or until bleeding slows or stops.
4. Do not lift bandage to check bleeding. If blood soaks through, apply another bandage on top. Remember to keep pressure firm on wound.
5. Raise injured part above level of victim's heart (unless you suspect broken bones).
6. Stay with the client until help arrives.

BURNS

Burns are very painful and, in extreme cases, can even be life-threatening. To determine the severity of the burn, you will need to know the degree of injury involved.

1st degree—Red and painful, like a sunburn

2nd degree—Red and painful, with blistering

3rd degree—May be black or white; there may or may not be pain involved

What to Do

1. If at all possible, "stop the burning." This is done by removing the source of burn, i.e., hot iron.
2. Immerse burned area in cold water. If this is not possible, apply cold water directly to area with a cloth, sponge, etc.

3. *Do not* apply oil, butter, or ointments to burn (this holds heat in).
4. *Do not* break blisters.
5. Place clean wet dressing on area (use sterile cloth if available).
6. Call the health care provider or emergency room for further instructions. Stay with the client until help arrives.

CHOKING

When a client is choking, you must act quickly; seconds count and can mean the difference between life or death. Figure 1 shows the universal sign for choking.

1. If the client can speak, wheeze, or moan, encourage him or her to cough out the object.
2. If client is coughing, encourage him or her to keep coughing until object is actually dislodged.
3. If client is unable to make any noise, do abdominal thrusts:
   - Stand directly behind client.
   - Reach both your arms around client's waist.

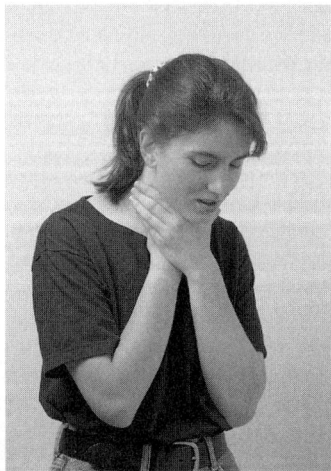

Figure 1 The person is choking. She cannot speak, cough, or breathe.

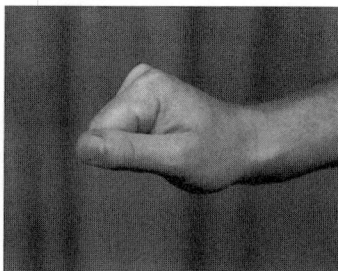

A

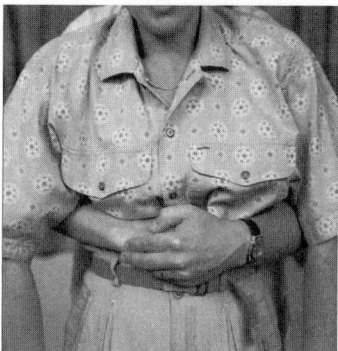

B

Figure 2 Abdominal thrust.

- Make a fist with one hand, keeping thumb straight (Figure 2A). Place fist, thumb side in, against abdomen slightly above navel.
- Grasp hold of fist with other hand (Figure 2B); press fist inward and upward, using short, quick movements.
- Procedure should be repeated until object is dislodged or person becomes unconscious.

POISONING
Swallowed

When you suspect someone may have swallowed poison, the three most important things you can do are:

1. Find out exactly what was taken (you will need to know name, ingredients—if listed—and amount swallowed).

2. Call your local poison control center (PCC) or hospital emergency room.
3. Follow the instructions they give you.

(Do not give antidotes or induce vomiting unless specifically told by PCC to do so.)

Inhaled

1. Get fresh air for client—preferably outdoors.
2. Call PCC or activate EMS.

Skin

1. Flush with water at least 10 minutes.
2. Call PCC or activate EMS.

SHOCK

Shock can be life-threatening, and requires immediate attention. Symptoms may include:

Pale, cool, moist, or sweaty skin. Client may be restless or drowsy, may have rapid and irregular heartbeat and breathing, may complain of nausea and chills; may have bluish discoloration of lips and nailbeds. Pupils may be enlarged or dilated.

Activate EMS Immediately

1. Induce client to lie down.
2. Elevate legs (unless you suspect fracture).
3. Cover with light blanket.
4. Keep client quiet and comfortable (be reassuring).
5. Do NOT give anything by mouth.

HEART ATTACK/STROKE

Heart attacks and strokes are both serious medical conditions that require immediate attention.

Heart attack symptoms may include chest pain (described as pressure, or like something sitting on the chest), nausea, indigestion, vomiting, profuse sweating, or pain radiating into arm or jaw.

What to Do (If Victim Is Conscious)

1. Activate EMS in your area.
2. Tell EMS your exact location.
3. Stay with client and remain calm.
4. Do not take client to hospital yourself or allow client to refuse treatment.
5. If you are trained in CPR, be prepared to start procedure immediately if symptoms require CPR.

Stroke symptoms may vary, but the most common symptoms are sudden weakness or numbness in the face or arm or one side of the body, loss or slurring of speech, difficulty understanding speech of others, consistently falling to one side, or unexplained unsteadiness.

Because stroke is diagnosed by history and physical examination, prompt medical treatment is necessary and should be sought immediately.

APPENDIX B

Prefixes and Suffixes Commonly Used in Medical Terminology

a-, an-: without, not

ab-: from, away

ad-: to, toward

adeno-, aden-: gland, glandular

-algia: pain

ambi-: both

angio-: vessel, duct

ante-, pre-: before

anti-, contra-: against

arthro: joint

audio-: sound, hearing, dealing with the ear

auto-: self

bi-, bis-: twice, double

bio-: life

brady-: slow

bronch-, bronchi-: air tubes in the lungs, bronchi

cardi-, cardia-, cardio-: pertaining to the heart

-cide: causing death

crani-, cranio-: pertaining to the skull

cyst-, cysto-, cysti-: bladder, bag

-cyte, cyt-: cell

derm-, derma-, dermo-, dermat-: pertaining to skin

dia-: through, between, apart

dorsi-, dorso-: to the back, back

dys-: difficult, painful

ecto-, ex-, exo-: outside of, external

-ectomy: surgical removal of

endo-: within, innermost

entero-. intestine, pertaining to the intestine

gastro-, gasti-: stomach

-genetic, -genic: origin, producing

genito-: organs of reproduction

glyco-, gly-: sugar

gyn-, gyno-: women, female

hema-, hem-, hemo-, hemato-: blood

hemi-: half

hepato-: liver

hetero-: other, unlike, different

homo-, homeo-: same, like

hydro-: water

hyper-: over, increased, high

hypo-: under, decreased, low

hystero-, hyster-: uterus

inter-: between, among

intra-: within, into

-itis: inflammation, inflammation of

leuko-, leuco-: white

-logy, -ology: study of, science of

mal-: abnormal, disordered

mast-, masto-: breast

micro-: small

mono-: one, single

multi-: many, much, a large amount

myo-: muscle

neph-, nephro-, ren-: kidney

neuro-, neur-: nerve or nervous system

-ology: study of a science

ophthalm-, ophthalmo-: eye

-ostomy: creation of an opening by surgery

ot-, oto-: ear

-otomy: cutting into

path-, patho-, pathy, -pathia: disease, abnormal condition

ped-, pedia-: child

peri-: around

plasty: surgical replacement

-plegia: paralysis

pnea-: respiration/breathing

pneum-: lung, pertaining to the lungs

post-: after

proct-, procto-: rectum, rectal

pseudo-: false

psych-, psycho-: pertaining to the mind

sclerosis: hardening

scopy: visual examination

sep-, septic-: poison, rot

sub-: less, under, below

super-, supra-: above, upon, over

tachy: fast

therm-, thermo-: heat

-toxic, -tox: poison

tracho-: trachea, windpipe

-uria: urine

INDEX